# Welcome to Essential Skills

**G-W** Goodheart-Willcox Publisher

# Essential Skills
## for Health Career Success

Jacquelyn Rhine Marshall

*Contributing Editor*
**Kay Lynette Stevens**

*Essential Skills for Health Career Success*

Marshall
Stevens, *Contributing Editor*

**G-W** PUBLISHER

# Begin Preparing for Your Healthcare Career Today!

# Learn the Basic Skills Needed to Succeed

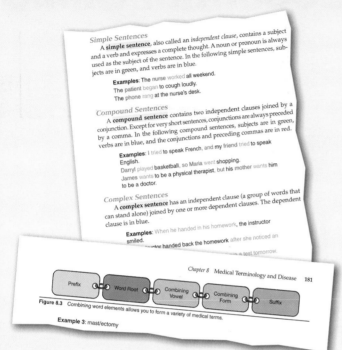

### Simple Sentences

A **simple sentence**, also called an *independent clause*, contains a subject and a verb and expresses a complete thought. A noun or pronoun is always used as the subject of the sentence. In the following simple sentences, subjects are in green, and verbs are in blue.

**Examples:** The nurse worked all weekend.
The patient began to cough loudly.
The phone rang at the nurse's desk.

### Compound Sentences

A **compound sentence** contains two independent clauses joined by a conjunction. Except for very short sentences, conjunctions are always preceded by a comma. In the following compound sentences, subjects are in green, verbs are in blue, and the conjunctions and preceding commas are in red.

**Examples:** I tried to speak French, and my friend tried to speak English.
Darryl played basketball, so Maria went shopping.
James wants to be a physical therapist, but his mother wants him to be a doctor.

### Complex Sentences

A **complex sentence** has an independent clause (a group of words that can stand alone) joined by one or more dependent clauses. The dependent clause is in blue.

**Examples:** When he handed in his homework, the instructor smiled.
The instructor handed back the homework after she noticed an error.

Chapter 8 Medical Terminology and Disease 181

**Figure 8.3** Combining word elements allows you to form a variety of medical terms.

**Example 3**: mast/ectomy

Examples help you apply academic concepts to situations found on the job.

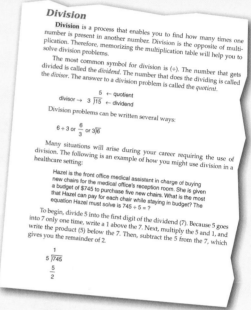

### Division

**Division** is a process that enables you to find how many times one number is present in another number. Division is the opposite of multiplication. Therefore, memorizing the multiplication table will help you to solve division problems.

The most common symbol for division is (÷). The number that gets divided is called the *dividend*. The number that does the dividing is called the *divisor*. The answer to a division problem is called the *quotient*.

$$\text{divisor} \rightarrow 3\overline{)15} \begin{array}{l} 5 \leftarrow \text{quotient} \\ \leftarrow \text{dividend} \end{array}$$

Division problems can be written several ways:

$$6 \div 3 \text{ or } \frac{6}{3} \text{ or } 3\overline{)6}$$

Many situations will arise during your career requiring the use of division. The following is an example of how you might use division in a healthcare setting:

Hazel is the front office medical assistant in charge of buying new chairs for the medical office's reception room. She is given a budget of $745 to purchase five new chairs. What is the most that Hazel can pay for each chair while staying in budget? The equation Hazel must solve is 745 ÷ 5 = ?

To begin, divide 5 into the first digit of the dividend (7). Because 5 goes into 7 only one time, write a 1 above the 7. Next, multiply the 5 and 1, and write the product (5) below the 7. Then, subtract the 5 from the 7, which gives you the remainder of 2.

$$5\overline{)745} \begin{array}{l} 1 \\ \underline{5} \\ 2 \end{array}$$

Walk through sample math problems to learn each step of the arithmetic and why it's done.

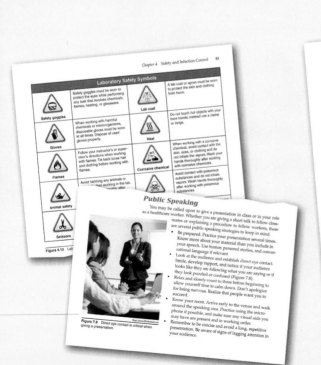

Chapter 4 Safety and Infection Control 81

#### Laboratory Safety Symbols

| | | | |
|---|---|---|---|
| **Safety goggles** | Safety goggles must be worn to protect the eyes while performing any task that involves chemicals, flames, heating, or glassware. | **Lab coat** | A lab coat or apron must be worn to protect the skin and clothing from harm. |
| **Gloves** | When working with harmful chemicals or microorganisms, disposable gloves must be worn at all times. Dispose of used gloves properly. | **Heat** | Do not touch hot objects with your bare hands; instead use a clamp or tongs. |
| **Flames** | Follow your instructor's or supervisor's directions when working with flames. Tie back loose hair and clothing before working with flames. | **Corrosive chemical** | When working with a corrosive chemical, avoid contact with the skin, eyes, or clothing and do not inhale the vapors. Wash your hands thoroughly after working with corrosive chemicals. |
| **Animal safety** | Avoid harming any animals or yourself when working in the lab. | **Poison** | Avoid contact with poisonous substances and do not inhale vapors. Wash hands thoroughly after working with poisonous substances. |
| **Scissors** | | | |

**Figure 4.12** Lab

#### Public Speaking

You may be called upon to give a presentation in class or in your role as a healthcare worker. Whether you are giving a short talk to fellow classmates or explaining a procedure to fellow workers, there are several public speaking strategies to keep in mind.

- Be prepared. Practice your presentation several times. Know more about your material than you include in your speech. Use humor, personal stories, and conversational language if relevant.
- Look at the audience and establish direct eye contact. Smile, develop rapport, and notice if your audience looks like they are following what you are saying or if they look puzzled or confused (Figure 7.8).
- Relax and slowly count to three before beginning to allow yourself time to calm down. Don't apologize for being nervous. Realize that people want you to succeed.
- Know your room. Arrive early to the venue and walk around the speaking area. Practice using the microphone if possible, and make sure any visual aids you may have are present and in working order.
- Remember to be concise and avoid a long, repetitive presentation. Be aware of signs of lagging attention in your audience.

**Figure 7.8** Direct eye contact is critical when giving a presentation.

Practical skills are included to ensure you are well-prepared for your future career.

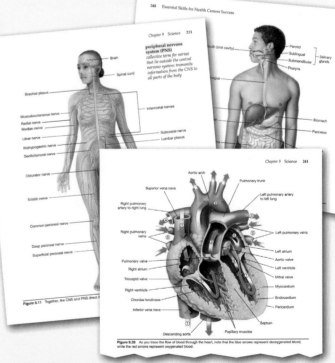

248 Essential Skills for Health Careers Success

Chapter 9 Science 231

**peripheral nervous system (PNS)** collective term for nerves that lie outside the central nervous system; transmits information from the CNS to all parts of the body

Brain
Spinal cord
Brachial plexus
Musculocutaneous nerve
Radial nerve
Median nerve
Ulnar nerve
Iliohypogastric nerve
Genitofemoral nerve
Obturator nerve
Sciatic nerve
Common peroneal nerve
Deep peroneal nerve
Superficial peroneal nerve
Intercostal nerves
Subcostal nerve
Lumbar plexus

**Figure 9.11** Together, the CNS and PNS direct

Mouth (oral cavity)
Parotid
Sublingual
Submandibular
Salivary glands
Pharynx
Esophagus
Stomach
Pancreas

Chapter 9 Science 241

Aortic arch
Superior vena cava
Pulmonary trunk
Right pulmonary artery to right lung
Left pulmonary artery to left lung
Right pulmonary veins
Left pulmonary veins
Pulmonary valve
Left atrium
Right atrium
Aortic valve
Tricuspid valve
Left ventricle
Right ventricle
Mitral valve
Chordae tendineae
Myocardium
Inferior vena cava
Endocardium
Pericardium
Descending aorta
Septum
Papillary muscles

**Figure 9.20** As you trace the flow of blood through the heart, note that the blue arrows represent deoxygenated blood, while the red arrows represent oxygenated blood.

Detailed anatomical illustrations convey important information without including unnecessary complexity.

# Put Your Skills to the Test

Special features, end of chapter review material, and Additional Practice sections allow you to put your knowledge to the test and improve retention.

---

### Real Life Scenario
*Calculating Volunteer Hours and Student Loans*

1. Madison is a high school senior who wants to be an LPN (licensed practical nurse). Madison's school counselor recommends volunteering at a hospital to observe the daily responsibilities of an LPN. The volunteer program at the local hospital requires a commitment of 100 volunteer hours to complete the program. If Madison volunteers for 5 hours a week, how many weeks will it take her to complete her volunteer commitment?

2. Steven decides he wants to become an EMT. He will need a student loan to pay for the required classes. The cost of an EMT program is $1,195 with additional fees for textbook rentals of $240. After training, he will have to pay back the loan at $100 a month. How many months will it take Steven to pay back the loan?

 *Check Your Understanding*

1. $100 \times 10 =$
2. $325 \times 35 =$
3. $220 \div 20 =$
4. $1,425 \div 5 =$
5. $15.20 \times 9 =$
6. $457 \div 3 =$
7. $547.89 \times 40 =$
8. $546.20 \div 4 =$
9. $10,439 \times 426 =$
10. $40,200 \div 9 =$

---

## Additional Practice

### Basic Math Review

*If you are confident in your math abilities and are able to answer these questions correctly, skip ahead to the Data Analysis section. These questions can also be used as review upon completing the chapter.*

**Values**

*Identify the value of each digit in the following numbers.*

1. 210
2. 3
3. 203,987
4. 1,244,765
5. 66,789

**Addition**

*Find the sum of the following addition problems without using a calculator.*

6. $213 + 456 + 342 =$
7. $4,500 + 97 + 456 =$
8. $43 + 345 + 1,234,679 =$
9. $45 + 678 + 1,908 =$
10. A student studying to be a hospital dietician is told by her instructor that a diet should not contain large amounts... The student is...

16. $546 + 3,467 + 237,689 + 34 + 7 + 90,458 =$
17. $34 + 345 + 1,234 + 12,608 + 214,896 =$

**Subtraction**

*Find the difference without using a calculator.*

18. $23 - 12 =$
19. $245 - 239 =$
20. $1,200 - 36 =$
21. $534 - 315 =$
22. Dr. James told an obese patient that he needed to enroll in a weight loss program. The patient initially weighed 320 pounds; today the patient weighs 245 pounds. How much weight has he lost?
23. Javier's physician has told Javier that he needs to lose 15 pounds... in at 210...

**Multiplication**

*Find the product without using a calculator.*

31. $22 \times 10 =$
32. $56 \times 8 =$
33. $120 \times 60 =$
34. $28 \times 28 =$
35. A registered nurse is giving a patient 225 mg of penicillin 4 times a day. How many mg of penicillin does the patient receive each day?
36. On average, Juanita processes 35 insurance claims per day. How many claims does she process in a two-week period (assuming she works 5 days a week)?
37. $1,466 \times 599 =$

**Multiplication Using a Calculator**

*Use a calculator to find the product in each of the following multiplication problems.*

38. $23 \times 234 \times 543 =$
39. $6,846 \times 414 =$
40.

**Division Using a Calculator**

*Use a calculator to find the quotient in each of the following division problems.*

51. $125 \div 15 =$
52. $400 \div 200 =$
53. $1,456 \div 56 =$
54. $54,320 \div 245 =$
55. $23,000 \div 15 =$

**Fractions**

*Solve the following fraction equations without using a calculator.*

56. $\frac{1}{10} + \frac{2}{10} + \frac{6}{10} =$
57. $\frac{4}{16} + \frac{3}{16} + \frac{10}{10} =$
58. $\frac{5}{9} \div \frac{2}{7} =$
59. $\frac{4}{5} \times \frac{1}{3} =$

...triplets were born yesterday at Eastridge Hospital. Each baby was weighed at birth. The three girls weighed: 3½ pounds (lbs), ...lbs, and 3¼ lbs. How much did they weigh all together?

... $\frac{1}{2}$

... $\frac{25}{5}$

*...following questions without using a...*

$127 + 2,130.02 + 54.5 =$

...off each of the following numbers ...nearest tenth.

---

## Chapter Review and Assessment

### Summary

Many of the skills you will master by using this textbook overlap. For example, effective studying depends on excellent reading skills. To read, write, and study well, an adequate vocabulary is necessary. Increasing your vocabulary requires discipline and will help improve your reading skills.

Active reading means concentrating while reading. Strategies like the SQ3R reading system will help you become an active participant in your reading. These strategies are also designed to increase your reading comprehension.

You will be required to take a variety of courses throughout your education. Different courses may require that you adapt certain strategies to read the materials specific to that subject matter. Improving your retention of information can be achieved by highlighting passages of importance, as well as underlining, writing in the margins of the text, and defining new words.

Reading dense, difficult material for a class or for your job can be made easier by strategies such as skimming, summarizing, and working with study groups. You can overcome reading problems by maintaining a positive attitude.

Dyslexia is a genetic learning disorder that can be managed, but will present a challenge throughout a person's life. To learn more about dyslexia, you can find information online or by consulting your school counselor.

Some students may have a desire to increase their reading speed—a goal that can be accomplished by relaxing, timing yourself, and being flexible in your reading speed and habits. Finally, eye strain can present a challenge to reading. Adopting the practices presented in this chapter can help alleviate this problem.

### Review Questions

**Short Answer**

1. Identify three benefits of reading.
2. Name four ways to improve your vocabulary.
3. What is active reading?
4. What are some advantages to using an e-reader?
5. What does SQ3R stand for?
6. Identify three strategies that will help you read difficult material.
7. How might reading for a social science course be different from reading for a literature course?
8. Describe dyslexia.
9. How might highlighting and note taking improve your reading skills?
10. Name three ways to decrease eye strain while studying.

**True/False**

11. *True or False?* Dyslexia is easily cured.
12. *True or False?* Never write in your textbooks, even if you own them.
13. *True or False?* Expanding vocabulary is an important goal for the student and the healthcare worker.
14. *True or False?* You can read rapidly and still understand what you are reading.
15. *True or False?* Retention means being able to retrieve information you read from your memory.
16. *True or False?* Active reading occurs when you have skimmed a passage but recall nothing of what you just read.
17. *True or False?* When reading your history textbook, all you need to remember are the dates of historical events.
18. *True or False?* Before you begin reading a challenging chapter, it is helpful to skim the material for key phrases and terms.

**Multiple Choice**

19. The SQ3R reading system includes each of the following steps, *except* ___.
   A. survey
   B. quantify
   C. read
   D. recite

20. Which of the following statements about eye strain is false?
   A. Eye strain problems have increased as workers spend many hours in front of a computer screen.
   B. Eye strain cannot be prevented.
   C. Eye strain is particularly problematic when the air is dry.
   D. Eye strain can be helped by using eye drops to add moisture to the eye.

21. What is a good method for identifying important or hard-to-understand material in your textbook?
   A. Put a Q next to material you don't understand.
   B. Mark particularly important concepts with an asterisk (*).
   C. Circle or underline terms you do not understand.
   D. All of the above.

22. When reading difficult material, it may be helpful to ___.
   A. summarize what you have read
   B. scan the document for key words and headings
   C. physically change positions
   D. All of the above.

23. When highlighting your notes or textbook, try to highlight less than ___ of the material.
   A. 50%
   B. 5%
   C. 15%
   D. 10%

24. Identifying common themes to help put dates and facts in order is helpful when reading a ___ textbook.
   A. social science
   B. math
   C. science
   D. history

25. ___ is the process used to break down words into recognizable units.
   A. Comprehending
   B. Deciphering
   C. Decoding
   D. Articulating

26. To improve your reading speed, it is helpful to ___.
   A. skim for main ideas
   B. time yourself
   C. relax
   D. All of the above.

27. When reading for a ___ course, it is important to explain theories in your own words.
   A. literature
   B. social science
   C. math
   D. history

28. ___ indicates a possible decoding problem.
   A. Reading with great expression
   B. Reading out loud at a slow pace
   C. An inability to recognize words out of context
   D. B and C only.

### Critical Thinking Exercises

29. Take a minute to think about your personal vocabulary. How would you rate your vocabulary? Does it need improvement? Does texting affect how you express yourself? Do you find yourself using excessive amounts of slang or swear words when trying to get your point across? Do you think people who use big words are pretentious?

30. What challenges have you faced when completing reading assignments? Would any of the strategies presented in this chapter make you a more efficient reader? Explain your answer.

31. How much reading do you do every week? Track your reading time and create a chart listing how long you read, what material you read, and if you experienced any challenges while reading.

32. What is your favorite material to read? Do you enjoy fiction or nonfiction? Would you prefer reading magazines or novels? Have you used e-books downloaded on your computer or tablet? After considering your reading preferences, review the chart you created for question 31. Did you read mostly for pleasure, school, or work in the past week?

# Reinforce Concepts

**Think It Through**

What techniques do you use to memorize information before an exam? Do you use any of the methods listed in this chapter? Are there any methods not mentioned in the text that you have found useful? What is the most effective memorization technique that you use?

✓ *Check Your Understanding*

1. Why is it important to never run i[n a] care facility?
2. Explain the importance of hospital emerge[ncy]
3. What information should you include when writing an incident report?
4. What is the purpose of OSHA?
5. What is a material safety data sheet (MSDS)?

Critical thinking and review questions will keep you engaged as you read and help you check your progress along the way.

## Real Life Scenario

### Needle Safety and Procedures

Isabella just started her job as a phlebotomist at North Haven Hospital. It is her first week drawing blood, and her supervisor is very strict about procedures. Isabella already feels that her supervisor does not have much faith in her abilities.

Isabella's next patient is a male adult who admits to being afraid of needles, increasing Isabella's anxiety. Isabella's hands are shaking, and she worries that her supervisor will come into the drawing room to watch, so she hurries through the blood draw. She is able to draw the blood quickly, but in her haste to put away the needle she sticks herself with it.

Isabella immediately decides that she won't tell anyone about the needlestick for fear of getting in trouble, or possibly fired.

What could be the possible consequences of Isabella's failure to report this incident? Do you think her supervisor should fire her? What if her patient has a bloodborne disease? What would you do?

Practical application helps connect the topics presented with scenarios you may encounter in your future career.

## Extend Your Knowledge

### Burn Degrees

Burns are classified in degrees. The three degrees of burns that are most relevant to the healthcare worker include first-, second-, and third-degree burns.

First-degree: the skin is usually red and very painful, and heals in 3–5 days.

Second-degree: blisters can be present, wound will be pink or red in color, painful, and appear to be wet. These burns will take several weeks to heal.

Third-degree: All layers of the skin are destroyed, extending into tissue. Areas can be black or white, and dry. Third-degree burns may take months to heal, and could require skin grafts—the surgical transfer of healthy skin to the burned area.

Dive further into the material at hand to improve your understanding.

**Did You Know?** *Cramming and Pulling All-Nighters*

Cramming and pulling all-nighters are not effective study methods. Reviewing materials over several study sessions gives you time to adequately absorb the information. Students who study regularly remember the material far better than those who did all of their studying in one last-minute session. Remember that being well-rested makes learning much easier.

Interesting facts about the topics at hand will keep you focused on the text.

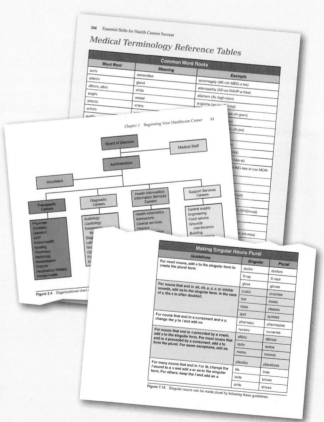

Numerous charts and tables help you plan your future career and understand important concepts.

# Explore Digital Learning Tools

## Extensive Digital Offerings

*The textbook—printed or online*

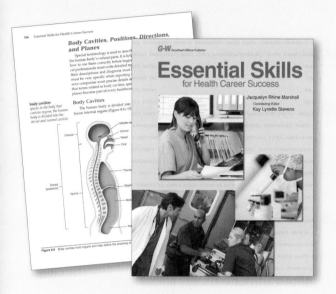

### Student Textbook and Online Textbook

Available as a printed textbook or interactive digital text, *Essential Skills for Health Career Success* offers a wonderful learning experience. Written in easy-to-understand language and supported with exceptional activities and assessment opportunities, this text will help you hone the skills needed to succeed in your future healthcare career.

www.g-wonlinetextbooks.com

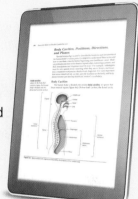

### Companion Website

The companion website provides additional resources including interactive art review and labeling, vocabulary review and practice, posttests, and colorful animations. You can e-mail answers to the additional assessments provided online to yourself or directly to your instructor for grading.

www.g-wlearning.com/healthsciences

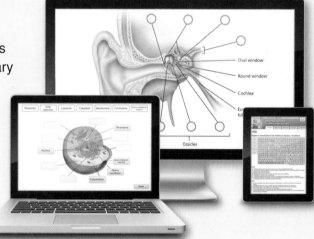

### Mobile Site

Study on the go with the mobile site. E-flash cards enable you to quiz yourself on the key terms presented in the text. Also included are posttests designed for self-assessment.

www.m.g-wlearning.com

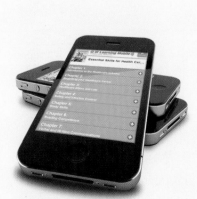

# Goodheart-Willcox
# Welcomes Your Comments

We welcome your comments or suggestions regarding *Essential Skills for Health Career Success*. Please send any comments you may have to the editoral director of our Health and Health Sciences Editorial Department. You can send an e-mail to healthsciences@g-w.com or write to:

Editorial Director—HHS
Goodheart-Willcox Publisher
18604 West Creek Drive
Tinley Park, IL 60477-6243

# Essential Skills
## for Health Career Success

First Edition

Jacquelyn Rhine Marshall, BA, CLS, MA

Kay Lynette Stevens, BA, MA, RN

*Contributing Editor*
Department Chair, Medical Assistant Program, Insurance
    and Coding
Saddleback College
Mission Viejo, California

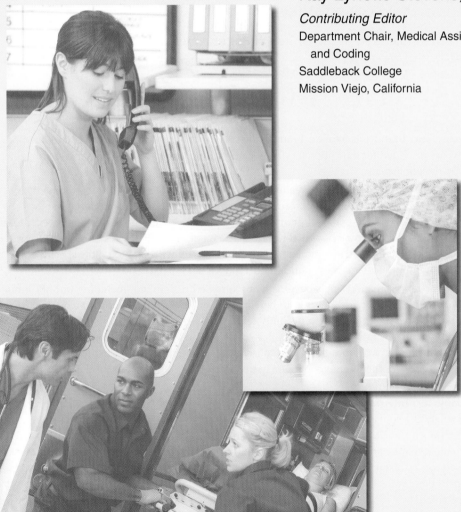

Publisher
**The Goodheart-Willcox Company, Inc.**
Tinley Park, Illinois
www.g-w.com

# About the Author

For 35 years, **Jacquelyn Rhine Marshall**, BA, CLS, MA, has been a medical professional; a medical careers instructor for Regional Occupational Programs, California; a medical writer; and a consultant/writer for the Center for Occupational Research and Development in Austin, Texas. Ms. Marshall has authored several textbooks and written medical course curriculum for the state of California. She has also developed several instructor guides and has edited or contributed to three medical series. Ms. Marshall holds degrees from the University of California, Berkeley; California State University, Hayward; and Notre Dame de Namur University.

**Kay Lynette Stevens**, Contributing Editor, BA, MA, RN, is a professor and Department Chairperson of the Medical Assistant Program, and Insurance and Coding at Saddleback College in Mission Viejo, California. Prior to joining the faculty at Saddleback College, she worked at hospitals as a critical care nurse and clinical educator. She also worked as a Program Coordinator teaching a variety of allied health courses to high school students and adults. She was a Professional Development Consultant and a Health Careers Master Teacher Trainer for the California State University Consortium and California Polytechnic University for 10 years. She has authored a textbook and has been the creator/editor of several additional texts in the Health Sciences.

## Dedications

To my husband Darryl, whose contributions to this textbook were invaluable.

Jacquelyn Marshall

I would like to dedicate this to my husband, Jim, in appreciation of his love and support during the creation of this textbook.

Kay Stevens

# Reviewers

Goodheart-Willcox Publisher, the author, and the contributing editor would like to thank the following instructors who reviewed selected manuscript chapters and provided valuable input into the development of this textbook program.

Glenda Algaze, BS, Med, CDA, CPht, NBCT
National Board Certified Teacher
Miami Lakes Educational Center
Miami Lakes, FL

Gwen Barnett, BS, MT (ASCP)
Health Science Education Instructor
Southern Indiana Career and Technical Center
Evansville, IN

Karen Beilman, RN, BSN
Allied Health Instructor
Wallenpaupack Area High School
Hawley, PA

W. Lynne Clarke, RN, Ed.S.
Health Science Department Chair
AR Johnson Health Science and Engineering
    Magnet School
Augusta, GA

Shelley Dougherty, MS Ed
Director of Educational Programs
Oregon Pacific Area Health Education Center
Lincoln City, OR

Linda Essick, RN, BSN
Allied Health Sciences Instructor
Concord High School
Concord, NC

Beverly Felder, RN, BSN, MPA
Health Professions Retention Specialist
Elgin Community College
Elgin, IL

Dolly Horton, CMA (AAMA), M.Ed
Dean, Allied Health and Public Service
Asheville-Buncombe Technical
    Community College
Asheville, NC

Laura Ing, RN
Certified Nurse Assistant Instructor
Mt. Vernon Township High School
Mt. Vernon, IL

Kurt Krahenbuhl
CTE Teacher
Rochester STEM High School
Rochester, NY

Rebecca Laidig
CTE Teacher
Paradise Valley High School
Phoenix, AZ

Monique Maskell, RN, BSN
Allied Health Instructor
Weymouth High School
Weymouth, MA

Sharon Musser, BS, RN
LPN Instructor, BOOST Instructor
Mercer County Technical Schools Health
    Career Center
Trenton, NJ

Shannon Niaves, CNMT
Health Science Teacher
DeBakey High School for Health Professions
Houston, TX

Kelly Rogers, MS Ed
CTE Teacher
Riverside High School
Buffalo, NY

Davion White
Math, PE, and Health Science Teacher
California Academy of Math and Science
Carson, CA

# Contents in Brief

# Contents

## Chapter 5

## *Study Skills* . . . . . . . . . . . . . . . . . . . . . . . . . . . . . . . . . . **96**

## Chapter 6

## *Reading Competence* . . . . . . . . . . . . . . . . . . . . . . . . . . **120**

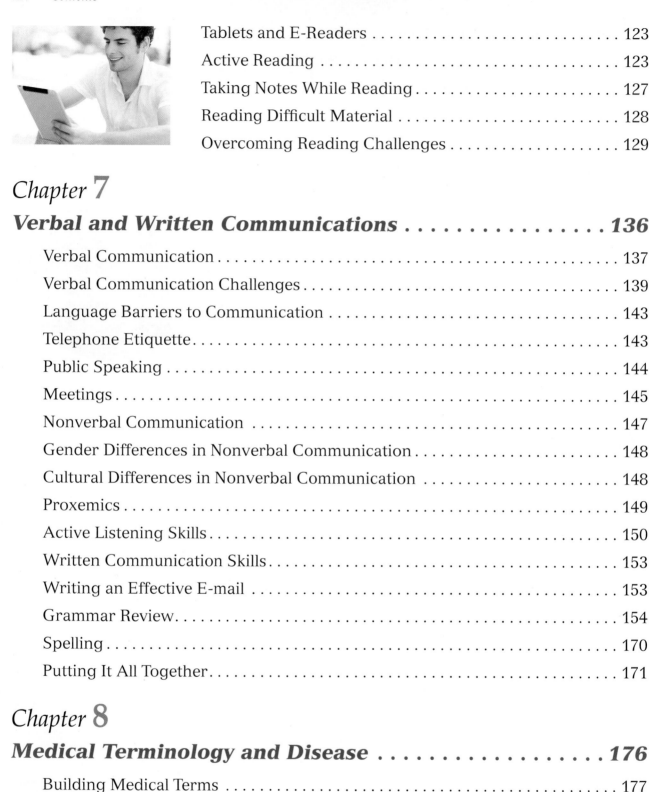

## Chapter 7
# Verbal and Written Communications . . . . . . . . . . . 136

## Chapter 8
# Medical Terminology and Disease . . . . . . . . . . . . 176

# Chapter 9

## Science . . . . . . . . . . . . . . . . . . . . . . . 216

# Chapter 10

## Math . . . . . . . . . . . . . . . . . . . . . . . . . . 262

# Chapter 11

## Healthcare Technology . . . . . . . . . . . . . . . . . . . . . 302

# Chapter 12

## Employability Skills . . . . . . . . . . . . . . . . 328

### Extend Your Knowledge

## *Real Life Scenario*

# To the Student

As you begin planning for a career in healthcare, are you concerned about job security after you complete an educational program? According to the United States Department of Labor, in the last decade, growth in health-related occupations has soared above almost all others. The future for healthcare occupations looks bright! With the aging baby boomer generation and the expansion of medical technology, health careers offer secure, well-paying employment.

One challenge employers face is finding entry-level employees who have the basic skills needed to succeed in the healthcare world. Every healthcare worker must be proficient in the following areas: oral and written communications, math, reading, study skills, and computing skills. Are you confident about your abilities in these areas, or would you welcome some review? This textbook is designed to provide students who desire a healthcare career, an opportunity to enhance these skills before embarking on a career pathway.

Additionally, this textbook will introduce you to medical terminology; healthcare ethics and law; safety and infection control in the healthcare environment; and body structure, function, and disease. Information about obtaining and maintaining a satisfying job in the healthcare field is also provided. Special features are also included to provide opportunities to review and apply what you have learned, while also delivering a more detailed discussion of the topic at hand.

*Essential Skills for Health Career Success* will provide opportunities to critically think through challenges you may face as a healthcare employee. This textbook will also introduce you to a wide range of healthcare careers from which you can choose. We believe that through your study you will find that a career in healthcare can be exciting, rewarding, and long-lasting.

Jacquelyn Rhine Marshall

Kay Lynette Stevens

1

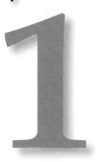

# Chapter 1

# *Introduction to the Healthcare Industry*

## Terms to Know

Affordable Care Act
anesthesia
antibiotics
caduceus
diabetes
epidemics
Hippocratic Oath
health maintenance
  organizations (HMO)
hospice

Medicaid
Medicare
microscope
National Healthcare Skill
  Standards Project
pathogens
preferred provider
  organizations (PPO)
psychoanalysis
vaccination

## Chapter Objectives

- Discuss the contributions of various cultures to the advancement of medicine.
- Identify the importance of the Hippocratic Oath.
- Describe the significant medical advancements made during the Renaissance and the Industrial Revolution.
- Discuss the significance of vaccinations.
- Explain the importance of hand washing, hygiene, and sterilization in healthcare facilities.
- Identify the significance of Louis Pasteur's discovery of microbes.
- Compare and contrast Medicare and Medicaid.
- Discuss two common models of managed care.
- List and describe the various healthcare facilities in the United States.

Reinforce your learning with additional online resources
- **Practice** vocabulary with flashcards and interactive games
- **Assess** with posttests and image labeling
- **Expand** with activities and animations

www.g-wlearning.com/healthsciences

Companion
G-W Learning

**Study on the Go**
Use a mobile device to practice vocabulary terms and review with self-assessment quizzes.

www.m.g-wlearning.com

Mobile
G-W Learning

According to the United States Department of Labor, growth in two areas of employment—computer-related jobs and healthcare occupations—has soared above all others in the last decade. The future looks bright for those hoping to obtain excellent, challenging occupations in the healthcare industry. With the aging baby boomer generation (those born during the population increase following World War II) and the expansion of medical technology, health professions offer secure, well-paying employment.

The Patient Protection and Affordable Care Act (commonly called *The Affordable Care Act* or *Obamacare*), was passed into law in 2010 by the US Congress. This act is the most significant government expansion and regulatory overhaul of US healthcare since the passage of Medicare and Medicaid in 1965. The Affordable Care Act is designed to provide affordable healthcare insurance coverage for all Americans, and reduce the overall costs of health care.

**Affordable Care Act**
*passed into law in 2010 for a major regulatory overhaul of US healthcare*

The United States Department of Education has developed the **National Healthcare Skill Standards Project** to address a critical shortage of highly skilled healthcare professionals. This project developed skill standards for today's labor force based on an understanding of core academic subject matter. Healthcare workers must be knowledgeable in several academic areas (including reading, writing, math, life sciences, medical terminology, and the history of healthcare) to succeed in this industry. This textbook focuses on each of these academic areas, as well as

**National Healthcare Skill Standards Project**
*system developed by the United States Department of Education to address a critical shortage of highly skilled healthcare professionals*

- oral and written communications;
- employability skills;
- legal and ethical responsibilities;
- safety practices;
- teamwork;
- health maintenance practices; and
- information technology skills.

Health career programs are competitive and demanding. This textbook will help the entry-level student review and improve the basic skills listed above. By mastering such skills, the student will be prepared to enter into a meaningful, challenging program leading to a rewarding career.

Some healthcare careers are stepping-stones to other careers. Because the healthcare field grows and changes so rapidly, careers that do not exist today may materialize tomorrow.

## *A Brief History of Healthcare*

All societies have medical beliefs providing explanations for birth, death, and disease. Throughout history, illness has been attributed to witches, demons, astrological influences, or the gods making mischief. In many cases, the rise of scientific medicine over the past millennium has altered or replaced such mysticism.

Many people greatly influenced what we know as our healthcare industry today. Their contributions to modern medicine were often both significant and lasting. Reading about these pioneers may inspire you to conduct further research (either individually or with a group) to learn how these innovative and determined individuals made such discoveries.

## The Chinese

Ancient Chinese doctors made many advancements in the practices of acupuncture, or the strategic insertion of small needles into the body to treat disease and pain. The effectiveness of acupuncture is sometimes called into question, but it is still used today, often as a treatment for chronic pain and infertility. The Chinese were also the first to study the pulse as a means of diagnosis. They believed that examining the characteristics of a patient's pulse—its strength, rate, and regularity, for example—could help determine the severity of an illness.

## The Egyptians

Ancient Egyptians (and the Babylonians—people who lived in what is present-day Iraq and made great advances in agriculture and science) developed a system of medicine that was quite advanced for that time period. The Egyptians began the practice of medical examinations and introduced the concepts of diagnosis (the process of determining the cause of the disease) and prognosis (forecasting the probable course and outcome of a disease). Figure 1.1 shows hieroglyphics, which the ancient Egyptians used to record their history and accounts of medical procedures.

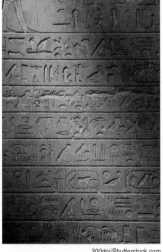

*300dpi/Shutterstock.com*

**Figure 1.1** Ancient Egyptians recorded their history, including medical practices and developments, using hieroglyphics.

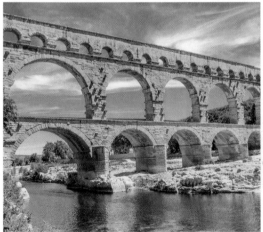

*Berti123/Shutterstock.com*

**Figure 1.2** Aqueducts were built with a slight downward slope from the water source, allowing fresh water to flow into cities by the force of gravity.

## The Greeks

One of the biggest challenges to ancient medicine was sanitation. Ancient people did not understand germs and their role in transmitting disease. The Greeks, however, realized that some diseases were caused by poor sanitation, particularly contaminated water. They built aqueducts to bring clean water into cities and sewers to carry away waste (Figure 1.2).

Hippocrates was a Greek physician who described many diseases and conditions in the fifth century BCE (before the Common Era). Hippocrates is credited with being the first person to believe that diseases were caused naturally and not as a result of superstition or the gods. He separated the discipline of medicine from religion, believing and arguing that disease was not a punishment inflicted by the gods, but rather the product of environmental factors, diet, and living habits.

Hippocrates has been credited with writing the **Hippocratic Oath**, a promise to practice medicine honestly, that physicians still make today. Although credited to Hippocrates, authorship of the oath has never been proved. A portion of the Hippocratic Oath states, "I will follow that method of treatment which according to my ability and judgment, I consider for the benefit of my patient and abstain from whatever is harmful or mischievous." Many people today consider Hippocrates to be the father of western medicine.

Another Greek physician, Galen, was one of the greatest surgeons of the ancient world. Galen performed brain and eye surgeries that were not attempted again until 2,000 years after his death.

An emblem of the medical profession, the **caduceus**, has also been traced back to ancient times (Figure 1.3). The caduceus originally symbolized peace and was carried by Hermes, the messenger of the Greek gods. In the early 1900s, the caduceus was mistakenly adopted as the symbol of the US Army Medical Corps. Officials had confused it with the staff of Aesculapius, a Greek god of medicine. The staff of Aesculapius is a branch with a single snake wrapped around it, which resembles the caduceus (Figure 1.4). Today, both the caduceus and staff of Aesculapius are used to represent the medical profession, although the caduceus is used more commonly in the United States.

**Hippocratic Oath**
*a promise of professional behavior made by physicians beginning their careers; promises ethical and honest practice of the medical profession*

**caduceus**
*an emblem of medicine in the United States*

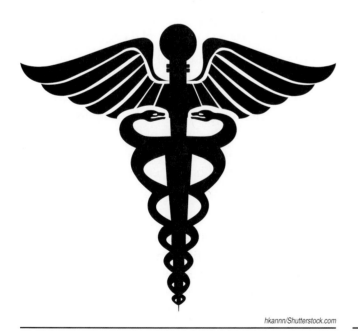

hkannn/Shutterstock.com

**Figure 1.3**   The caduceus has been used as a symbol for various medical groups, including the US Army Medical Corps and Nurse Corps.

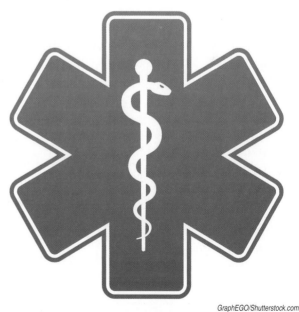

GraphEGO/Shutterstock.com

**Figure 1.4**   The staff of Aesculapius appears on the Star of Life, a common medical symbol.

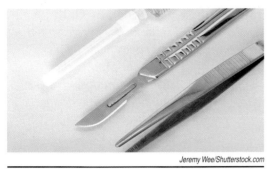

**Figure 1.5**  First developed by the Romans, scalpels, forceps, and surgical needles are basic tools used in healthcare today.

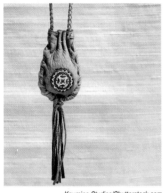

**Figure 1.6**  Native American healers often carried medical bags containing items they believed held spiritual healing powers.

**epidemics**
*diseases that affect many people and spread rapidly by infecting a certain area or population*

**antibiotics**
*drugs that slow the growth of, or destroy bacteria; used to treat infections*

**vaccination**
*the use of medicines that contain weakened or dead bacteria or viruses to build immunity and prevent disease*

# The Romans

The Romans were one of the first societies to use organized medical care. For example, Roman armies were accompanied by physicians, who carried medical equipment to care for wounded soldiers. Hospitals were created in Roman times, when physicians set aside a room in their houses to care for the ill. Eventually, separate buildings were built to accommodate the sick. The Romans also invented many surgical instruments such as forceps, scalpels, and surgical needles (Figure 1.5). Cataract surgery of the eye was first performed by Roman surgeons.

# Native Americans

Native Americans were some of the earliest and most effective practitioners of the medical arts. Healers date back 40,000 years in North America. Because tribes did not have a written language, traditions were passed on orally from healer to healer. Healers believed that they should honor the patient's wishes and never force treatment on a patient.

Both the Navajo and Cherokee tribes used herbs and natural pain relievers (Figure 1.6). In many tribes, a person who recovered from a serious illness was thought to have supernatural powers after their recovery. Several tribes prayed to the spirits to intervene with a cure for the sick.

# Dark and Middle Ages (400 CE to 1400 CE)

When the Roman Empire came under the rule of northern nomads called the Huns around 400 CE (Common Era), progress in the study of medical science slowed dramatically. For the next thousand years, medicine was practiced only in monasteries and convents. The Roman Catholic Church taught that life and death were in the hands of God, and there was little interest in learning how the body functioned or in curing disease by man's hands. Prayer was the preferred method of healing and curing disease. Physicians as we know them did not exist.

Terrible **epidemics** (the bubonic plague, in particular) killed millions of people during this period. Other serious diseases without cures were smallpox, syphilis, tuberculosis, and diphtheria. Today, the plague, syphilis, and tuberculosis—which are all caused by different bacteria—can usually be cured by **antibiotics** and other antibacterial agents. According to the World Health Organization, smallpox has been officially eradicated, or done away with completely. This was done through a global effort involving **vaccinations** and quarantines (isolating infected individuals). Today, diphtheria is controlled by vaccinations.

The Islamic civilization rose to prominence in medical science during the Middle Ages. Arab physicians made significant contributions to medicine in disciplines such as anatomy, ophthalmology, pharmacology, physiology, surgery and the pharmaceutical sciences. The Arabs were influenced by the Greeks, Romans, and the progress people in India had made. Like the Romans before them, Arab societies established hospitals dedicated to the care of the sick and injured.

Maimonides (1135–1204) was an extremely important Jewish philosopher and one of the most prolific and inventive biblical scholars and physicians of the Middle Ages. In his many writings, he described numerous medical conditions including asthma, diabetes, hepatitis, and pneumonia. Maimonides emphasized the importance of moderation and a healthy lifestyle. His writings influenced generations of physicians.

**Did You Know?**

## *Bubonic Plague*

Bubonic plague is a disease transmitted by small rodents who are infested with fleas. Bubonic plague is caused by a bacterium called *Yersinia pestis* (Figure 1.7). This bacterium is very sensitive to antibiotics we have today and can easily be destroyed with proper treatment. Without antibiotics, an infected person can die within six days of contracting the bubonic plague.

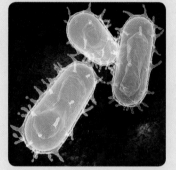

*MichaelTaylor/Shutterstock.com*

**Figure 1.7**  Yersinia pestis bacteria

Bubonic plague bacteria invade the lymphatic system, causing *buboes*, or swollen and painful lymph nodes throughout the body. As the bacteria spread, the bloodstream can become infected, causing a condition called *septicemic plague*. When the lungs become infected, the condition is then called *pneumonic plague*. Together, these three infections are known as the *Black Death* or the *Black Plague*. In the fourteenth century, the Black Death killed approximately 25 million Europeans, which amounted to approximately 30% to 60% of the European population.

## *The Barber-Surgeon*

In the Middle Ages, a barber cut more than just hair. Barbers could also practice surgery, dentistry, and bloodletting (a procedure thought to rid the body of disease-causing substances circulating in the blood). The barber-surgeon also traveled with armies and often performed amputations.

Barber poles placed outside the home of a barber-surgeon were red, white, and blue. The red represented blood, the white bandages (or the tourniquet used to raise veins), and blue for the veins (Figure 1.8). The pole itself represented the stick squeezed by the patient to dilate, or enlarge, the veins.

During the Middle Ages, physicians first became licensed after completing formal training with an experienced physician. Surgeons, like the barber-surgeons, had different training than physicians. Women were not allowed to practice medicine, but were allowed to be nurses and midwives.

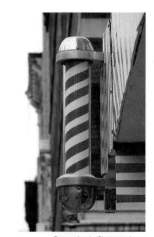

*Danger Jacobs/Shutterstock.com*

**Figure 1.8**  Placed on the outside of buildings, the barber pole has long signified the presence of a barber, or barber-surgeon, within.

Religion continued to play an important role in healthcare. In the Middle Ages, Christian and Muslim teachings encouraged members of their religions to care for those in need, including the sick. Prayer and rest continued to be prevalent treatments in many places.

> **Did You Know?**
>
> ## Bloodletting
>
> The practice of bloodletting as a medical treatment came to North America on the Mayflower. This medical practice was incredibly popular in the eighteenth and early nineteenth centuries. In fact, President George Washington died in 1799 after being drained of nine pints of blood within 24 hours in an attempt to cure him of a sore throat and cold. By the end of the nineteenth century, the use of bloodletting as a medical treatment for minor illness was proved ineffective and considered quackery.

## The Renaissance

There were many developments in healthcare during the Renaissance, a period that began in the fourteenth century and lasted until the seventeenth century. The invention of the printing press made it possible to mass produce books, allowing information about new medical discoveries to spread quickly. During the sixteenth century, scientists began to use the scientific method. Instead of guessing what made people sick, scientists could use the scientific method to make accurate conclusions based on observation and careful note-taking. You will learn more about the scientific method in Chapter 9, *Science for Healthcare Careers*.

**microscope**
*an instrument that uses a lens to magnify objects too small to be seen with the naked eye*

Another dramatic development during the Renaissance was the invention of the **microscope**. During the first century CE, some Romans experimented with making images larger by using crude lenses. It was not until 1,500 years later that a Dutch dry goods store owner, Anthony Van Leeuwenhoek (1632–1723), used lenses to magnify and count threads in cloth. Van Leeuwenhoek became fascinated with making lenses and successfully produced magnifications up to 270×. Van Leeuwenhoek later developed the device we know today as the microscope.

Van Leeuwenhoek observed specimens no person had ever seen before—bacteria, yeast, red blood cells, sperm, and tiny microorganisms swimming in a drop of pond water. Leeuwenhoek has been called the "father of microscopy." Robert Hooke (1635–1703), an Englishman who is sometimes called the "English father of microscopy," also spent much of his life working with microscopes and improved their design and capabilities.

## The Industrial Revolution

The Industrial Revolution of the mid- to late-eighteenth and nineteenth centuries brought great changes to industry, communication, and travel. Inventions such as the telegraph and railroad lines were developed to make communication and travel faster (Figure 1.9). Ideas could now be exchanged easily and more quickly.

Factories were developed using better technologies, allowing for the mass production of more sophisticated medical equipment such as finer syringe needles and microscope lenses. Considerable progress was made in the field of medicine with the invention of the stethoscope, which enabled medical professionals to listen to a patient's chest cavity, heart, and pulse points without an invasive procedure.

With the advent of industrialization, rural residents moved in great numbers to the cities to find work. The results of this mass exodus from the country to the city brought overcrowded conditions in which people lived close together, spreading infectious diseases in great numbers. During this period, development of public health laws began to control the spread of disease.

## Vaccination

An English doctor named Edward Jenner (1749–1823), developed the practice of vaccination. Vaccination is the administration of dead or weakened microorganisms of a disease that increases a person's immunity, or resistance, to a particular disease.

Jenner observed that people who worked around cows and horses developed cowpox (a virus causing sores), but did not generally get a similar disease called *smallpox*. Smallpox was a highly infectious, and often fatal, disease caused by a poxvirus. The symptoms of smallpox included

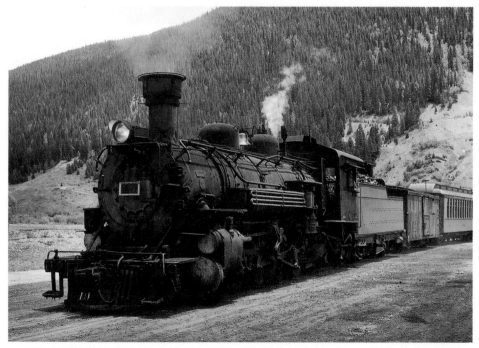

*Paul Dempsey/Shutterstock.com*

**Figure 1.9**   Steam engines transported goods, people, and ideas.

fever, headache, and inflamed skin sores. Jenner vaccinated people with the fluid from the cowpox blisters, which protected people from smallpox.

Throughout this period, vaccinations were developed for other diseases such as cholera, anthrax, rabies, tetanus, diphtheria, typhoid fever, and various plagues.

### Pain Management

**anesthesia**

*loss of feeling with or without the loss of consciousness*

Before the nineteenth century, pain was a serious problem, especially during surgery. **Anesthesia** was not invented until the nineteenth century. Ether was first available as an inhalable anesthetic, followed by nitrous oxide and chloroform. Today, with the advent of more advanced methods of putting patients in deep sleep, anesthesia makes painless surgery possible.

**Did You Know?**

### Early Pain Relief

In the early days of medicine, physicians used herbs, hashish (a product of cannabis), and alcohol to relieve pain during surgery. Some physicians choked patients into unconsciousness to stop pain. Many patients died from the terrible pain and shock caused by surgery.

### Women in Medicine

Before the Industrial Revolution, women played only a minor role in organized medical care, serving as cleaning women and midwives. However, the work of a few pioneering individuals opened up possibilities for women throughout the healthcare field.

**Florence Nightingale.** The work of Englishwoman Florence Nightingale (1820–1910) increased the participation of women in medical care (Figure 1.10). Nightingale demonstrated the critical role of nurses in the formerly male-dominated medical profession. Her goal was to reduce patient mortality that resulted from lack of hygiene and nutrition.

Nightingale came to prominence during the Crimean War, when she tended to wounded soldiers, saving many through the use of proper hygiene. Nightingale felt that disease was caused by an unclean environment. In hospital wards, she insisted that bed linens be changed frequently, rooms be well ventilated, chamber pots be emptied often, and the walls and floors be scrubbed regularly.

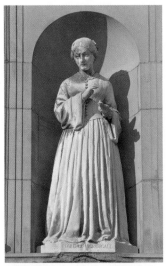

*Guy Erwood/Shutterstock.com*

**Figure 1.10** This statue of Florence Nightingale was erected in Derby, England to recognize her contributions to the field of nursing.

Nightingale also laid the foundation for professional nursing with the establishment of her nursing school at St Thomas' Hospital in London in 1860. Nightingale's school was the first secular (nonreligious) nursing school in the world. The role of the nurse has expanded greatly since Nightingale's time, producing several levels of nurses' training. You will learn more about nurses' training in Chapter 2, *Beginning Your Healthcare Career*. Today, the nurse's role has evolved into a professional and technological one, especially in acute care units.

**Elizabeth Blackwell.** In 1849, Elizabeth Blackwell (1811–1910) graduated with her medical doctor (M.D.) degree, becoming the first woman to formally study and practice medicine in the United States. Blackwell's sister, Emily, followed in her footsteps as the third woman to earn a medical degree in the United States. The sisters worked together at the New York Infirmary for Indigent Women and Children for over 40 years. In 1868, the sisters founded the Women's Medical College in New York.

**Clara Barton.** In 1881, Clara Barton (1821–1912) formed the American Red Cross, which has become one of the largest humanitarian organizations in the world (Figure 1.11). During her life, Barton was first a teacher and then a clerk. However, during the Civil War, she dedicated herself to caring for soldiers on the front, gathering supplies from all over the country. After the war, Barton was recognized as a hero all over the world, receiving the Iron Cross, the Cross of Imperial Russia, and the International Red Cross medal.

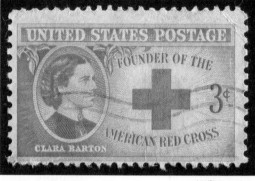

*rook76/Shutterstock.com*

**Figure 1.11**   This stamp from the late 1940s honors Clara Barton for her role as the founder of the American Red Cross.

### Pathogens and Sterilization

In 1847, Hungarian physician Ignaz Semmelweis (1818–1865) noticed a dramatic difference between the death rate of women who had babies at home and women who had babies in hospitals. In hospitals, mothers often came down with childbed fever, a severe vaginal or uterine infection. At the time, surgeons did not wash their hands before treating women in childbirth. Surgeons might deliver a baby after working with diseased patients, without first washing their hands. Semmelweis faced hostility from his fellow physicians for a time, until they began to realize the health benefits of hand washing.

Louis Pasteur (1822–1895), a French chemist, carried out experiments that helped develop the modern science of microbiology. Microbiology is the study of infectious microscopic organisms such as bacteria, viruses, fungi, and parasites. Pasteur developed the first vaccine for rabies and anthrax and developed the pasteurization (application of heat to destroy pathogens) of milk and wine.

Considered the father of antiseptic surgery, the British surgeon Joseph Lister (1827–1912) insisted on using soap to disinfect instruments and clean hands before doctors moved from patient to patient. Today, sterilizing surgical equipment, disinfection, and hand washing are rigorously practiced as a way to prevent infection in hospitalized patients.

During the Industrial Revolution, German physician Robert Koch (1843–1910) discovered that some diseases are caused by microorganisms called **pathogens**. The discovery of pathogens confirmed Lister's insistence upon maintaining medical asepsis (the practice of keeping things free of pathogens to prevent infection).

> **Think It Through**
>
> Why do you think that colleagues of Dr. Semmelweis were skeptical of his research on the benefits of hand washing?

**pathogens**
*disease-producing microorganisms*

# *The Twentieth Century and Beyond*

In 1928, Scottish physician Alexander Fleming (1881–1955) discovered a mold that contained antibacterial secretions. Fleming's discovery, which he called *penicillin*, became the first antibiotic to treat bacterial infections. By 1943, mass production of penicillin had begun. The importance of penicillin was fully realized during World War II, when it prevented thousands of deaths by treating infected wounds. Along with other antibiotics, penicillin revolutionized healthcare, dramatically reducing death rates and giving birth to the modern pharmaceutical industry.

The development of X-ray technology by German physicist Wilhelm Roetgen (1845–1923) at the end of the nineteenth century opened up new and exciting possibilities in healthcare. X-ray technology has inspired the development of other noninvasive means of diagnosis using computers, such as magnetic resonance imaging (MRI) and computerized axial tomography (CT scans). An X-ray only produces a two-dimensional view of the body, but a computer can create a three-dimensional image, leading to more informed diagnoses. Another tool developed to monitor internal organs was the electrocardiogram (ECG or EKG). The electrocardiogram was developed by Willem Einthoven (1860–1927) in 1903 to monitor heart function.

## Discovering Radium, Insulin, and DNA

Radium was discovered by French scientists Marie and Pierre Curie at the beginning of the twentieth century (Figure 1.12). After her husband died, Marie Curie dedicated herself entirely to the development of X-ray use in medicine, as well as therapeutic uses for radiation, including cancer treatment.

**diabetes**

*an incurable metabolic disease that results in an increased level of glucose, or sugar, in the blood*

Insulin, an injectable hormone used to manage **diabetes** symptoms, was discovered in 1922 by Canadian physician Frederick Banting and his student, Charles Best. These two men isolated the internal secretions of the pancreas, the organ that creates insulin, and were able to harvest insulin from these secretions.

Insulin is used to regulate levels of glucose (a sugar) in the blood. Diabetics experience an inadequate production or utilization of insulin, resulting in excessive amounts of glucose in the blood and urine. Today, insulin is produced synthetically.

The discovery of deoxyribonucleic acid (DNA), the molecule that carries genetic information from one generation to the other, took place in April 1953. Although three men—James Watson (1928–), Francis Crick (1916–2004), and Maurice Wilkins (1916–2004)—were credited with the discovery of DNA, the research of Rosalind Franklin (1920–1958) helped them make their discovery. However, in 1962, Watson, Crick, and Wilkins were awarded the Nobel Prize in Physiology or Medicine for their discovery.

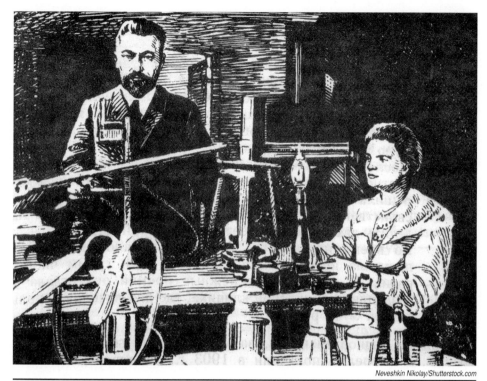

*Neveshkin Nikolay/Shutterstock.com*

**Figure 1.12**   Working together, Marie and Pierre Curie discovered the elements radium and polonium, which was named for Madam Curie's home country of Poland.

## Medical Machines and Electronics

Machines can now serve as substitutes for certain organs such as dialysis machines that replace the function of kidneys and heart-lung bypass machines that take over the heart's function during surgery. The first heart-lung bypass machine, which was invented by American physician John Gibbon (1903–1973), was used on a human in May of 1953.

Organ transplantation continues to be increasingly successful. The first organ transplant was a kidney transplant performed in 1954 by Dr. John P. Merrill. Today, combination heart-lung, bone marrow, stem cell, and liver transplants are possible. Antirejection drugs have improved to counter the body's reaction to foreign tissue introduced by an organ transplant.

Electronics and computer science have changed clinical medicine. One such change comes from the development of tiny robotic devices that assist in microsurgery. These devices view internal tissues during surgery. Fully mobile robots with computer screens for "heads" and video cameras for "eyes" and "ears" can be operated by a physician using a joystick and wireless technology. Using this kind of robot, physicians can perform examinations on patients while being far away from them.

Robots are also used in hospital pharmacies. Pharmacists enter prescriptions into a computer. The robot collects the dosages by scanning the barcode on a medication container and then packages a proper amount of

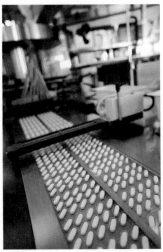

oknoart/Shutterstock.com

**Figure 1.13** Mechanized tablet packaging at a pharmaceutical company.

**psychoanalysis**
*a method of analyzing and treating mental and emotional disorders through sessions in which the patient is encouraged to talk about personal experience and dreams*

the medication. The robots ensure that the correct medication reaches the correct patient. Pharmaceutical companies also use automated systems to package their medications (Figure 1.13).

## Treating Mental Illness

Significant progress has been made in treating mental illness. At the beginning of the twentieth century, **psychoanalysis**—a method of treating mental and emotional disorders—became known to the medical community. Psychoanalysis is based on the concepts and theories of Sigmund Freud (1856–1939), an Austrian neurologist. Freud was known for his sessions during which the patient is encouraged to speak freely about personal experiences, particularly about his or her early childhood and dreams. Later in the twentieth century, psychoanalysis became a popular form of therapy for mental illness.

Before the twentieth century, mentally ill patients were placed in asylums, which are called *mental hospitals* today. After World War II, soldiers received increased psychiatric attention, thanks to the development of a new psychiatric manual for categorizing mental disorders.

Psychiatric medication gradually became prevalent during the twentieth century. Such medications were used to treat anxiety and depression. Some of these medications caused unpleasant side effects and dependency. New antidepressants known as SSRIs (selective serotonin reuptake inhibitors) became some of the most widely prescribed drugs in the world.

### ‖*Extend Your Knowledge*‖

*Controlling Healthcare Costs*

Research the national debate on how to control healthcare costs. What do you think would help lower healthcare costs? What roles do insurance companies play in healthcare costs?

### Think It Through

How has treatment of the mentally ill changed over time? In particular, what changes have been made in the United States? Do you think that there is prejudice against the mentally ill?

## *The United States' Healthcare Industry Today*

Medical care in the United States receives an abundance of media attention today. The developments taking place in the healthcare industry are undoubtedly contributing to the larger history of healthcare. As a future healthcare employee, you should understand some of the components of our current healthcare system. This section will present a snapshot of the healthcare industry in the United States today.

### Health Insurance

In contrast to most European countries, the United States depends primarily on a privatized system of healthcare. Almost 60% of US citizens have private (commercial) health insurance or are covered under a managed care plan (see below). Fewer than 30% of residents have coverage under public (government) programs. The remaining 10% of US residents have no health insurance.

## Government Insurance Programs

The two largest public health insurance programs run by the government are **Medicare** and **Medicaid**. Medicare is a government-funded insurance program for individuals over the age of 65 and people with disabilities or illnesses that prevent them from working, such as permanent kidney failure. Medicare is funded by taxes, and eligibility is determined by the federal government. Many people who qualify for Medicare also have a supplemental insurance policy for costs not covered by Medicare, such as many prescription medications and portions of medical bills.

Medicaid is an insurance program for people with low incomes and very few personal assets other than a home. It is a combined federal and state government insurance program, which means that it is paid for by state and federal taxes. States determine who is eligible for the program by following federal guidelines (Figure 1.14).

The Military Health System (TRICARE) is the program within the United States Department of Defense responsible for providing healthcare to active duty and retired US military personnel and their dependents.

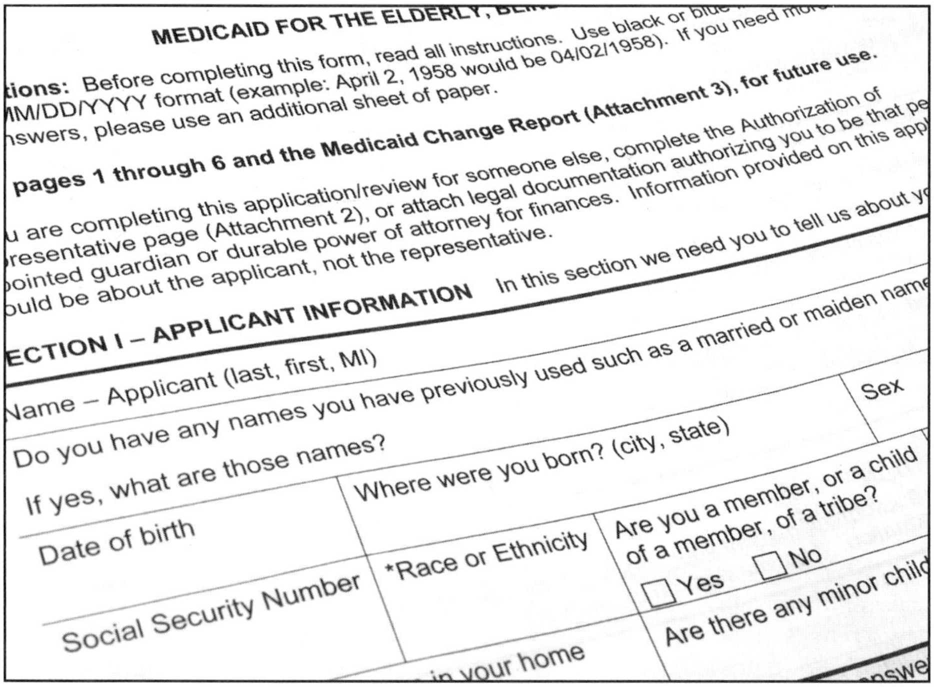

**Medicare**
*a federal health insurance program for persons 65 or older and disabled individuals*

**Medicaid**
*a program jointly-funded by state and federal taxes that provides medical aid for low-income individuals of all ages; managed by the states*

*Keith Bell/Shutterstock.com*

**Figure 1.14**  In order to receive Medicaid assistance, candidates must first apply and be found eligible for this insurance program.

**health maintenance organizations (HMO)**
*managed care organizations that provide prepaid, comprehensive healthcare at a flat rate and for a fixed period of time through a network of participating healthcare professionals and hospitals; policyholders select a primary care physician (PCP) and referrals from the PCP must be obtained to see a specialist*

**preferred provider organizations (PPO)**
*health insurance organizations that contract with a network of preferred providers from which the policyholder can choose; often involves an annual deductible payment for service, but patients do not have a designated primary care physician and may self-refer to specialists*

## Managed Care Plans

*Managed care* is a general term for any healthcare plan that emphasizes wellness and provides healthcare through a network of physicians, hospitals, and other healthcare providers at predetermined rates. There are several models of managed care, each with its own variations. The most common models are the **health maintenance organizations (HMOs)** and the **preferred provider organizations (PPOs)**.

The Health Maintenance Organization Act of 1973 caused a rapid increase in the number of health maintenance organizations. HMOs are set up so that you receive most, or all, of your healthcare from a network provider. You select a primary care physician who is responsible for managing and coordinating your healthcare. If you choose to have medical treatment outside of the HMO network, you will most likely pay the entire bill. If you cannot reach a network provider when outside the network area, you will probably be covered by your insurance for the out-of-network care you received. Most HMOs require a co-payment at the time of a visit.

PPOs contract with a network of preferred providers from which you can choose. Under this plan, you do not have to select a primary care physician. Instead, you will have a choice of doctors, hospitals, and other providers within the PPO network. But if you choose an out-of-network healthcare provider, you will pay more. Instead of a co-payment, PPOs may require an annual deductible payment for services.

There are many controversies surrounding health insurance today. Although most people agree that pre-existing conditions such as diabetes should be covered when you apply for insurance or change insurance companies, or that children should be covered by their parents' insurance until age 26, there is much debate over healthcare mandates. Healthcare mandates are government-issued laws that require individuals to buy health insurance. If mandates are put in place, the government, rather than private companies, will become the major players in the healthcare industry.

## Real Life Scenario

### Insurance Choices

Kevin is a twenty-six year old student who has no medical insurance. His part-time job doesn't have any benefits, and his heavy academic load does not allow him time to get a full-time job with benefits. Kevin has been debating whether or not to buy medical insurance now that he is no longer covered by his parents' insurance. He decides that his tight budget won't stretch to cover the cost of health insurance, and he'll worry about health insurance when he is older.

Has Kevin made a wise choice for this time in his life? Does he have any options for affordable health insurance? Is Kevin taking a risk living without health insurance?

# Types of Healthcare Facilities

When illness or injury occurs, patients have several types of healthcare facilities they can turn to in the United States. Remember that there are many options for employment in such institutions. The following are some of the most common healthcare facilities you might encounter in a city setting. Rural areas may only have a general hospital with few specialties.

## Hospitals

There are over 6,500 hospitals in the United States today. Hospitals are often described as short-stay or long-term care facilities, depending on the length of time a patient stays before discharge.

Short-stay hospitals are also referred to as acute-care facilities, where patients are admitted to treat acute, or severe, medical problems. However, these facilities are very expensive, and insurance companies only cover a certain amount of days of the patient's stay before requiring their transfer to a long-term care facility.

Emergency departments are most often found in acute-care hospitals. Patients are taken to the emergency department for treatment when they have life-threatening symptoms related to stroke, severe trauma, excessive bleeding, chest pains, and other serious situations (Figure 1.15). People without insurance or an established primary care physician often go to emergency departments for treatment of noncritical problems. The wait time for treatment may be lengthy and the cost may be higher than what patients would normally pay. If the patient is not able to pay for this treatment, the hospital absorbs the cost through government subsidy programs.

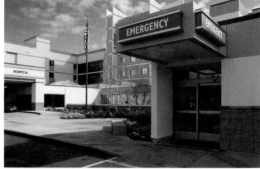

Galina Barskaya/Shutterstock.com

**Figure 1.15** Emergency rooms often have separate entrances so that people recognize where to go to obtain rapid medical treatment.

---

## ⊣‖Extend Your Knowledge‖

### Hospitals

What do you know about the hospital you use or would use if you needed a serious medical procedure? How would you proceed if you wanted to gather information about what services your local hospital offers? How can you find out if this hospital is the best one for your needs?

---

## Long-Term Care Facilities

These facilities generally house elderly or disabled patients who have a medical problem or problems that keep them from being able to take care of themselves. While family members remain the primary caretakers of elderly, dependent, or disabled patients, the growing elderly population is increasing the demand for long-term care facilities. The number of long-term facilities—often called *convalescent hospitals* or *nursing homes*—

has gone up in recent years. Many patients have a short recovery stay at a nursing home after receiving treatment at an acute hospital. Others may live in long-term care for the rest of their lives.

### Trauma Centers

Many hospitals are designated as trauma centers, which means that they are set up to handle the most serious of emergencies. Trauma surgeons and physicians trained in treating serious injuries are on staff at these centers. Highly sophisticated medical diagnostic equipment and treatment rooms designed for trauma injuries are available. The leading causes of traumatic injuries are motor vehicle accidents, assaults, and falls.

### Surgical Centers

Surgical centers are also called *ambulatory surgery centers*. These centers are designed to perform routine surgical procedures that do not require an overnight stay in the hospital. Minor surgeries such as biopsies, hernia repair, and cosmetic surgeries are performed in these centers.

### Doctors' Offices

Doctors' offices can be found in almost every area of the country. Physicians often have family practices that focus on providing healthcare to people of all ages. These doctors provide continuing care such as annual checkups for all family members. Some doctors' offices focus on specialties such as orthopedics, pediatrics, cardiology, and obstetrics and gynecology. Physicians in these offices are often affiliated with a hospital where they will send their patients if necessary, or perform surgery.

Urgent care centers often serve as family practices as well. These facilities treat injuries or illnesses that are not life-threatening, but require intervention within a few hours of occurrence or on the same day as they occur. Urgent care centers usually do not take appointments, so the wait time may be significant, but not as long as an emergency room. Urgent care facilities are often less expensive than an emergency room visit. Treatments at an urgent care center might cover eye, ear, throat, and bladder infections; stomachaches; flu; asthma attacks; or broken bones and sprains. Both adults and children can be treated at urgent care centers.

### Walk-In Clinics

Walk-in clinics are found in some department stores, pharmacies, or shopping centers. There is much variation in the staff of these clinics—some are staffed by physicians, while others are staffed by nurse practitioners with a specialty in this line of work. These clinics are designed for the convenience of patients. Some are affiliated with hospitals. Most of these clinics treat colds, sinus infections, strep throat, muscle sprains, and other minor problems. Some walk-in clinics can also provide vaccinations, routine physicals, and pregnancy tests.

## Mental Health Facilities

These facilities provide mental health care for a variety of patients. Some of these patients are severely mentally ill, but may be able to function normally with treatment. Others are mentally disabled (such as accident victims and patients with developmental disabilities) or suffer from chronic mental disabilities and do not respond to treatment. Mental health facilities are often very expensive as funding for mental health services in the United States is declining.

## Home Healthcare

Home healthcare is a popular alternative to long, costly hospital stays. Home healthcare agencies provide a wide variety of services for patients at home, from help with bathing, light housekeeping, and meal preparation, to skilled nursing care. Caregivers include registered nurses, practical nurses, and home health aides. Other caregivers may include physical therapists, social workers, and speech pathologists.

## Hospice Care

Facilities that offer care for terminally ill (dying) patients are called **hospice** facilities, or *palliative care*. Hospice care focuses on relieving patients' pain and symptoms of their terminal illness without seeking to cure the illness. Hospitals can arrange for hospice services to be provided at the patient's home.

**hospice**
*a type of care designed to relieve pain and reduce suffering in terminally ill patients*

## Kidney Dialysis Centers

Kidney dialysis is the process of removing waste products and excess fluid from the body (Figure 1.16). Dialysis centers provide comprehensive treatment for patients with chronic kidney disease. Patients visit the kidney dialysis center 3–4 times a week where machines serve as replacement kidneys.

Dialysis involves a machine that removes impurities and toxins from a person's blood, which would normally be filtered and excreted from the body by the kidneys. People who undergo regular dialysis treatment usually have end-stage kidney disease and no more than 10–15% kidney function remaining. Dialysis patients are often waiting for a kidney transplant.

## Rehabilitation Centers

Rehabilitation centers are facilities where patients work to reestablish or relearn abilities they lost because of a serious injury or illness, such as a stroke. Physical therapy helps with movement or previous loss of movement. Occupational therapy focuses on relearning activities of daily life or finding ways to perform them despite a disability.

## Freestanding Laboratories and Radiology Facilities

For the convenience of patients, freestanding laboratory facilities are available for routine tests and blood drawing. Some of these facilities have

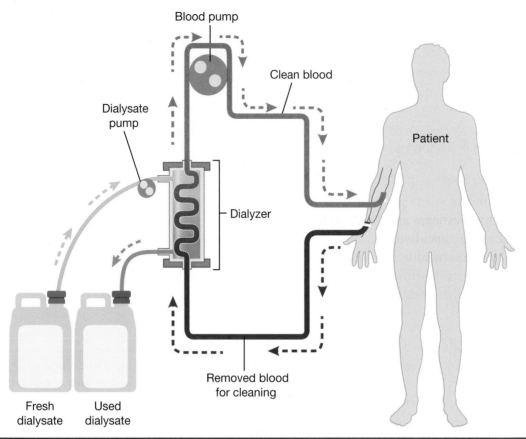

**Figure 1.16**   The most common type of dialysis is hemodialysis, a process by which blood is withdrawn from the body, filtered using a machine called a dialyzer, and then pumped back into the body. The filtering solution used by the dialyzer is called dialysate.

the ability to produce rapid test results such as complete blood counts and throat cultures. Doctors often send their patients to freestanding laboratories when their own offices do not have the space for a lab. There are also radiology facilities separate from hospitals that perform routine radiology procedures.

 *Check Your Understanding*

1. What facility would a person go to after a serious car accident?
2. Where would you go if you needed a routine blood test done?
3. What facility would be appropriate for a terminally ill person with no hope of a cure?
4. Where would you go if your kidneys failed?
5. What type of facility would be appropriate if you needed an appendectomy (appendix removal)?

# Rules and Regulations in Healthcare

It is important to understand the rules and regulations connected to healthcare. Chapter 3, *Healthcare Ethics and Law* details the legal and ethical responsibilities of a professional healthcare employee. Depending on what state you live in and the type of facility in which you are employed, you will be given an employee handbook with all the rules and regulations you will be required to follow.

Generally, there are rules and regulations that cover

- treating persons with disabilities;
- patient rights;
- eligibility for Medicare and Medicaid;
- reporting facility accidents;
- reporting communicable diseases;
- how different facilities are run;
- treating patients with dignity; and
- maintaining confidentiality.

# The Future of Healthcare

As healthcare in this country becomes more expensive, there will be continuing controversy over how to control costs. Should there be a national health plan? Are healthcare mandates acceptable to the American public? Should we keep our healthcare system the way it is?

The average life expectancy in the United States has dramatically increased since 1900, when the average life expectancy was 46.3 years for men, and 48.3 years for women (Figure 1.17). In the first decade of the 21st century, the average had risen to 75.7 for men and 80.6 for women.

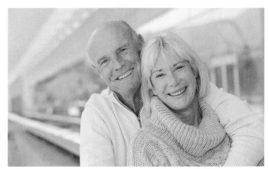

*Goodluz/Shutterstock.com*

**Figure 1.17**   Thanks in part to medical advancements, the average life expectancy in the United States continues to rise.

Hopefully, the future will bring cures for diseases like AIDS, and a decrease in cases of malaria, influenza, leprosy, and other diseases prevalent in third world countries. Much research is being done to cure genetically transferred diseases such as muscular dystrophy and cerebral palsy. Researchers are working aggressively on cures for heart disease, cancer, and Alzheimer's disease. In the future, new and exciting drugs will be developed that we cannot imagine at present.

There is still much to accomplish in the field of healthcare. Brilliant, innovative minds are continually at work in the spirit of such innovators as Hippocrates, Pasteur, Florence Nightingale, and the Curies. Medical technology continues to grow, with countries like the US and Japan developing innovative medical devices to advance the healthcare industry. Hardworking healthcare workers will continue to provide outstanding care to the suffering as well. Perhaps someday you, too, will contribute to this worthy cause.

# Chapter Review and Assessment

## Summary

Healthcare has developed and changed dramatically throughout history. The Chinese, Egyptian, Greek, Roman, Islamic, and Native American cultures, among others, all made healthcare discoveries that shaped the history of medicine and medical treatment around the world. The development of the printing press and the scientific method during the Renaissance allowed medical ideas and advances to spread quickly throughout the world.

The Industrial Revolution brought about more effective communication tools and factories that developed sophisticated medical equipment. Vaccines were developed for smallpox, cholera, and tetanus. The introduction of anesthesia was an incredibly important contribution to the practice of surgery. With the help of a few fearless female leaders, the profession of nursing became more respected and critical to improvements in healthcare. The importance of hand washing as part of medical practice was also realized and promoted.

Many brilliant scientists in the late nineteenth and twentieth centuries discovered the role of microorganisms in infection. Antibiotics were discovered and promoted, as was insulin. The discovery of DNA allowed researchers to begin unlocking the mysteries of heredity and further advances in computers and electronics changed how clinical medicine is practiced.

The medical industry is continually growing and changing. Today, health insurance is a huge part of the healthcare industry. In the United States, health insurance is a mixture of private programs, managed care plans (HMOs and PPOs), and government insurance programs such as Medicare and Medicaid.

Several types of healthcare facilities are available in communities across the country. The various facilities each have a unique set of rules and regulations and many are designed with a spcified purpose or patient in mind. When hired for a position at a healthcare facility, you will be given an employee handbook with all the rules and regulations you must follow.

## Review Questions

*Answer the following questions using what you have learned in this chapter.*

### Short Answer

1. What are the areas of focus for the US Department of Education's *National Healthcare Skill Standards Project*?
2. What important contribution did Hippocrates make to healthcare?
3. What is the significance of a caduceus?
4. What causes bubonic plague?
5. What important invention did Anthony Van Leeuwenhoek develop?
6. How did the development of aqueducts affect the people of ancient Greece?
7. What kinds of surgical instruments were developed by the Romans?
8. What is an antibiotic?
9. Describe the practice of vaccination.
10. How has treatment of the mentally ill changed over time?

### True or False

11. *True or False?* The first vaccine developed was for polio.
12. *True or False?* Louis Pasteur was the first scientist to develop a rabies vaccine.
13. *True or False?* Elizabeth Blackwell was the first woman to study and practice medicine in the United States.
14. *True or False?* Clara Barton started the American Red Cross.
15. *True or False?* PPOs and HMOs are both examples of managed care programs.
16. *True or False?* Psychoanalysis is a method of treating mental and physical disorders.
17. *True or False?* The caduceus and the staff of Aesculapius both feature two snakes wrapped around a staff.

18. *True or False?* The Hippocratic Oath is a promise of professional behavior made by physicians at the beginning of their careers.

## Multiple Choice

19. _____ is credited with the discovery of DNA.
    A. Marie and Pierre Curie
    B. James Watson, Francis Crick, and Maurice Wilkins
    C. Clara Barton and Alexander Fleming
    D. None of the above.

20. Which of the following is *not* a type of healthcare facility?
    A. rehabilitation facility
    B. emergency department
    C. urgent care clinic
    D. yoga studio

21. Which of the following health insurance plans is available in the United States?
    A. Medicare
    B. Medicaid
    C. Military Health System
    D. All of the above.

22. What are pathogens?
    A. harmless microorganisms
    B. vaccinations
    C. disease-producing organisms
    D. hand washing antiseptics

23. What is hospice care?
    A. a facility that rehabilitates addicts
    B. a physical therapy facility
    C. a facility that cares for the dying
    D. a long-term care facility

24. Many exciting inventions were made during the Renaissance, including the _____.
    A. forceps
    B. surgical needle
    C. microscope
    D. scalpel

25. Developments such as telegraph and railroad lines during the _____ enabled people to quickly and easily share ideas.
    A. Middle Ages
    B. Dark Ages
    C. Renaissance
    D. Industrial Revolution

26. Edward Jenner successfully vaccinated people for _____ using fluid from cowpox blisters, a symptom of a similar disease.
    A. cholera
    B. chicken pox
    C. smallpox
    D. rabies

27. _____ is the father of antiseptic surgery.
    A. Joseph Lister
    B. Louis Pasteur
    C. James Watson
    D. Alexander Fleming

28. _____ is a program jointly-funded by state and federal taxes that provides medical aid for low-income individuals of all ages.
    A. Medicare
    B. TRICARE
    C. Medicaid
    D. HMO

## Critical Thinking Exercises

29. Research the effects of the bubonic plague in the Dark and Middle Ages. Why isn't the bubonic plague a huge problem for the world today?

30. Imagine your neighbor is a new mother confused by the conflicting information she hears through the media about vaccinations. She asks you for your opinions about vaccinating very young children. Research the pro and con arguments surrounding the vaccination of infants and children. How would you present your findings to your neighbor?

31. Select an important person from the past who played a critical role in the development of medical advances and healthcare. Research this person and wexplain what special qualities the person possessed to make such discoveries.

32. Imagine you are just starting a new job, and you're meeting with the human resources representative about your health insurance options. She tells you that you can choose either a PPO or HMO. Which plan do you think would best suit your needs? Why?

# Chapter

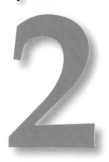

2

# *Beginning Your Healthcare Career*

## Terms to Know

associate's degree
bachelor's degree
career ladder
certification
diagnostic-related groups
  (DRGs)
diagnostic services
doctorate
electronic medical
  records (EMR)

health informatics
  services
job shadowing
licensure
master's degree
nosocomial infections
support services
therapeutic services

## Chapter Objectives

- Understand the importance of self-assessment before embarking on a health career exploration.
- Identify the different levels of education required for various health careers.
- Compare and contrast licensure and certification for healthcare workers.
- Discuss the differences among therapeutic, diagnostic, health informatics and information services, and support services in a healthcare setting.
- Identify possible careers in biotechnology research and development.

Reinforce your learning with additional online resources
- **Practice** vocabulary with flashcards and interactive games
- **Assess** with posttests and image labeling
- **Expand** with activities and animations

www.g-wlearning.com/healthsciences

**Study on the Go**
Use a mobile device to practice vocabulary terms and review with self-assessment quizzes.

www.m.g-wlearning.com

There are many career paths from which to choose, particularly in the healthcare field. Before selecting a future career, you might first ask yourself if you are suited for a career in healthcare. It is important to assess your goals and needs before you put time, energy, and money into pursuing a career. This chapter includes self-assessment questions as well as educational requirements and brief descriptions for many careers.

## *Planning for a Career in Healthcare*

Many factors influence a person's choice of career. Some people pursue a career based on family expectations or suggestions of others. However, it's important not to take this decision lightly. You need to give serious thought to your talents, limitations, and goals for success before settling on a career. If you decide that your talents and goals are best suited for the healthcare field, you will need to choose a specific career path within the field. The following are tips for narrowing your desired career path in healthcare.

### Self-Assessment

Since the medical field offers a wide variety of career paths to choose from, it's important to consider what type of position would be best for you. Many factors will help you make this decision. As you begin researching careers in the medical field, ask yourself the following questions. Your answers to these questions will help guide you toward your ideal career:

- Do you like being with people of all ages (Figure 2.1)?
- Do you enjoy working as a team player, or do you prefer to work alone?
- Do you enjoy working with computers more than interacting with others?
- Do you find helping others to be rewarding?
- Is job security an important consideration for you?
- Do you want to work only a nine-to-five, weekday job?
- Are you comfortable supervising the work of other people?
- Do you like to be creative in your work, or are you more comfortable with having one way to do things?
- Do you imagine yourself advancing up the career ladder quickly?
- Do you see yourself as a high wage earner?
- Do you enjoy being in school?
- Do hospitals and sick people make you feel queasy?
- Would you rather work outside, or inside a healthcare facility?

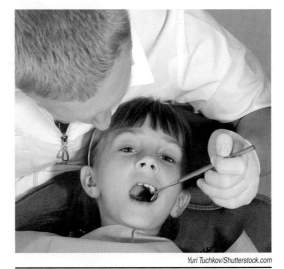

Yuri Tuchkov/Shutterstock.com

**Figure 2.1** Some healthcare careers require working with patients of all ages.

It is critically important to find a career that matches your interests and abilities. Your school counselor should be able to help you identify a potential career path using career assessment testing (Figure 2.2). These tests are not perfect but may give you a starting point when looking for a career that will best suit you.

In addition to seeking the help of your guidance counselor, you can also access free career inventory tests online. Some helpful career assessments include the Holland Codes, the Myers-Briggs Type Indicator, and the Enneagram of Personality. Another useful tool for researching a career is the *Occupational Outlook Handbook*, published by the US Bureau of Labor Statistics. The *Occupational Outlook Handbook* provides information about different careers, including working conditions, the training and education required, salary, and the job outlook for hundreds of different occupations.

## Job Shadowing

**job shadowing**
*a job exploration tool that involves following an employee completing the tasks of a job you find interesting*

Another valuable resource that may be available to you is **job shadowing**. Before making a commitment to a particular career and its related courses, you may want to shadow a person who already has that job.

Job shadowing allows you to follow an employee completing the tasks of a job you find interesting. This allows you to see for yourself what the job entails. You might find that your concept of the career was not accurate, or

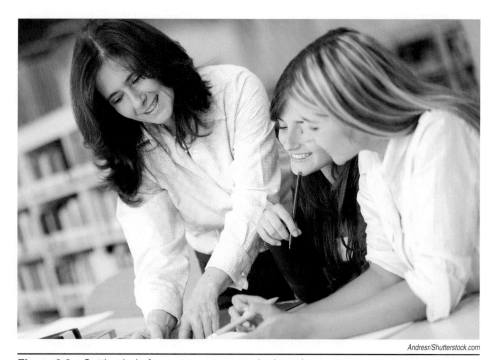

Andresr/Shutterstock.com

**Figure 2.2**   Getting help from a career counselor is an important way to assess your goals and needs for a career.

that you are not suited for the day-to-day demands of the position. Another perk of job shadowing is that it exposes you to the sights, sounds, and even smells that you may encounter in the healthcare world.

Your school counselor can help you set up job shadowing opportunities, or you can even contact a healthcare facility yourself and ask about job shadowing possibilities.

## *Choosing a Career Path*

Once you have identified your personal strengths, talents, likes, and dislikes, you can begin to research the type of career you would like to pursue. In addition to evaluating your personality needs, you need to decide how much education you are willing to complete, what kind of salary you want, and what type of workplace environment you would prefer. You will want to make sure there are plenty of opportunities available in the healthcare field you are researching.

The *Occupational Outlook Handbook* is a very useful starting point for researching a career. The Internet also has a great deal of information about healthcare careers, but you need to be aware of how current or accurate this information is. The United States government produces many publications related to jobs, such as guides for writing résumés, finding federal government jobs, and how to act while on a job interview. These publications can be found online. The National Institutes of Health (NIH), a government organization, also offers excellent Internet resources that discuss medical careers.

Many healthcare associations publish journals that include valuable career information. You can find these journals at your school or local library. Such journals include *The Journal of the American Medical Association (JAMA)*, *The Journal of Medical Ethics*, *The American Journal of Nursing*, *The Online Journal of Issues in Nursing*, and *The Journal of Physical Therapy*. Some communities also have a medical library, which is especially helpful when looking for specific periodicals and research materials that focus on medical issues and career possibilities. The career counselor at your school may be able to help you with your search.

## Educational Requirements

As you begin to explore a career in healthcare, you should research how much education will be required for various careers. The amount of education you need varies from career-to-career and state-to-state. You need to ask yourself how much education you are prepared to pursue. You may not enjoy classroom work and find that on-the-job training would better suit you. Conversely, you might really enjoy classroom work and wish to take a variety of classes to satisfy your academic curiosity and explore different fields.

> **Think It Through**
>
> Make a list of the five things you want most from a career. For example, a flexible schedule, good insurance benefits, or a high salary might be at the top of your list. Then list five of your strongest abilities, such as people skills, advanced math abilities, or organizational skills. Next, answer the questions from the self-assessment section of this chapter. Compare your list of career qualities, personal abilities, and self-assessment answers. What does this information tell you about yourself?

### High School

A high school education will prepare a student for an entry-level position after graduation. Most occupations require at least a high school diploma. Specific classes that explore health careers or health occupations would be particularly helpful to take. Some high schools offer certification programs at the high school level. Graduates may start an entry-level career immediately following high school.

### On-the-Job Training

During high school or after graduation, you can receive training to help advance your career. This training can be available for many careers such as home health aide, medical receptionist, food service worker, or central services worker. Though on-the-job training can be beneficial, further advancement will come through more formal education.

### Technical Schools

Sometimes referred to as *vocational, trade,* or *proprietary schools,* technical schools provide training for specific careers beyond high school. Technical schools can be more expensive than training at a community college because technical schools are privately owned and operated. However, scholarships and loans are often available to cover these educational costs.

Technical degrees and certifications are available, and some schools offer four-year degrees and higher degrees as well. Job placement guarantees are often a part of a technical school's offerings. Many of these schools have agreements with local companies to place students in unpaid internships. Then companies are able to assess potential employees before making employment commitments. In turn, companies work with the schools to ensure their students are exposed to the skill sets they require of their employees.

### Community College

A community college usually offers a two-year degree, called an **associate's degree**, in a specific course for a healthcare career. Students can use an associate's degree to transfer to a four-year college, where they can work toward a bachelor's degree. There are also many certificate programs at the community college level. Such programs might include emergency medical technician, medical assistant, health information technology, medical laboratory technician, and nursing.

Internships are often a part of community college programs. Internships (also known as *the community classroom, externship,* or *clinical rotation*) involve placement and training in a healthcare facility. Internships are usually unpaid and require completion of a specified number of hours. These experiences give students the opportunity to observe and practice the skills learned in class.

---

**Think It Through**

What attracted you to a career in healthcare? Did a family member who works in healthcare inspire you to explore the field? Do you have a mentor who encouraged you to follow this path? Are you motivated by a desire to help people?

---

**associate's degree**
*a two-year college degree, often offered through a community college and awarded after completing 60 credit hours or more when on a semester system*

## Four-Year College or University

Some healthcare careers require students to obtain a **bachelor's degree** and complete further training before starting a career. This training may include a clinical internship in which the student or recent graduate undergoes supervised training before becoming licensed or certified. Some clinical internships are unpaid, while others offer a small stipend (money given to offset costs such as transportation) during training. If you are taking classes full-time, a bachelor's degree typically takes about four years to complete.

Some professional-level careers may prefer candidates who have earned a further degree such as a **master's degree**. A master's degree can take one or two additional years of education to earn.

High-level positions often require an advanced degree called a **doctorate** degree. Several professional schools offer such degrees. A student can earn a professional doctoral degree in medical fields such as medical doctor (MD) and veterinarian (DVM), or an academic doctorate such as a doctor of philosophy (PhD). Each of these doctoral degrees can take several years to attain.

Figure 2.3 shows the various levels of employment and the education they require, and provides examples of job titles found at each level.

## Continuing Education

In many healthcare occupations, your education continues after you are hired. Some employers or government agencies require you to take additional courses to maintain professional status in your career. These requirements vary from state-to-state and among careers. In today's world, where changes and discoveries continually occur, continuing education is critical. Opportunities for continuing education may be offered at your place of employment; online; or through courses offered by schools, colleges, or private vendors.

**bachelor's degree**
*a four-year college degree awarded after 120 credit hours or more when on a semester system*

**master's degree**
*academic degree awarded by a college or university to those who complete from one to two years (depending on the degree) of prescribed study beyond the bachelor's degree*

**doctorate**
*a degree awarded after two to six years of education beyond the bachelor's degree; available in many disciplines*

| Healthcare Employment Levels | | |
|---|---|---|
| *Level* | *Educational Requirements* | *Example* |
| **Professional** | four-year degree; advanced degree; clinical training | physician; registered nurse practitioner; registered nurse; pharmacist |
| **Technologist** | three to four years of college; clinical training | laboratory technologist; radiologic technologist |
| **Technician** | often associate's degree; clinical training; possible licensure | X-ray technician; health information technician; licensed vocational nurse |
| **Assistant** | up to one year of classroom and clinical training | physical therapy assistant; medical assistant; nursing assistant |
| **Aide** | high school diploma; on-the-job training | laboratory aide; central services aide |

**Figure 2.3**   Healthcare careers vary by level and educational requirements. Continuing your education is one way to advance in your healthcare career.

## Licensure and Certification

In addition to educational requirements and training, some careers require **licensure** and **certification**. By obtaining licensure or certifications, employees ensure they have met all of the standards required for that particular healthcare career.

### Licensure

**licensure**
*recognition given by a state agency when a person meets the qualifications for a particular occupation; given after the person passes a licensure examination; required in order to practice*

**certification**
*recognition given for completing a course of study*

Licensure is awarded by a state agency when a person meets the qualifications for a particular occupation. People seeking licensure must pass a licensing exam. For instance, laboratory technologists must take a state examination and pass with a certain percentage before obtaining a license to work as a technologist. Registered nurses and licensed vocational nurses must pass a state board examination and receive a license to practice in a particular state.

### Certification

Certification is given as recognition for completing a specific course of study or passing a certification exam. For instance, a phlebotomist (a person who draws blood) may earn a certificate after completing the clinical training hours required in the course of study. A health information technician must have an associate's degree and pass an examination given by a certifying agency to become a registered health information technician (RHIT).

In some occupations, certification is voluntary. An individual may chose to take a certification exam for professional advancement. In other cases, certification is required and is considered equivalent to licensure.

# Exploring Healthcare Careers

Do you follow the latest technology trends and enjoy working with computers? Are you interested in encouraging healthy lifestyles and helping promote wellness in patients of all ages? Does using your knowledge and training to diagnose and treat injuries and diseases appeal to you? Imagine being in a position to save someone's life—what an amazing feeling that would be!

If the job situations listed above appeal to you, then a career in healthcare is something to explore. To choose a specific path in the healthcare field, you should research and compare a variety of careers. In this section you will learn about several of these healthcare careers. These careers are divided into four pathways—therapeutic services, diagnostic services, health informatics services, and support services.

There is no right or wrong way of presenting these services, but this chapter covers major career opportunities that exist in a full-service healthcare facility. Figure 2.4 illustrates the four areas of employment presented in this chapter. A fifth career pathway includes biotechnology research and development careers. This pathway is not discussed in detail because it

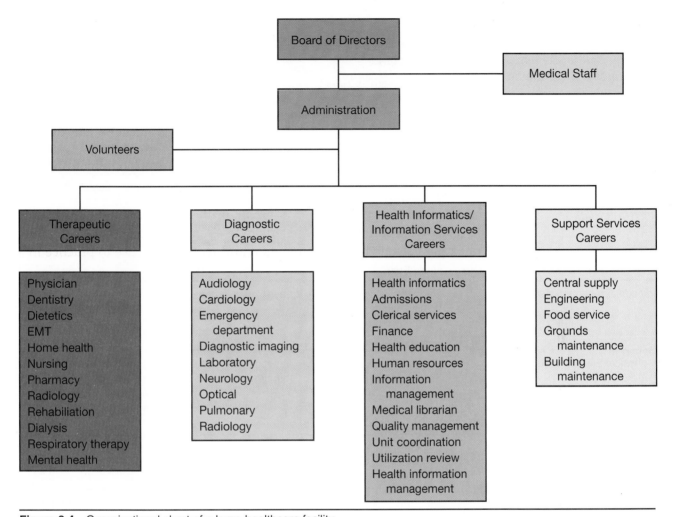

**Figure 2.4**   Organizational chart of a large healthcare facility

includes careers that are highly scientific—people in this field would work mostly in laboratories separate from hospital environments.

It is important for students to be aware of their options before embarking on a path that may not be suitable for their long-term needs. This is when job shadowing and talking with a career counselor are very important steps to take.

## Therapeutic Services Careers

The **therapeutic services** pathway offers many career possibilities ranging from driving an ambulance to working with a child who has speech problems. Do hands-on experiences with patients seem like something you would enjoy? If so, being in the therapeutic services might be a rewarding career path for you. Figures 2.4 and 2.5 both illustrate some therapeutic services careers, along with their educational requirements. Use these references to begin exploring careers that interest you.

**therapeutic services**
*career path that offers hands-on experience with patients and focuses on changing the health status of a patient over time*

| Educational Requirements for Common Therapeutic Careers | | | |
|---|---|---|---|
| High School Diploma/Industry Certification/On-the-Job Training | Associate's Degree | Bachelor's Degree | Master's or Professional Degree |
| home health aide; certified nursing assistant (CNA); patient care technician (PCT) | registered nurse (RN) | registered nurse (RN, BSN) | nurse practitioner (MSN, FNP); registered nurse (RN, BSN, MSN); doctorate of nursing practice (DNP) |
| respiratory therapist aide | respiratory therapy technician | respiratory therapist (RRT) | pulmonologist (MD) |
| emergency medicine tech (EMT) | paramedics | [required for admittance into advanced degree programs] | exercise physiologist |
| medical receptionist; file clerk | administrative front office; clinical back office medical assistants; office manager | physician assistant (PA) | physician (MD); physician assistant (PA) |
| physical therapy assistants; sports medicine aide | physical therapy assistant; sports medicine assistant | athletic trainer; physical therapist | speech and language pathologist; physiatrist, MD; physical therapist (MPT); doctorate of physical therapy (DPT) |
| dental assistants | dental laboratory technicians; dental hygienists | [required for admittance into advanced degree programs] | dentists (DDS) |
| pharmacy clerk | pharmacy technician | [required for admittance into advanced degree programs] | pharmacist (PharmD) |
| mental health aide | mental health technician; substance abuse counselor | counselor | counselor; psychologist; psychiatrist (MD) |
| veterinarian assistant | veterinarian technician | [required for admittance into advanced degree programs] | veterinarian (DVM) |
| occupational therapy aide | certified occupational therapy assistant (COTA) | occupational therapist (OT) | Masters of Science in Occupational Therapy (MOT) |

**Figure 2.5** Many fulfilling career opportunities exist in therapeutic services. These careers vary greatly based on education.

Careers in the therapeutic services pathway are focused primarily on changing the health status of a patient over time. Health professionals in this pathway work directly with patients by providing care, treatment, counseling, and health education information. The amount of education required for therapeutic services careers varies.

As Figure 2.5 shows, there is much room for career advancement in this pathway. For instance, you can train on-the-job for an assistant or aide level career, and then go back to school to get an associate's degree in a related field. If you want to further advance your career to one with better pay and more responsibility, you can get a four-year degree or higher.

## Nurses

Nursing is an exciting field that offers many opportunities for employment as well as advancement (Figure 2.6). For example, you may begin your career as a certified nursing assistant but eventually decide you would like more responsibility. To become a registered nurse, you must obtain an associate's degree in nursing. Depending on the school, the name of the associate's degree may change; possibilities include associate's degree in nursing (AN), associate's degree of applied science in nursing (AAS), or an associate's degree in nursing (ADN) from a community college.

Further professional development might lead you to pursue a bachelor's degree (BSN), a master's degree (MSN), or a doctorate degree (DPN) in nursing. These advanced degrees will allow you to become a nurse manager, an instructor, or a nurse practitioner. Some nurses eventually go to medical school and become physicians. There are many opportunities to climb the **career ladder** and receive a promotion in the medical field.

Nurses are employed in many types of healthcare facilities. If you would prefer to work in a small healthcare facility, there are many therapeutic career options in clinics, physician offices, and nursing homes. Figure 2.7 is a sample of the organization and hierarchy of the medical staff in a smaller facility. For current information about the careers mentioned in this organizational chart, see your school's job counselor or conduct further research online.

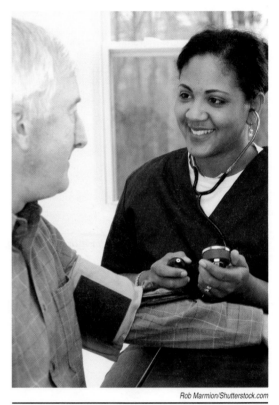

Rob Marmion/Shutterstock.com

**Figure 2.6** Nurses must be comfortable working closely with patients.

**career ladder**
*term for the progression from an entry-level position to higher levels of pay, skill, and responsibility*

## Physicians

Becoming a physician (otherwise known as a *doctor* or *MD*) requires many years of hard work that includes earning admission into colleges, universities, and medical school; studying; testing; writing; researching; and training. In order to achieve optimal success as a doctor of medicine, you should start preparing as early as possible, preferably in high school. The required education can take about 10 to 15 years after high school to complete, depending on what specialty (the specific area of medicine to be practiced) you choose. Although physicians are listed under the therapeutic careers, they are equally involved in diagnostic services.

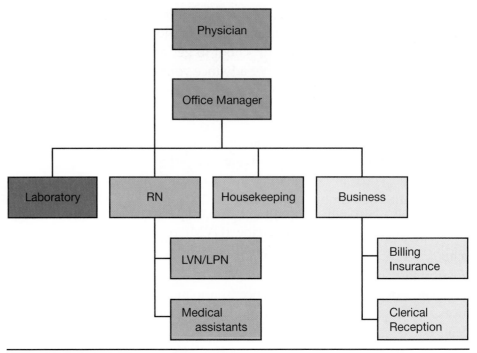

**Figure 2.7**    Medical office organization chart

## Dentists

Dentistry is the branch of medicine that involves the study, diagnosis, prevention, and treatment of diseases, disorders, and conditions of the oral cavity and nearby structures (Figure 2.8). Individuals who have graduated from dental school are called dentists, or *doctors of dental surgery* (*DDS*).

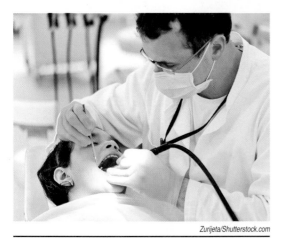

*Zurijeta/Shutterstock.com*

**Figure 2.8**    It takes many years of education to become a dentist.

After earning a bachelor's degree, candidates for dental school take the Dental Admissions Test (DAT) to ensure they are prepared for dental school training. The DAT is a multiple choice examination that includes sections focused on the sciences (especially biology and chemistry), math, reading comprehension, and perceptual ability testing (the test taker's spatial visualization skills). In order to prepare for the DAT, future dentists should take courses in these areas during their undergraduate education.

Dental schools should be fully accredited, or *recognized*, by the American Dental Association's (ADA) Commission on Dental Accreditation. Dental school usually lasts four years, and graduates earn a doctor of dental surgery (DDS).

## Veterinarians

Veterinarians care for animals by diagnosing, treating, or researching their medical conditions and diseases. In their practice, veterinarians treat pets; livestock; and animals found in zoos, racetracks, and laboratories (Figure 2.9).

Students who wish to enter a veterinary program typically obtain a bachelor's degree in a science-related area such as zoology, molecular biology, chemistry, animal science, or biochemistry. In some instances, veterinary programs do not require students to hold four-year degrees. However, students may experience difficulty gaining admittance into veterinary programs as these schools are extremely competitive, even with a degree.

Veterinary students are required to complete a four-year doctor of veterinary medicine (DVM) program in addition to earning their bachelor's degree. These professionals are also required to obtain licensure to practice in the profession.

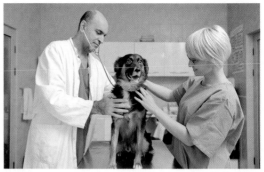

*dotshock/Shutterstock.com*

**Figure 2.9**   Veterinarians are trained in animal medicine, surgery, and behavior.

### Respiratory Therapists and Respiratory Care Workers

Helping patients with their breathing is a critical part of healthcare. Without proper breathing, patients can suffer brain damage within a few minutes, with death following soon after.

Respiratory care workers perform many tasks to help patients who are having trouble with their breathing. Respiratory therapists test the patient's lung capacity and check oxygen and carbon dioxide levels in his or her blood. These workers give patients treatments and teach patients with chronic lung conditions to care for themselves. Respiratory therapists also provide emergency care to patients who have suffered strokes, electrical shock, heart failure, and other life-threatening conditions. As part of their responsibilities, respiratory therapists take care of their equipment and do a great deal of record keeping.

If you refer back to Figure 2.5, you will see there is definite potential for moving up the career ladder in this field. By continuing their education, respiratory care workers can advance from an aide to a technician-level position, or become a respiratory therapist after earning their bachelor's degree. Respiratory therapists might even advance to the level of pulmonologist, a physician who specializes in the care and treatment of the lungs.

### Physical Therapy and Occupational Therapy Workers

Physical therapists and physical therapy aides assist and direct patients in the process of rehabilitation. A physical therapist's goal is to reduce pain and restore physical function and promote healing. Occupational therapy workers interact with people who are physically, mentally, developmentally, or emotionally disabled. These workers plan and develop programs that help restore, maintain, or develop the patient's ability to manage activities of daily living (ADL). The goal of these careers is to help patients be able to function independently by showing them ways to compensate for disabilities. These careers require creativity and flexibility while working with patients to find the right equipment and tools to help the varying needs of each individual.

Workplaces for physical and occupational therapists include hospitals, schools, nursing homes, outpatient clinics, rehabilitation centers, and mental health facilities and agencies.

### Emergency Medical Service Providers

Peoples' lives often depend on the quick reaction and competent care of emergency medical technicians (EMTs) and paramedics (Figure 2.10). Incidents as varied as automobile accidents, heart attacks, slips and falls, childbirth, and gunshot wounds require immediate medical attention. EMTs and paramedics provide this vital service as they care for and transport the sick or injured to a medical facility.

In an emergency, EMTs and paramedics are typically dispatched to the scene by a 911 operator. When they arrive on the scene, EMTs and paramedics often work alongside police and firefighters. EMTs and paramedics immediately assess the nature of the patient's condition, while trying to determine whether the patient has any preexisting medical conditions. Following protocols and procedures, these workers provide emergency care and transport the patient to a medical facility. EMTs and paramedics perform their duties in emergency medical services systems in which a physician provides medical direction and oversight.

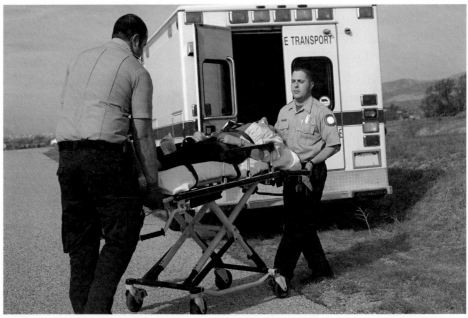

**Figure 2.10**   Emergency medical technicians must remain calm when dealing with life and death situations.

## Medical Assistants

Medical assistants work primarily in physicians' offices, clinics, and other outpatient medical facilities. They perform the administrative and clinical duties needed to assist physicians in providing patient care. Medical assistants may work with physicians who provide either general or specialized care.

Clinical, or back office, medical assistants assist the physician with examinations, treatments, and diagnostic procedures. In many states, clinical medical assistants are allowed to give injections and draw blood.

Administrative, or front office, medical assistants manage the reception area. They also complete clerical duties, such as managing insurance claims, collections, and electronic medical records. Many medical assistants study to become comprehensive medical assistants, skilled in both administrative and clinical procedures.

Many community colleges, adult schools, and proprietary schools offer medical assistant programs. Although no license is required to practice as a medical assistant, most employers want medical assistants to be certified.

### ✔ Check Your Understanding

When disasters occur, EMTs and paramedics are among the first responders to the site. Do you have disaster drills in your school? Do you have an escape route planned if a fire or other disaster should happen in your home?

## Diagnostic Services Careers

When you choose the **diagnostic services** healthcare career path, you become an integral part of the diagnosing process. These careers involve procedures that determine the causes of diseases or disorders. Some workers have direct contact with patients, but others do not.

Some careers are not only considered diagnostic, but fall into the therapeutic services category as well. An example of this is a cardiologist who diagnoses heart-related problems, but also works with patients and recommends therapies.

Diagnostic careers focus on planning services for patients as well as performing tests accurately. Those in this career path are responsible for quality control, which involves implementing a system for verifying and maintaining a desired level of quality in a product or process, use of proper equipment, continued inspection, and corrective action as required. If you are engaged in any testing procedures, you *must* produce accurate results and report them in a timely manner. Record keeping is also very important in this area.

**diagnostic services**
*a healthcare pathway offering careers in implementing procedures to determine causes of diseases or disorders*

When you work in diagnostic services, your attention to detail is critical. Sloppy handling of specimens to be tested, failure to correctly enter results into a computer, and inability to deal with deadlines can all lead to possible termination. Remember, an incorrect test result could adversely affect the treatment of a patient. As with many healthcare fields, diagnostic services offer a variety of jobs depending on your level of education. As you read through the job descriptions in Figure 2.11, think about what diagnostic careers interest you the most.

### The Clinical Laboratory

The clinical laboratory, often called the *medical laboratory*, is a separate section of a healthcare facility. The laboratory is the place where blood, urine, sputum (mucus coughed up from the lung), stool (feces), and tissues are analyzed in a precise, accurate, and timely manner. The results of these analyses give physicians valuable information about a patient's medical condition. A number of conditions can be rapidly diagnosed by the laboratory, including heart attack, diabetes, and strep throat.

Many tests in the clinical laboratory are very complicated and involve complex machines that require high levels of training to operate (Figure 2.12). Clinical laboratory technologists train other staff members on the use of laboratory machines. Tests that are relatively simple and may not require the use of complex machines can be accomplished by the clinical laboratory technician or clinical laboratory aide. Each state has its own requirements for performing clinical laboratory tests.

| Educational Requirements for Common Diagnostic Careers | | | |
|---|---|---|---|
| *High School Diploma/Industry Certification/On-the-Job Training* | *Associate's Degree* | *Bachelor's Degree* | *Master's Degree or Professional Degree* |
| clinical laboratory aides; phlebotomists; venipuncture technicians; clinical laboratory clerical worker | clinical laboratory technicians; cytologist; histologist | clinical laboratory technologist | clinical laboratory supervisor; laboratory administrator; chief technologist; pathologist |
| EKG technician | cardiovascular technologist | [required for admittance into advanced degree programs] | cardiologist |
| X-ray technician*; radiology aide | CT scan technologist* | radiologic technologist; diagnostic medical sonographers; radiologic technologist chief | radiologists; radiation oncologists |
| ophthalmology aide | optician | [required for admittance into advanced degree programs] | optometrists; ophthalmologists |

*Note: An advanced degree may be required by some states.

**Figure 2.11**   Advancement in diagnostic service careers can come from continuing education.

There are many work environments available to clinical laboratory workers, such as acute care hospitals, private laboratories, physician office complexes, clinics, health maintenance organizations (HMOs), and research facilities. In a healthcare facility, the clinical laboratory continually interacts with almost every other department, providing critical services for inpatients and outpatients served by the facility.

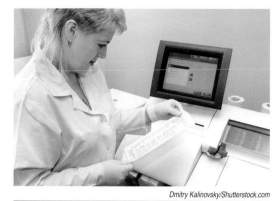

Dmitry Kalinovsky/Shutterstock.com

**Figure 2.12**   Clinical laboratory professionals must be able to work with sophisticated, often automated machinery.

**Clinical Laboratory Technologist.** The clinical laboratory technologist (also called a *clinical laboratory scientist* or *medical technologist*) typically has a bachelor's degree in a science discipline and has completed a yearlong internship in a healthcare facility. Today, the clinical laboratory technologist often supervises one of the departments in the clinical laboratory, and is responsible for all test results produced in her department. With proper training, these workers are legally able to perform all tests in the clinical laboratory.

**Phlebotomists.** Lab workers who are trained to draw blood from a live person or animal for tests, transfusions, donations, or research are called *phlebotomists*. Phlebotomists collect blood primarily by performing venipuncture, a surgical puncture in which blood is extracted from a vein, or by taking small quantities of blood from the finger. Blood may be collected from infants by means of a heel stick, a procedure in which the infant's heel is pricked by a needle. Blood is then collected in a pipette (narrow tube) or on special paper. Some counties, districts, or states require phlebotomy personnel to be licensed or certified.

### *Real Life Scenario*

*Argumentative Patients*

Daisy is a phlebotomist who works in the outpatient laboratory at Eastridge Hospital. A very nervous woman, Mrs. Rice, comes to her blood drawing station. Mrs. Rice's physician wants her to have several blood tests, which requires Daisy to draw four vials of blood from Mrs. Rice.

Mrs. Rice is very upset that she has to have her blood drawn and immediately tells Daisy that she will not cooperate, and gets up to leave. Imagine that you are Daisy; what would you do in this situation?

A. Do you insist that Mrs. Rice sit down and give you her arm, not taking no for an answer?

B. Do you try to talk Mrs. Rice into having her blood drawn?

C. If Mrs. Rice still refuses to have her blood drawn, do you let her leave and then call her doctor to explain why no blood has been drawn?

**Pathologist.** Although pathologists are physicians, they do not treat patients of their own. Instead, pathologists conduct laboratory tests to diagnose diseases in the patients of other physicians. They perform or review tests on body tissues, secretions, and other specimens to see whether a disease is present and, if so, to determine its stage.

### Vision Care

Half of the people in the United States currently need some sort of vision care and 96% of people over the age of 65 have vision problems. As a result, there are many different types of vision care workers whose job it is to provide treatment for this high-demand area of healthcare. Due to our aging population, vision care will be a growing industry in the coming years.

There are three categories of eye care professionals—ophthalmologists, optometrists, and opticians. Vision care professionals need a great deal of scientific training, including anatomy and physiology, pharmacology (the study of drugs), mathematics, and other science disciplines. There is also considerable patient interaction in this field. Career opportunities include working in clinics, large medical facilities, private practice offices, and even retail stores (many have an eye care section).

**Ophthalmologists.** Ophthalmologists are medical doctors who have received training beyond medical school with a specialty in vision care and eye diseases. They are licensed to diagnose, write prescriptions for, and treat all eye problems.

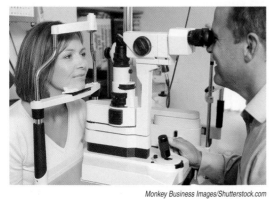
*Monkey Business Images/Shutterstock.com*

**Figure 2.13**  Optometrists are required to complete four years of graduate education.

**Optometrists.** After obtaining their bachelor's degree, optometrists complete four years of graduate education at a college of optometry. They then receive a doctor of optometry (OD) degree and are able to examine patients for eye problems, and fit eyeglasses and contact lenses. In some states, optometrists can prescribe and administer drugs to diagnose and treat eye diseases (Figure 2.13).

**Opticians.** Opticians fit and dispense glasses and contact lenses after receiving a prescription written by other professionals. Optician training varies from state to state. Becoming an optician requires a high school diploma or an approved GED equivalent, followed by formal education and training, or an apprenticeship.

Many opticians go to college to earn a two-year associate's degree in optometry, which involves coursework in basic anatomy, eye anatomy, algebra, trigonometry, optical physics, and administration.

### Radiology Workers

Today, X-ray departments are also called *diagnostic imaging departments*. Radiology employees operate X-ray equipment to take pictures of internal parts of the body. X-rays can be used to diagnose lung diseases such as cancer or tuberculosis  as well as blood clots, ulcers, and fractures. As

| Advanced Radiology Machines | | |
| --- | --- | --- |
| *Diagnostic Imaging Technique* | *Description* | *Operator* |
| **Ultrasound** | transmission of sound waves at high frequencies into a patient's body, resulting in an image called a sonogram; often used for prenatal care and for cardiology | ultrasound technologists; sonographers |
| **Magnetic Resonance Imaging (MRI)** | used to visualize detailed internal structures; provides good contrast between the different soft tissues of the body, making it especially useful in imaging the brain, muscles, the heart, and tumors | magnetic resonance technologist |
| **Computer Axial Tomography (CT Scans)** | an X-ray procedure that combines many X-ray images with the aid of a computer to generate cross-sectional views or three-dimensional images of the internal organs and structures of the body; used to define normal and abnormal structures in the body or assist in procedures by helping to accurately guide the placement of instruments or treatments | CT scan technologist |
| **Mammography** | a low-energy X-ray machine used to examine the breasts; helps to diagnose and screen for breast cancer, typically through detection of masses or calcium deposits in the breasts | mammographer |

**Figure 2.14**   Advanced radiology machines can be used for a variety of purposes.

Figure 2.14 shows, sophisticated imaging technology is increasingly being used to make more detailed diagnoses. Such technology includes ultrasound, computerized axial tomography (CT) scans, and magnetic resonance imaging, or *MRI* (Figure 2.15).

When working with radiation, it is imperative to exercise caution and take the appropriate safety measures. Exposure to radiation can cause cell damage. A protective barrier should always be placed between the equipment operator and the source of radiation. Lead is the most common shielding material, and is embedded in walls, gloves, aprons, partitions, and other protective items in X-ray rooms. Radiology workers must also maintain a safe distance of at least six feet from the radiation source.

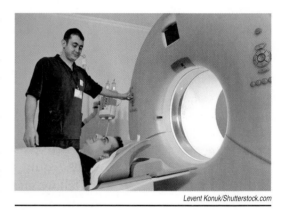

*Levent Konuk/Shutterstock.com*

**Figure 2.15**   An MRI machine can be used to create detailed images of internal structures.

Radiation badges called *dosimeters* monitor radiation exposure over a period of time. Employees working with radiation must wear dosimeters at all times to ensure that they are not being exposed to dangerous levels of radiation. Results of this monitoring are sent wirelessly to a computer.

Proper protection and adherence to safety guidelines ensure that radiation is not a problem for radiology employees. However, people under the age of 18 are not allowed to work around radiation because the tissues in their bodies are still growing and are more susceptible to injury from radiation. Because it is so important that people are aware of radiation, an

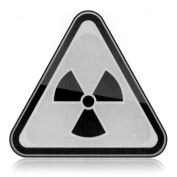

vector illustration/Shutterstock.com

**Figure 2.16** This symbol alerts patients and health-care workers that radiation is present.

**health informatics services**

*career field considered to be a bridge between medicine and technology, and which provides critical support to all other medical services; includes positions such as medical clerical worker, human resource workers, and medical records workers*

internationally-recognized symbol alerts people to its presence (Figure 2.16). This is discussed more completely in chapter 4.

Excellent career opportunities exist in radiology. To qualify for most technician positions in this career path, you will need to learn to use sophisticated equipment. Much more education is required for positions such as radiologist or radiation oncologist.

**Radiologists.** Radiologists are medical doctors who specialize in the use of diagnostic imaging to diagnose and treat disease. Agents such as dyes are often administered to the body to help radiologists see imaging results more clearly. Radiologists also diagnose findings seen on X-rays.

**Radiation Oncologists.** Radiation oncologists are doctors who specialize in cancer treatment using radiation. A radiation oncologist determines a tumor treatment plan for each patient. Beams of radiation are directed at cancerous cells or tumors to destroy or inhibit the cancerous cells' ability to grow.

## Health Informatics and Information Services Careers

**Health informatics services** is one of the fastest growing fields in the healthcare industry today. This field serves as a bridge between the worlds of medicine and technology. Health information service workers such as hospital admitting department workers, various medical clerical positions, human resources workers, health unit coordinators, and medical records workers provide critical support to all other medical services in a healthcare setting.

There are many positions in this field that offer secure employment with excellent benefits. These positions vary greatly in a few key aspects—some require a high level of expertise with computers, some do not include contact with patients, and some deal directly with patients. All of these positions require people skills, whether or not you are working with patients or fellow employees. These careers also require exceptional attention to detail. Figure 2.17 lists some careers in health informatics and information services. Again, the requirements for these careers may vary among states.

### Health Informatics

Health informatics is an exciting health career field today. This area includes the knowledge, skills, and tools that enable information to be collected, managed, used, and shared to support the delivery of healthcare and to promote health.

Careers in health informatics involve incorporating advanced technology into patient care and facility operations. As technology continues to change, these professionals are needed to help implement these changes in healthcare settings. Jobs that fall under the health informatics category range from a health information assistant with an associate's degree, to a member of health informatics management with a master's degree. Many

| Educational Requirements for Common Health Informatics and Information Service Careers | | | |
|---|---|---|---|
| *High School Diploma/Industry Certification/On-the-Job Training* | *Associate's Degree* | *Bachelor's Degree* | *Master's or Professional Degree* |
| health information file clerk | health information assistant | certified medical informatics specialist | medical and health services manager; informatics consultant for information systems |
| health information management clerk | registered health information technician (RHIT) | Registered Health Information Administrator (RHIA) | |
| unit secretary; health unit coordinator; medical transcriptionist | manager of health unit coordinators; medical transcriptist | | |
| medical clerical worker: | medical office manager; medical records and health information technician | hospital admitting officer | |
| human resources assistant | human resources technician | human resources generalist | human resources manager |

**Figure 2.17**   Various health informatics and health information service careers are available to you depending upon your education level.

career opportunities will exist for individuals with health information technology expertise to conduct or provide training for physicians and nurses as they adopt new electronic healthcare systems.

Jobs in health informatics are growing at a rapid rate. According to the Bureau of Labor Statistics, employment in health information careers is expected to increase by 20%—much faster than the average for all occupations—through 2018. Job prospects are very good, especially for technicians with strong computer software skills. This is one healthcare occupation in which there is no hands-on patient care.

Applicants for jobs in this area usually have at least an associate's degree. A master's degree in health informatics prepares you for a number of careers. Career titles include the following:

- certified health information specialist
- chief information officer
- clinical informaticist
- informatics consultant
- medical and health services manager
- medical informatics specialist
- nursing information officer

Employment in the field of health informatics can be found in both rural and metropolitan areas in hospitals, clinics, universities, biomedical research facilities, and many other places.

## Medical Clerical Workers

Medical clerical workers serve as support to all other medical services. These workers handle complaints, interpret and explain policies, prepare payrolls, resolve problems with billing, and collect overdue accounts. The following list includes some positions in the healthcare field of information services that may require on-the-job training or participation in a one- or two-year training program through a community college or vocational education program:

- appointment scheduler
- bill collector
- claim representative
- data processor
- insurance processor
- material or purchasing clerk
- payroll or timekeeping clerk
- personnel clerk
- medical receptionist
- administrative medical assistant

Medical clerical workers ensure that the everyday operations of healthcare organizations run smoothly and efficiently, while working to provide excellent customer service. Some of these workers deal directly with patients and their families, while others may not see patients.

## Health Information Specialists

Detailed records are kept every time a patient receives care or interacts with a healthcare professional. Prescriptions, treatment plans, test results, diagnoses, the patient's medical history, and the description of symptoms are included in these records. These records are the primary responsibility of the health information technician, a position that was formerly called the *medical records technician* (Figure 2.18).

A traditional patient record is on paper and stored in medical facilities. However, electronic record keeping is quickly becoming the norm. Problems with paper medical records, such as illegible handwriting, can lead to serious errors in diagnosis, treatment, and billing. Also, there is only one copy of a paper record, leading to problems with sharing patient information and the likelihood of misplacing a record. There can also be a time delay between the

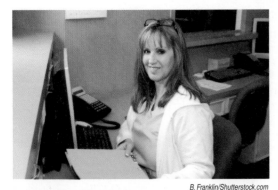

B. Franklin/Shutterstock.com

**Figure 2.18** Keeping accurate medical records, whether computerized or on paper, is critical for the correct diagnosis and treatment of patients.

examination and completion of a doctor's notes. In some small doctor's offices and noncomputerized or partially computerized healthcare facilities, paper records are still used.

**Electronic medical records (EMR)** are now being used in many medical offices. The use of EMR has been encouraged by HIPAA and the federal government. Universal adoption of EMR will ideally have taken place no later than 2014. Today's health information department employee must be able to work with both paper and electronic medical records, making sure that the information recorded is correct and complete.

**electronic medical records (EMR)**
*digital versions of a paper chart that contains a patient's medical history*

**Did You Know?**

**HIPAA**

The Health Insurance Portability and Accountability Act (HIPAA) is an act that was approved by the US Congress in 1996. The act resulted in the creation of a law that included a privacy provision for patient health records, to be fully enforced in 2006. Under this act, patients must be aware of this privacy policy and be notified when their information is shared. Staff must be trained to respect the privacy of patients. Chapter 3, *Healthcare Ethics and Laws*, discusses patient confidentiality in greater detail.

The career ladder in this field includes

- health information clerks, who have completed a vocational education program;
- registered health information technicians (RHIT), who have graduated from a program accredited by the Commission on Accreditation for Health Informatics and Information Management of Education (CAHIM) and have passed a national certification exam; and
- registered health information administrator (RHIA), who have attained a bachelor's degree, have received a passing grade on a certification examination given by the American Health Information Management Association (AHIMA) and usually act in a supervisory or consulting capacity.

The responsibilities of a health information technician depend largely on the size of the institution in which he is working. Smaller facilities may employ an experienced health information technician to supervise the entire records department, while medium-sized and larger departments usually have technicians specializing in one area of healthcare. For example, a large records department might employ a medical coder who specializes in coding patient information for reimbursement purposes.

**Diagnostic Coding Specialists.** There are several hundred **diagnostic-related groups**, or *DRGs*, that health information technicians use. DRGs group patients by diagnosis. A code is assigned to each diagnosis and medical procedure.

**diagnostic-related groups (DRGs)**
*a system that categorizes patients according to their diagnosis*

Coding specialists are known as *health information coders*, *coding specialists*, *medical record coders*, or *coder/abstractors*. These are occupations that are related to medical records and require completion of a community college program or a course offered in a technical school. Employment settings for these occupations may include acute-care hospitals, long-term care hospitals, physician's offices, public health departments, health information systems manufacturers, and insurance companies.

### Health Unit Coordinators

The health unit coordinator (HUC), also referred to as the *unit secretary*, is often the first person you encounter when you enter a hospital nursing unit. The health unit coordinator, stationed at the desk on a nursing unit, coordinates activities on the unit and handles telephone calls. The health unit coordinator reports to the nurse manager or unit manager (Figure 2.19).

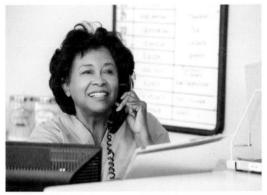

The person in this position interacts directly with the public, including patients, families, and various staff members. In addition to copying information into charts and transcribing handwritten physician orders, the health unit coordinator requisitions laboratory tests and other diagnostic orders, and files reports on patient charts. Excellent computer skills are necessary to succeed in this career path.

Today's health unit coordinator often completes a vocational education program for a unit secretary or health unit coordinator. There is also a national certification examination for health unit coordinators. The National Association of Health Unit Coordinators, or NAHUC, provides continuing education and other membership benefits for people in this field. National certification is available through an examination given by NAHUC.

*Monkey Business Images/Shutterstock.com*

**Figure 2.19**   Health unit coordinators interact directly with staff, patients, family, and visitors.

## Health Facility Support Services

In any healthcare environment, the main focus is always the safety of the patient and employees in the facility. Workers in the **support services** occupy a variety of jobs throughout a healcare facility.

**support services**
*a sector of the hospital that plays a critical role in providing a clean, safe environment for all who enter a healthcare facility*

Employees in the support services include housekeepers, central service workers, food service workers, grounds and building maintenance workers, and biomedical technicians. Some support services jobs, and their educational requirements, are listed in Figure 2.20. These are only a few of the jobs available in this field.

### Housekeeping Services

A health facility's housekeeping services workers are responsible for the cleanliness of the healthcare environment (Figure 2.21). Their labors

| Educational Requirements of Common Support Services Careers | | | |
|---|---|---|---|
| **High School Diploma/Industry Certification/On-the-Job Training** | **Associate's Degree** | **Bachelor's Degree** | **Master's Degree or Professional Degree** |
| support services aide; support services attendant; support services crew leader | support services technician | director of support services | director of support services and central services |
| food service worker | dietetic technician | dietetic intern; registered dietitian | administrative dietitian |
| central service worker | central services technician | central service supervisor/coordinator | |
| biomedical equipment technician aide | biomedical equipment technician (BMET) | health technology manager (HTM), biomedical technologist | |

**Figure 2.20**   Many rewarding careers are available in the areas of support services.

help prevent the spread of infection, creating a more pleasant, safe environment for everyone who enters the hospital, including patients and staff. Hospital housekeepers have many job opportunities in acute-care hospitals, long-term care facilities, and clinics.

Healthcare facility cleaning requires specialized training and compliance with various local laws and regulations, some of which dictate how to clean up potentially infectious materials. **Nosocomial infections** are a reality in any healthcare facility. Housekeeping employees work continually to see that patients' rooms and the general environment of the facility are free from infectious agents. You will learn more about safety and infection control in chapter 4.

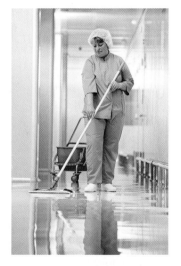

*Dmitry Kalinovsky/Shutterstock.com*

**Figure 2.21**   The housekeeping staff plays a critical role, ensuring the safety of patients, visitors, and staff.

## ‖*Extend Your Knowledge*‖

### *Dietary Needs*

Do you know someone who is on a special diet because of a health problem? Research what constitutes a healthful diet. You might want to refer to the United States Department of Agriculture (USDA) website. Discuss your findings in class.

**nosocomial infections**
*hospital-acquired infections*

### *Food Services*

Employees in food services are responsible for providing patients with safe, nutritional meals. Food service workers plan special diets such as low-sodium, low-fat, and restricted-carbohydrate meals. Food service employees also bring menus to patients, prepare food trays, and deliver food to the patients. Hospitals typically have cafeterias where staff and visitors may eat their meals.

There are many career options in food services, including food service workers, dietetic technicians, dietetic interns, and registered dietitians. All of these employees provide a critical service to make sure patients are given balanced meals to help the recovery process.

**Dietitians.** Dietitians have degrees in nutrition, dietetics, public health, or a related field from accredited colleges and universities. Registered dietitians have successfully completed internships and passed an examination for their credentials. Dietitians also work with patients newly diagnosed with a disorder that requires a special diet, such as heart disease, diabetes, kidney failure, and many other conditions.

### Central Services

Another support service occupation is the central processing services worker. These workers keep an inventory of supplies and equipment for the facility in which they work. Supplies and equipment must be properly packaged, cleaned, and sterilized. Central service workers play a key role in making sure patients are not exposed to infectious diseases and ensuring that doctors and nurses have proper, sterile equipment with which they can perform various procedures. Jobs in central services can be found in acute-care hospitals and large outpatient clinics.

### Biomedical Equipment Technician

A biomedical equipment technician (BMET) is responsible for medical equipment maintenance. This job is also referred to as a *biomedical electronics technician* or *biomedical engineering technician*. A BMET maintains, installs, and repairs a wide variety of healthcare technology and equipment (Figure 2.22). They may work on ventilators, X-ray or ultrasound machines, or medical laboratory equipment. A BMET also trains health facility staff to ensure they understand how to properly operate biomedical equipment.

Technology is a critical component of patient care that improves medical outcomes and safety. Highly skilled and trained biomedical equipment technicians are increasingly sought by hospitals, the medical equipment industry, and many other healthcare employers to ensure medical equipment is up-to-date and functioning efficiently and safely for optimal patient care.

A biomedical equipment technician is required to earn an associate's degree or a bachelor's degree in a related field, such as electronic technology. Some employers may only require a high school diploma and provide on-the-job training.

**Think It Through**

Jason is not comfortable around sick people and prefers working with computers instead of interacting with others. Jason's father and grandfather are physicians. Jason's family is pressuring him to become a third-generation physician. What might be some other healthcare career options for Jason?

# Biotechnology Research

The biotechnology research and developmental careers pathway includes jobs that are highly scientific. In general, these employees do not work in healthcare facilities, but instead work in laboratories. Many of these employees are biologists and chemists.

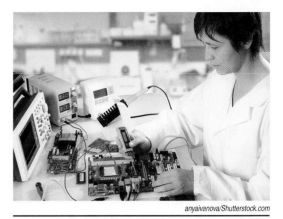

*anyaivanova/Shutterstock.com*

**Figure 2.22**   The biomedical equipment technician is a highly skilled and trained position.

To enter this field, a person needs a strong background in and love of science. This field also requires excellent communication skills. Many of the tasks involved in this job consist of sharing research results through speeches, articles, and reports. Chapter 7 discusses many of the important the verbal and written communication skills you will need in your healthcare career.

Positions in biotechnology research include assistants, technicians, educators, researchers, or scientists. Individuals may work in the food industry, agriculture, pollution control, pharmaceuticals, government agencies, water treatment plants, or education. Educational requirements range from a two-year technical degree from a community college to 8–12 years of study in order to earn a doctoral degree, or PhD.

Careers in biotechnology research include

- biological and medical scientist;
- biostatistician;
- microbiologist;
- quality assurance technician; and
- toxicologist.

## Extend Your Knowledge

### Deep Brain Stimulation for Parkinson's Disease

Parkinson's disease (PD) is a degenerative disorder that affects the nervous system. People with Parkinson's disease experience tremors that often affect their coordination and speech, among other bodily functions.

An exciting biomedical therapy has emerged to treat the symptoms of Parkinson's. Deep brain stimulation is performed by electrodes that are surgically inserted into the brain. These electrodes are connected to a pacemaker placed under the skin of the chest, near the collarbone.

The pacemaker sends continual electrical impulses to the areas of the responsible for producing the tremors. These electrical impulses work to prevent the debilitating tremors associated with Parkinson's.

# Chapter Review and Assessment

## Summary

It is important to assess your goals and needs before you put time, energy, and money into pursuing a career. In exploring a career in healthcare, you will find that there are many career pathways from which to choose. Therapeutic, diagnostic, health informatics and information services, support services, and biomedical research all contain wonderful positions with impressive career ladders.

Only a fraction of the careers in healthcare are discussed in this chapter. Making the correct choice means matching your needs and interests with a career. Your career decision will include how much education you are willing to complete, how much time you can dedicate to your education, your budget, and the availability of your chosen career where you live. Be sure to see the job counselors at your school, take career inventory tests, volunteer in a healthcare facility where you can observe career professionals at work, and interview someone who has a career about which you are curious. Remember also that your state may have different educational requirements for such careers.

## Review Questions

*Answer the following questions using what you have learned in this chapter.*

### Short Answer

1. Make a list of three occupations that appeal to you in the healthcare world.
2. Name five healthcare careers in therapeutic services.
3. Name five healthcare careers in diagnostic services.
4. Name five careers in health informatics and information services.
5. Name three careers in healthcare facility support services.
6. What kind of student would be attracted to jobs in the biomedical technology field?
7. List six strengths you have that will serve you well for a career in healthcare.
8. What does health informatics mean?
9. What is a career ladder?
10. Name three types of degrees that might be required of a healthcare professional.

### True or False

11. *True or False?* Becoming an optometrist only requires a bachelor's degree.
12. *True or False?* You must take a licensing exam in order to receive a license for certain healthcare professions.
13. *True or False?* Respiratory therapists help patients walk after surgery.
14. *True or False?* Phlebotomists draw blood from patients' veins.
15. *True or False?* Dosimeters are what patients use to call the nursing station.
16. *True or False?* All healthcare facilities have computerized medical records.
17. *True or False?* There are many jobs in healthcare facilities for biotechnology research and development.
18. *True or False?* Being a nurse is a diagnostic services position.
19. *True or False?* Continuing education opportunities after being hired as a healthcare worker are restricted to doctors.
20. *True or False?* HIPAA is an organization for physical therapists.

### Multiple Choice

21. Which of the following statements can be used to describe the responsibilities or qualifications of a hospital dietitian?
    A. plans balanced meals for patients
    B. earns a degree in nutrition, dietetics, public health, or a related field from an accredited college or university
    C. becomes licensed as a dietitian
    D. All of the above.

22. Which of the following careers is *not* considered a therapeutic career?
    A. physical therapist
    B. dental assistant
    C. nurse
    D. medical laboratory technician

23. Which of these machines is used in the radiology department?
    A. MRI
    B. CT scan
    C. mammography
    D. All of the above.

24. Which of the following healthcare professions does *not* require at least a bachelor's degree?
    A. medical doctor
    B. dentist
    C. paramedic
    D. nurse practitioner

25. What career is categorized under diagnostic services?
    A. physical therapist
    B. dental laboratory technician
    C. pharmacist
    D. medical doctor

26. Which of the following occupations does *not* work in the clinical laboratory of a healthcare facility?
    A. phlebotomist
    B. laboratory aide
    C. radiologist
    D. pathologist

27. Nosocomial infections can be described as _____.
    A. problems with the nose
    B. hospital-acquired infections
    C. the flu
    D. the common cold

28. Support services in a healthcare facility include _____.
    A. food service workers
    B. central service workers
    C. biomedical equipment technician
    D. All of the above.

29. Which of the following certifications is granted in the area of health information?
    A. PA
    B. DPT
    C. RHIT
    D. DDS

## Critical Thinking Exercises

30. Take career aptitude tests through your school counselor or online. Remember, these tests are simply a tool to help you assess what careers might best suit your personality and abilities. Analyze your results. Do your results seem to accurately reflect your interests?

31. Consider the time, money, and effort you would like to invest in your education. How much education do you wish to complete in order to realize your career goals? on-the-job training? one to two years of training? associate's degree? bachelor's degree? advanced degree and training beyond a four-year degree? Why does a particular level of education appeal to you?

32. Choose an occupation in the medical field in which you are particularly interested. Answer the following questions in as much detail as possible:
    A. What are the educational requirements for this occupation?
    B. Are these jobs currently available in your community? Research projected job availability online. Using government resources like the Bureau of Labor Statistics might be a good place to start.
    C. What is the salary range for this job?
    D. If possible, interview one or two people who currently work in this position. Ask them what personality traits and skills are needed to do this job well.
    E. Do you think this is a job you might be interested in pursuing? Why or why not?

33. Based on the information in this chapter and your personal strengths, which careers do you think would be the best fit for you?

# Chapter

# 3

# Healthcare Ethics and Law

## Terms to Know

advanced directive (AD)
arbitration
civil law
confidentiality
criminal law
do not resuscitate (DNR) document
durable power of attorney
duty of care
emancipated minor
Good Samaritan laws
guardian
Health Insurance Portability and Accountability Act (HIPAA)
informed consent
malpractice
medical ethics
medical law
negligence
ombudsman
Patients' Bill of Rights
Patient Self-Determination Act
reasonable care
sexual harassment
standard of care
statute of limitations
values

## Chapter Objectives

- Discuss the difference between ethical and legal issues in healthcare.
- Understand the concept of values.
- Identify the importance of an ombudsman in a hospital setting.
- Understand important legal document terms, including *advanced directive*, *durable power of attorney*, *duty of care*, *emancipated minors*, *Good Samaritan laws*, *guardianship*, *medical malpractice*, *negligence*, *reasonable care*, and *statutes of limitation*.
- Explain why maintaining patient confidentiality in healthcare is critical.
- Identify the importance of patient consent forms.
- Explain how to recognize sexual harassment and other reportable behaviors in the workplace.

When you are sick or injured, or when a family member or a friend needs health care, you want to be certain that care is given in a safe, ethical, and legal manner. Many of us can think back on a time when a healthcare professional treated us with special care. Most healthcare workers perform their duties in an ethical manner, but you may have encountered a few who did not. Healthcare workers must be educated as to their ethical and legal responsibilities for the protection of patients, coworkers, employers, and themselves.

# Medical Ethics and Legal Responsibilities

When working in the healthcare industry, it is important to make legal and ethical decisions. **Medical ethics** are concerned with whether a healthcare worker's actions are right or wrong. **Medical law** focuses on whether a healthcare worker's actions are legal or illegal. These concepts can be related to one another as well. Illegal acts are always unethical; however, unethical behavior may or may not be illegal.

It is important to know that the application and impact of ethics and laws can vary widely depending on the facts involved in an incident, the institution's policies, and specific laws in each jurisdiction. Also, keep in mind that law is dynamic; it is constantly changing. This is especially true in health law. Courts and legislatures continually respond to issues and technologies that require a new interpretation of existing law or the creation of new laws.

**medical ethics**
*standards concerned with whether a healthcare worker's actions are right or wrong*

**medical law**
*standards concerned with whether a healthcare worker's actions are legal or illegal*

## Medical Ethics in the Workplace

Medical ethics have a long history, dating back to our earliest practicing physicians. You learned about Hippocrates in chapter 1. The oath written for physicians and attributed to Hippocrates implies that physicians should do no harm to their patients. Similar to the Hippocratic Oath, many healthcare organizations today have a code of ethics for physicians and other healthcare providers to follow.

## Ethical Behavior

Ethical behavior represents ideal conduct for a certain group. Medical ethics in the healthcare setting are established as a framework for describing ideal behavior for employees. Licensed healthcare professionals adopt a specific code of ethics when they become licensed. All healthcare workers at a facility are expected to know, understand, and comply with codes of ethics. Descriptions of workplace ethics are usually found in an employee handbook or a policy and procedure manual.

Examples of ethical behavior include treating all patients and coworkers with mutual respect and providing excellent service regardless of who the person is. As a healthcare professional, you are expected to

- be well groomed;
- respect the privacy of others;

- be aware of your limitations;
- avoid taking on tasks for which you are not trained; and
- be honest and trustworthy as you perform your job.

Unethical practices in the workplace include rude behavior toward any patient; being impatient with a patient who moves or talks slowly; arriving at work with dirty clothes and hair; gossiping about patients and coworkers; and lying about a mistake you made. It is also unethical for an employee to discuss salaries with coworkers. To do so can be cause for termination.

## Values

**values**
*the concepts, ideas, and beliefs important and meaningful to a person*

**Values** are the concepts, ideas, and beliefs that are important and meaningful to a person. Your values can be influenced by the people around you, and they help you make decisions by defining what you think is good or bad. Values greatly influence your behavior and serve as broad guidelines in all situations. Your employer may describe what values are important to perform your job and how to put them into practice. As you perform your job in a healthcare facility, your values and behaviors are a reflection of your ethics.

### Think It Through

Make a list of the values you believe should be most important to a healthcare worker. Then, make a list of the personal values that are important in your life. How do these two lists compare? Are the values you associate with a healthcare worker different than those you feel are important in your own life?

## *Medical Law*

Medical law governs the legal conduct of members of the medical professions. Medical law includes laws to be followed at the federal, state, and local levels. Breaking such laws subjects the offender to civil or criminal prosecution (Figure 3.1). **Civil law** (also known as *tort law*) refers to any laws that enforce private rights, not criminal behavior. **Criminal law** deals with criminal behavior that could have consequences such as imprisonment.

Breaking a medical law can lead to loss of a professional license, a fine, and even a prison sentence.

**civil law**
*directives that pertain to disputes between individuals, organizations, or a combination of the two in which monetary compensation is awarded; also known as tort law*

**criminal law**
*directives that pertain to a crime in which the guilty party is punished by incarceration and possible fines*

### *Real Life Scenario*

#### Ethics vs Legality

Scott works in the admissions office of a hospital. Scott admits Ben into the hospital and sees on Ben's paperwork that Ben is being admitted into the alcoholic rehabilitation unit. Scott does not approve of anyone who has an alcohol problem, so Scott is rude to Ben. That behavior is *unethical*. Scott then informs Ben's neighbors that Ben has checked into the alcoholic rehab unit. That behavior is *illegal*.

Diana is in a medical assistant program and is doing an internship in a medical office. Diana sees her friend's name on a medical record in the office. Out of curiosity, Diana sneaks a peek at her friend's chart and is surprised to learn that her friend has a sexually transmitted disease. Reading a chart out of curiosity is *unethical*. However, Diana also tells a mutual friend about their friend's condition. That action is *illegal*.

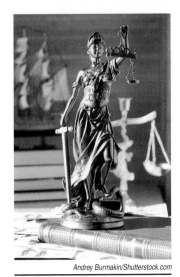

**Figure 3.1**   In this statue, a blindfolded Lady Justice holds the scales of justice. The blindfold she wears symbolizes the importance of impartiality.

---

## ⊣Extend Your Knowledge⊢

### Civil Law and Criminal Law

Civil law, also known as *tort law*, deals with the disputes between individuals, organizations, or a combination of the two, in which monetary compensation is awarded. An example of a civil law case related to healthcare is a healthcare worker telling a patient's employer that the patient has a disease that would keep him or her from being an effective employee. The patient then loses his or her job, resulting in a loss of wages. This case would be filed by a private party, and that party must present believable evidence that this patient has been injured by the healthcare worker.

Criminal law deals with a crime in which the guilty party is punished by incarceration (jail or prison), fines, or both. The state (prosecution) files the case and has the responsibility of proving the case "beyond a reasonable doubt." An example of breaking a criminal law in a healthcare setting would be a pharmacy technician stealing drugs and selling them.

---

# Legal Protection for Patients and Healthcare Workers

When a patient and a physician form a relationship, their relationship is considered a contract (Figure 3.2). The practice of medicine is carried out within a framework of laws that includes protections for patients, healthcare workers, and healthcare facilities. Knowledge of medical laws will help you avoid legal trouble while carrying out your duties as a healthcare professional. There are various legal protections in the healthcare world—some relate to the patient and some to healthcare workers.

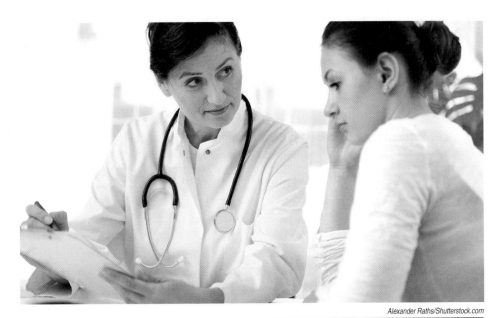

**Figure 3.2**   The patient and physician's relationship exists within a framework of laws.

# Patients' Bill of Rights

**Patients' Bill of Rights**
*summary of a patient's rights regarding fair treatment and appropriate information*

A **Patients' Bill of Rights** is a list of guarantees for those receiving medical care. It may take the form of a law or a nonbinding declaration. A patients' bill of rights guarantees patients information about medical decisions and fair treatment, among other rights. Today in the United States, there have been a number of attempts to create a universal patients' bill of rights and make it law. The Affordable Care Act of 2010 includes a listing of patient rights.

The American Hospital Association has developed a pamphlet highlighting the Patients' bill of rights, with the belief that it promotes more effective patient care. The pamphlet, which outlines how the patient should be treated by the staff, should be given to patients when they arrive at the healthcare facility. Hospitals are urged to adhere to rules about providing information regarding patient rights, as they apply to its medical staff, employees, and patients.

# Ombudsman

**ombudsman**
*a member of the healthcare team who ensures that patients are not abused and that their legal rights are protected*

The role of an **ombudsman** is to ensure that patients are not abused and that their legal rights are protected. An ombudsman may be a nurse, trained volunteer, or a social worker. In most facilities, there will be a person acting as an ombudsman, and a phone number is posted for employees to use when reporting violations of patients' rights. Employees can also discuss the issue with the ombudsman in person.

# The Patient Self-Determination Act

**Patient Self-Determination Act**
*a law passed by the US Congress in 1990 that requires most healthcare institutions to inform a patient about their rights at the time of admission*

The **Patient Self-Determination Act** was passed by Congress in 1990. This law requires that most healthcare institutions inform a patient about their rights, under state law, at the time of admission. These include the right to

- participate in and direct their healthcare decisions;
- accept or refuse medical or surgical treatment;
- prepare an advanced directive (see below);
- view information on the facility's policies about recognizing advanced directives; and
- know how the facility educates its staff regarding advanced directives.

# Advanced Directive (AD)

**advanced directive (AD)**
*a legal document in which a patient gives written instructions about healthcare issues in the event that the patient becomes unable to make such decisions in the future*

The **advanced directive (AD)** is a legal document in which a patient gives written instructions about healthcare decisions in the event that he or she becomes incapable of making such decisions in the future. An example of an advanced directive is a request by the patient to instruct his or her physician that "heroic measures," such as using feeding tubes and respirators, must not be taken if there is no expectation of patient recovery.

A **do not resuscitate (DNR)** document made by a patient is part of an advanced directive (Figure 3.3). This document indicates that if the patient stops breathing or the patient's heart stops, CPR or advanced cardiac life support (ACLS) should *not* be performed. The DNR document should be with the patient's medical chart. Some people also have a DNR document posted in their homes.

## Durable Power of Attorney

The **durable power of attorney** is a legal document that grants another person, or *agent*, the authority to make legal decisions for you. The Durable Power of Attorney for Health Care (DPAHC) allows the patient to express his or her healthcare decisions and outline how much authority the agent should be given. This power is often granted to a family member of an elderly relative.

## Duty of Care

Every patient is entitled to safe care. **Duty of care** is a legal obligation for healthcare personnel to take reasonable care of a patient to avoid causing harm. If this duty is not met, there may be a charge of negligence (see page 59) against the healthcare provider.

## Emancipated Minors

In most states, parents are required to sign medical consent forms for their children under 18 years of age. This is, however not the case for an **emancipated minor**. An emancipated minor is a person under 18 years of

**do not resuscitate (DNR) document**
*a legal document made by a patient, which states that CPR or other advanced cardiac life support should not be performed if a patient stops breathing or a patient's heart stops*

**durable power of attorney**
*a legal document that grants another person the authority to make legal decisions for you; the Durable Power of Attorney for Health Care includes patient instructions for healthcare decisions and gives another person the power to enforce such decisions*

**duty of care**
*a legal obligation for healthcare personnel to take reasonable care to avoid causing harm to a patient*

**emancipated minor**
*a person under 18 years of age who has legally established that he or she does not live with parents*

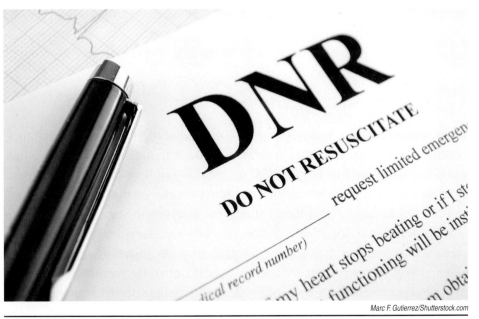

Marc F. Gutierrez/Shutterstock.com

**Figure 3.3**   Doctors and hospitals in all states accept DNR orders.

**Good Samaritan laws**
*laws that protect people from legal action after voluntarily giving emergency medical aid while using reasonable care*

**arbitration**
*a cost-effective alternative to litigation*

age who has legally established that he or she does not live with parents. The emancipated minor is financially and legally responsible for himself or herself, and can consent to treatment.

## Good Samaritan Laws

**Good Samaritan laws** are designed to protect people from legal action after they have given free emergency medical aid while using reasonable care. These laws are designed to encourage healthcare professionals to give first aid in an emergency situation without fear of being sued for negligence (Figure 3.4). Unfortunately, these laws are not always clearly written, sometimes creating confusion for healthcare professionals. Additionally, these laws differ from state to state. In some states, these laws apply to the general public as well as trained medical professionals.

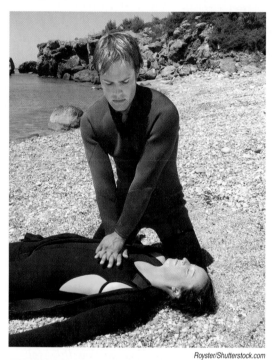

Royster/Shutterstock.com

**Figure 3.4**   A Good Samaritan will often perform CPR if properly trained.

**guardian**
*a court-appointed person who may make decisions for a patient who is mentally or physically incapable of making such decisions*

**malpractice**
*any misconduct or lack of skill that results in patient injury; also known as professional liability*

## Arbitration

**Arbitration** is a method of resolving disputes outside the courtroom. Rather than let the case go into litigation, or settled by a court of law, arbitration does not involve a trial. Hospitals, physicians, and other healthcare professionals often ask patients to sign arbitration agreements before care is provided. This protects the healthcare facility from entering a costly trial, should something go wrong.

## Guardianship

If a patient is not able to make his or her own decisions due to mental or physical incapacity, a court-appointed **guardian** may make decisions to protect the interests of the patient.

## Medical Malpractice

**Malpractice**, also known as *professional liability*, is defined as any misconduct or lack of skill that results in patient injury. When filing a malpractice claim, you must present information stating that a professional does not meet the standard of care. Most claims of this nature are filed against physicians or hospitals, but any medical employee can be named in a malpractice suit. Insurance policies may be purchased to protect healthcare employees against potential malpractice suits. Insurance policies often allow physicians to cover their employees, but other medical employees may also purchase their own policies. Some medical malpractice lawsuits must be settled in a court of law (Figure 3.5).

# Negligence

In the healthcare world, **negligence** refers to performing an act that a reasonable person would not have done. Negligence can also apply to failing to do something that a reasonable person would have done, resulting in injury or harm to a patient. An example of negligence is a nurse allowing a patient to develop an untreated bedsore while in a long-term care facility.

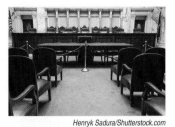
Henryk Sadura/Shutterstock.com

**Figure 3.5** While malpractice suits may end up in a courtroom, cases will often be settled out of court.

# Reasonable Care

**Reasonable care** is a legal protection for the healthcare worker. This protection applies if it can be proven that the worker acted reasonably as compared to actions that other members of the profession would take in similar circumstances. If the healthcare worker does not meet such a standard and the patient is harmed, negligence may be proven.

# Standard of Care

**Standard of care** refers to the skill and care that medical practitioners such as physicians, nurses, medical assistants, and phlebotomists must use as determined by their state license or certification. Such practitioners must perform a procedure in the way that someone with similar qualifications would have performed in the same or similar situation.

# Statute of Limitations

When a patient decides that something has been done to him or her that could lead to a lawsuit, there is a **statute of limitations**. The statute of limitations concerns the amount of time that can pass before any legal action is taken. After that time period, a lawsuit may not be filed.

---

 *Check Your Understanding*

When you pursue a career in healthcare, it is very important that you understand the laws that protect both patients and staff members in a healthcare facility. Which laws apply to the following situations?

1. A nurse performs CPR on a man who experiences cardiac arrest in a restaurant.

2. A patient is injured in the hospital by a worker who performed a procedure that met a standard set for other members of the worker's profession.

3. Rosie was disappointed that she couldn't sue her physician because too much time had passed since the incident.

4. A healthcare professional performed a procedure that wasn't in her job description and a patient was injured.

---

**negligence**
*performing an act that a reasonable person would not have done, or not doing something that a reasonable person would have done in the same or similar circumstance that results in harm to a patient*

**reasonable care**
*legal protection for the healthcare worker if proven that the worker acted reasonably as compared to other members of the profession in a same or similar situation*

**statute of limitations**
*the amount of time during which any legal action may be taken; after such time a lawsuit may not be filed*

**standard of care**
*reasonable and prudent care that a practitioner of similar qualifications would have performed in the same or similar situation*

## Confidentiality

**confidentiality**
*the practice of allowing only certain individuals the right to access information; ensures that others do not have the personal information of others*

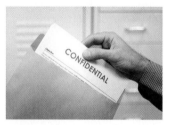

hafakot/Shutterstock.com

**Figure 3.6** Healthcare workers must protect patients by keeping their personal information confidential.

**Confidentiality** allows only certain individuals the right to personal information. Confidentiality protects a patients' personal information, ensuring others do not have access to such information. As a future healthcare worker, you are responsible for ensuring that confidentiality is upheld for patients. In a digital age in which privacy is increasingly threatened, the issue of confidentiality has never been more important.

Healthcare agencies and providers *must* provide confidentiality and privacy of any health-related information that is collected, maintained, used, or transmitted (Figure 3.6).

Confidentiality has been, and always should be, a critical aspect of the relationship between a patient and healthcare worker. Diagnoses or treatments could destroy the patient's reputation. Mental illness, drug or alcohol addiction, sexually transmitted diseases, and other types of problems can be misunderstood and unfairly judged by others. An example of this occurred when people first reacted to AIDS in the early 1980s. When word spread that someone had AIDS, ignorance caused employers to fire employees, insurance carriers to deny insurance to people with AIDS, and landlords to refuse to rent to someone with AIDS. Although laws are now in place to protect confidentiality of patients, problems still occur because of ignorance about many diseases and disorders.

**Did You Know?**

### Hippocrates

Hippocrates wrote about the importance of confidentiality approximately 2,500 years ago! Although there are many translations and versions of the Hippocratic Oath that vary slightly, one version states

"…Whatever, in connection with my professional service, or not in connection with it, I see or hear, in the life of men, which ought not to be spoken of abroad. I will keep this Oath unviolated, may it be granted to me to enjoy life and the practice of the art, respected by all men, in all times. But should I trespass and violate this Oath, may the reverse be my lot."

The American Medical Association's Code of Ethics also highlights the need for confidentiality:

"A physician shall respect the rights of patients, colleagues, and other health professionals, and shall safeguard patient confidences and privacy within the constraints of the law."

**Health Insurance Portability and Accountability Act (HIPAA)**
*an act approved by the US Congress in 1996 and fully enforced in 2006; created a law including a privacy provision for patient health records*

## HIPAA Privacy Protections

As you learned in chapter 2, Congress passed the **Health Insurance Portability and Accountability Act (HIPAA)** in 1996. One main purpose of the act was the continuation of health insurance coverage if a person changes jobs. It also provided standards for health information transactions, as well as confidentiality and security of patient data.

### HIPAA Privacy Rule

The HIPAA Privacy Rule has been enforced by the US government's Office of Civil Rights since April of 2003. This rule establishes national standards to protect individuals' medical records and other personal health information. It also gives patients rights over their health information, including rights to examine and obtain a copy of their health records, and to request corrections.

Violating the HIPAA Privacy Rule can result in civil penalties ranging from $100 per violation up to $25,000. Criminal penalties are also possible and may include a fine of $50,000 with the possibility of one year in prison if information is illegally disclosed. If there is intent to sell confidential information, there can be a maximum fine of $250,000 with the possibility of ten years in prison. Maintaining confidentiality is a serious business. Something as seemingly harmless as gossiping about a patient's condition can result in such penalties (Figure 3.7).

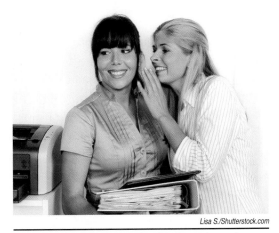

*Lisa S./Shutterstock.com*

**Figure 3.7**   Gossip can lead to breaches of patient confidentiality.

### Real Life Scenario

#### Confidentiality

Jane is a phlebotomist at Eastridge Hospital. One morning she is assigned to draw blood on the alcohol rehabilitation floor. One of her patients is a neighbor of Jane's sister. Jane knows that the patient is part of a car pool that takes Jane's niece and nephew to school. The possibility of an alcoholic driving children to school makes Jane very nervous. Jane adores her niece and nephew and is very concerned that they might be in danger. Should Jane tell her sister about the situation?

# Exceptions for Releasing Patient Information

Healthcare workers are both *ethically* and *legally* bound to protect the privacy and confidentiality of patient-physician interactions. Physicians may share information about patient confidences *only* if required by law. Breaches, or breaks, in confidentiality can result in a lawsuit against the physician and his or her employees, or against a healthcare facility.

A patient's medical record is a confidential, legal document and should not be discussed with anyone who does not have a need to know this information. Before information can be released for insurance billing purposes, a release-of-information form must be signed by the patient. As a healthcare employee, you will be exposed to a wide range of confidential information about many patients. Acting in a professional manner is *absolutely* mandatory.

**Think It Through**

Johanna and Emily are both working with a 1-year-old patient who was born with HIV. Both women want to discuss how they feel about this case, so they wait until they are in the hospital cafeteria to discuss their reactions. They didn't want to talk about it near their supervisor or the patient and her family. Are they right in waiting to talk in the cafeteria?

There are some exceptions for releasing patient medical information. Doctors are sometimes required by law to release medical information to authorities without the patient's consent. This situation may arise when authorities, including doctors, have concerns that a child or others may be at risk for immediate harm. Additionally, doctors must release medical information when ordered to by the court. Even so, privacy rules require a doctor to make reasonable efforts to disclose only the minimal amount of information necessary for the purpose requested. Rules about confidentiality are different in some healthcare agencies, schools, and social service agencies. You must be aware of specific rules of the facility in which you work.

## Patient Consent Forms

When a physician makes a diagnosis and recommends a specific treatment, the patient has the responsibility to decide whether or not to accept the diagnosis and method of treatment. The physician must inform the patient (or the patient's guardian), of the risk of the procedure, using words that the patient can understand. The benefits and risks must be explained to a patient or guardian before permission is given. If the patient is willing to accept the risks involved, a consent form—called an **informed consent**—is signed. You may be asked to prepare such a form. All signatures must be in ink and patients *cannot* be forced to sign a consent form.

**informed consent**
*a form given to a patient by a physician explaining the benefits and risks of a procedure; the patient accepts the risk by signing the informed consent form*

**sexual harassment**
*unwanted sexual advances and other forms of offensive sexual behavior; both men and women can be sexually harassed*

## Sexual Harassment

**Sexual harassment** can occur in any workplace. According to the United States Equal Employment Opportunity Commission (EEOC), sexual harassment is a form of sex discrimination. Employers must have a process in place to take immediate steps when they receive a sexual harassment complaint. Unwanted sexual advances or other forms of offensive sexual behavior should be reported immediately to a supervisor.

Both men and women can be sexually harassed. Your training manual or employee handbook should include definitions of sexual harassment, along with measures to stop the harassment. You may not realize that something you say in an offhanded way might be considered sexual harassment. An example of sexual harassment is a young man commenting to a woman that he really appreciated the tight blouse she wore to work yesterday.

Sexual harassment is considered unethical and, in most cases, illegal. You can be disciplined for such behavior and lose your job. For example, if an employer is found to deny a promotion to an employee because the employee did not return the employer's advances, that is illegal behavior.

## Real Life Scenario

### The New Employee

Mallory and Sadie are young, single women who work in the Financial Services Office of Eastridge Hospital. When a new employee, Mark, is hired to work with them, both women agree he is "hot." When Mark walks by Sadie and Mallory's desks, both women comment under their breath about Mark's physique so that Mark can hear. They also complement him on his trousers, giggling as they say that they could be tighter. Would this be considered sexual harassment? Why or why not?

# Recognizing Reportable Behavior

Healthcare workers are responsible for helping to protect everyone in the workplace. If you suspect that there is unethical or illegal behavior occurring in the workplace, or you have observed such behavior (not just relying on gossip), the incident must be reported. A reportable incident is an event that can affect the health, safety, or welfare of those around you. A few examples of reportable behavior include

- an employee harassing another employee;
- an employee slipping medication into his or her pocket;
- an employee making fun of a patient;
- evidence of misuse of hospital funds;
- a breach of confidentiality;
- a worker striking or otherwise harming a patient;
- an employee stealing property from the employer; or
- an employee stealing property from a patient or a coworker (Figure 3.8).

There should be instructions for reporting illegal and unethical conduct in your employee handbook. Your supervisor or human resources representative should be able to help you report such behavior if you are confused. If your supervisor is acting illegally or unethically, contact your human resources representative. Acting ethically and obeying laws that relate to the medical environment is essential to maintaining a high degree of professional behavior.

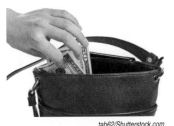

*tab62/Shutterstock.com*

**Figure 3.8** Stealing property from a coworker or a patient is reportable behavior.

## Real Life Scenario

### Acceptable Speech

Brad is a receptionist for Dr. Winston's dental practice. One day a new patient arrives in the reception area. This patient is an obese woman wearing unwashed clothes. After the patient is brought into an examination room, Jane—Dr. Winston's dental assistant—overhears Brad saying, "Wow! That patient is as big as a house and smells terrible! Someone should tell her how gross she is."

What should Jane do? Is this a reportable offense? Should Jane report Brad to Dr. Winston? Is Brad acting unethically or illegally? What would you do if you were Jane?

# Chapter Review and Assessment

## Summary

It is important for the healthcare worker to understand the concepts of medical ethics and medical law. A healthcare employee must make decisions that are both ethical and legal. Not following such guidelines may lead to termination of employment and even legal problems.

An employee must understand the various legal protections that exist for both patients as well as healthcare workers. These protections include advanced directives, durable power of attorney, duty of care, emancipated minors, Good Samaritan laws, guardianship, medical malpractice, negligence prevention, reasonable care, and statute of limitations.

The issue of confidentiality has never been more important than in this digital age, in which privacy is increasingly threatened. A healthcare worker must never discuss a patient's personal or medical information with anyone except a fellow employee involved in the patient's treatment and care.

Ethical behavior extends to relationships with any individual in the healthcare facility. Sexual harassment is a form of sexual discrimination. Other unethical and illegal behavior such as stealing, misuse of facility funds, or physical abuse must be reported to a supervisor or human resources representative.

Continual focus on ethical and legal issues is a necessity for truly professional behavior.

## Review Questions

*Answer the following questions using what you have learned in this chapter.*

### Short Answer

1. Explain what is meant by values.
2. Define medical law and medical ethics.
3. Why is confidentiality so important in a healthcare setting?
4. Explain what is meant by arbitration.
5. What is an advanced directive?

6. Define the following:
   A. medical malpractice
   B. duty of care
   C. Good Samaritan laws
   D. guardianship
   E. negligence
   F. standard of care
7. What does DNR mean?
8. What is another name for civil law?
9. What do the scales of justice symbolize?
10. What is the role of the ombudsman in a healthcare setting?

### True/False

11. *True or False?* Only a doctor can be sued for malpractice.
12. *True or False?* Telling your friends that your patient, Jane Maxwell, has a sexually transmitted disease is both unethical and illegal.
13. *True or False?* Breaking a medical law can lead to losing your professional license.
14. *True or False?* The standard of reasonable care protects the healthcare worker.
15. *True or False?* Confidentiality is a relatively recent concern for the medical world.
16. *True or False?* Breaking a civil law almost always results in imprisonment.
17. *True or False?* If something is illegal, it is always unethical.
18. *True or False?* Good Samaritan laws are the same in every US state.
19. *True or False?* If you hear "through the grapevine" that someone is being unethical, you should report the person immediately.

### Multiple Choice

20. Which of the following would be seen as unethical?
    A. being rude to a patient
    B. gossiping about a fellow team member
    C. ignoring supervisor requests
    D. All of the above.

21. Which scenario would be considered illegal?
    A. striking a patient
    B. revealing a patient's condition to someone outside the workplace
    C. coming to work with an illness
    D. Both A and B.

22. Which of the following could be considered sexual harassment?
    A. any unwanted touching by someone in the workplace
    B. a male employee telling a female team member that she has really "hot" legs
    C. telling a dirty joke
    D. All of the above.

23. The following are reportable incidents, *except* _____.
    A. an employee harassing another employee
    B. an employee stealing medication
    C. an employee making fun of a patient
    D. an employee taking a break

24. Which of the following statements is false?
    A. Every patient is entitled to safe care.
    B. An emancipated minor is a person over 18 years of age.
    C. Insurance policies can be purchased to protect employees from malpractice suits.
    D. Reasonable care is a legal protection for healthcare workers.

25. Professional liability is also known as _____.
    A. negligence
    B. malpractice
    C. reasonable care
    D. duty of care

26. _____ created a law including a privacy provision for patient health records.
    A. Civil law
    B. Durable power of attorney
    C. Good Samaritan laws
    D. HIPAA

27. Ethical behavior includes _____.
    A. treating all patients with respect if they show respect to you
    B. respecting the privacy of others
    C. understanding the limitations of your training
    D. B and C only.

28. The Patient Self-Determination Act of 1990 states that _____.
    A. health care institutions must inform the patient of rights under state law at the time of admission
    B. a patient can refuse medical or surgical treatment
    C. patients have the right to participate in healthcare decisions
    D. All of the above.

29. Which exception can be made for release of patient medical information?
    A. A woman's fiancé wants information about her surgery.
    B. A concerned citizen wants to know the diagnosis of her next door neighbor.
    C. A doctor is ordered by the court to reveal patient medical information.
    D. A reporter wants to know the status of a hospitalized celebrity.

## Critical Thinking Exercises

30. At your past jobs, did you ever see unethical or illegal behaviors? If so, did you report such behavior to a supervisor?

31. Do you think it is unethical to play games, send your friends personal e-mails, or shop online when using a work computer? What could you do on a work computer that would be considered illegal?

32. Research on the internet to find three cases in which healthcare workers were accused of unethical or illegal behavior. You may also find cases in newspapers as well. In your experience, have you found this type of behavior to be common or uncommon?

33. What is the difference between values and ethics? Give examples of each.

34. What would you do if you ever encounter an unethical or even illegal situation in a healthcare facility? Would there be any reason why you wouldn't report such a problem?

35. When can gossip become unethical or even illegal? Give two examples of cases where gossip can become damaging.

# Chapter

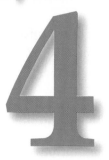

# Safety and Infection Control

## Terms to Know

autoclave
bacteria
biohazard sharps
    container
biopsy
bloodborne pathogens
body mechanics
carpal tunnel syndrome
Centers for Disease
    Control and Prevention
    (CDC)
chain of infection
disinfection
ergonomics
fire triangle
fungi
hand hygiene
hospital emergency
    codes
incident reports
infection control
isolation rooms
material safety data
    sheet (MSDS)
Methicillin-resistant
    *Staphylococcus aureus*
    (MRSA)

morphology
needlesticks
Needlestick Safety and
    Prevention Act
Occupational Safety and
    Health Administration
    (OSHA)
OSHA Bloodborne
    Pathogens Standard
OSHA Hazard
    Communication
    Standard
parasites
personal protective
    equipment (PPE)
potentially infectious
    materials (PIM)
protozoa
quality assurance
rickettsiae
sanitization
sharps
sterilization
viruses

## Chapter Objectives

- Understand the basic safety rules of a healthcare facility.
- Explain the role OSHA plays in a healthcare setting.
- Describe how to avoid chemical, electrical, radiation, and fire dangers in a healthcare facility.
- Discuss the proper responses to fires and other emergencies.
- List some ways to practice proper body mechanics when lifting objects and patients.
- Discuss the importance of proper hand washing.
- Explain the importance of infection control.
- List the parts of the chain of infection and explain how to interrupt it.
- Discuss the need for isolation procedures and how the procedures differ.

Reinforce your learning with additional online resources
- **Practice** vocabulary with flashcards and interactive games
- **Assess** with posttests and image labeling
- **Expand** with activities and animations

Companion
*G-W Learning*

www.g-wlearning.com/healthsciences

**Study on the Go**
Use a mobile device to practice vocabulary terms and review with self-assessment quizzes.

Mobile
*G-W Learning*

www.m.g-wlearning.com

Safety must be the primary concern of those who choose a career in healthcare. Maintaining safe conditions in healthcare facilities means avoiding danger, risks, injury, and infection for patients, healthcare workers, and visitors. **Infection control** encompasses any efforts made to avoid the spread of infection. Every effort must be made to maintain infection control in order to protect patients from further health problems and keep employees and their families healthy.

**infection control**
*term that describes any efforts made to avoid the spread of infection in a healthcare facility*

## Safety in Healthcare Facilities

Quality healthcare begins with strictly observing *all* safety procedures. Safety issues in a healthcare facility include risks related to patients, employees, visitors, and the environment.

### General Safety Rules

Some healthcare facilities have special safety regulations that apply to their specific environment, equipment, or patients. However, these are general safety rules that all healthcare workers should remember:

- **Walk on the right-hand side of a hallway**. Avoid walking alongside more than two people. Leave hallways open so that there are no "traffic" problems (Figure 4.1).
- **Always use handrails when using stairs**. If you are in a hurry and are not holding on to the railing, you may fall and injure yourself.
- **Never run in a hallway**. If you run, you can fall and injure yourself or may collide with another person or object. Running can also cause a panic. Walk, don't run!
- **Report any nonworking lighting that you observe in the facility**.
- **Cautiously open swinging doors**. Take care that someone is not on the other side of a swinging door. Otherwise, you can injure yourself or someone else.
- **Remove obstructions from floors and hallways**. Obstructions on floors and in hallways are possible tripping hazards. They might include spills, out-of-place equipment, or patients' personal items.
- **Do not prop open fire safety doors**. Keep all equipment away from these doors.
- **Wear sensible shoes**. Open-heel and open-toe shoes expose the foot to potential injury.
- **Store items in a safe, yet easily accessible manner**. Avoid placing items on the top of cabinets as they might fall off when you open the cabinet doors. Do not overfill shelves, as you do not want items falling off the shelves and posing a safety hazard. Heavier items should be stored close to the floor to allow everyone to reach and remove them safely.
- **Recognize and obey evacuation routes posted throughout the facility**. It is important to be familiar with evacuation routes and plans in the

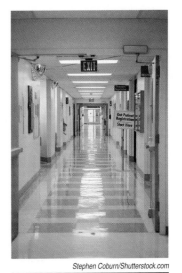

*Stephen Coburn/Shutterstock.com*

**Figure 4.1** Walk on the right-hand side of a hallway.

event of an emergency. Floor plans should also be posted with clearly marked exit routes.

- **Be aware of everyone around you**. If you see something that concerns you, or could be dangerous, say something.
- **Practice safety in your daily life**. It is easier to prevent accidents than to treat them. Be aware of potential hazards in your home and school environments.

## Safety Manual

Every healthcare facility has policies regarding safety and should have written safety instructions readily available to all employees. Instructions for following safety guidelines are part of in-service training given to all new employees. You will also be required to attend all staff training regarding patient safety issues. It is important that you follow all safety procedures in the safety manual of your facility.

Each department may have additional written safety rules specific to that department. For example, a department using hazardous chemicals will have plans for the safe handling of chemicals. The diagnostic imaging department will have manuals dealing with radiation safety.

## Hospital Emergency Codes

**hospital emergency codes**
*signals used in hospitals to alert staff to various emergencies; examples include code red (fire) and code blue (cardiac arrest)*

**Hospital emergency codes** are used in hospitals to alert staff to various emergencies. These codes quickly convey essential information while preventing stress and panic among patients and visitors to the hospital.

Although efforts have been made to establish uniform codes throughout the United States and the world, codes can still vary between facilities. This can cause confusion for employees, such as doctors, who work at different hospitals. When employed by a healthcare facility, employees must know the meaning of that facility's various codes.

Some frequently used hospital emergency codes are

- Code Red—fire in the facility;
- Code Blue—cardiac arrest;
- Code Pink—infant or child abduction;
- Code Orange—hazardous materials spill;
- Code Silver—dangerous person with a weapon; and
- Code Black—bomb threat.

When codes are announced, the location of the emergency is identified as well. An example of this is, "Code Blue, Cardiac Care Unit."

## *Patient Safety*

Caring for patients requires serious attention to detail to prevent accidents and provide competent care. As a conscientious healthcare worker acting in a professional manner, you are responsible for the safety of your patients. Even if you do not work directly with patients, you must still be observant. It is important that you act quickly if you see safety hazards in the facility, such as liquid spills, loose rugs, or confused and disoriented patients.

If you do work directly with patients, follow the guidelines of your facility. The following are some universal guidelines for patient safety:

- Always identify the patient before you interact with him or her. Check the patient's identification bracelet and your paperwork to make sure that you have the correct patient.
- Make sure your patient has privacy during all procedures (Figure 4.2). It is your responsibility to ensure the safety and comfort of a patient at all times.
- When leaving a patient, make sure the bed is in a low position with side rails up. The call button must be within reach of the patient.
- Be sure that the patient knows the location of the bathroom, call buttons, emergency call lights, handrails, and safety rails in the hospital room.
- Before performing a procedure, explain the entire procedure and make sure you have the patient's consent. For example, if a patient does not want you to take his or her blood and refuses permission, you must tell the nurse in charge that the patient has refused. Make sure that the patient understands you. If language is a barrier, your facility may have designated translators available to help. If the patient cannot understand you because of a medical challenge, make sure someone who can speak for the patient is there, such as a guardian or a close relative. *Always remember that the patient has the right to refuse treatment!* If an employee performs a procedure that the patient has refused, the employee may be sued for battery, or unlawful touching.

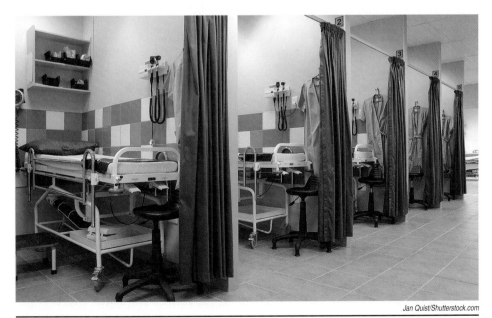

**Figure 4.2**  Respect the privacy of your patient and always close the curtain during examination.

- Never start a procedure that you are not trained to perform. Never take shortcuts such as skipping a time-consuming step because you are in a hurry. It would not be part of the procedure if it were not important.
- Immediately report safety hazards to a nearby supervisor. Such hazards can include tangled or frayed wires, any kind of liquid spill in the patient's room or hallway, hot beverages served to a patient who cannot manage the drink, the smell of smoke, and a patient who will not stay in bed when bed rest is required. A patient room crowded with equipment can become a hazard if the patient gets out of bed.
- Observe the patient carefully so that you may identify any changes in status. If you see increased coughing, changes in skin color, difficulty breathing, increased restlessness, change in the level of consciousness, unexpected bleeding, or accelerated pain, report these events to a supervisor as soon as possible. Do not leave a patient alone when you observe that he or she may be disoriented and confused. Again, report the situation to a supervisor to make sure the patient is safe.
- Patients can develop allergies to medications, food, as well as environmental conditions. Watch for signs of allergic reactions, which may include rash, difficulty breathing, coughing, sneezing, tightness in the throat, nausea, skin itching, tingling, redness, or swelling. Allergic reactions can be life-threatening if not treated quickly.
- Wash your hands upon entering and leaving a patient's room. Never wear gloves out of a patient's room. Discard them and wash your hands prior to leaving the room. Frequent hand washing is the best way to prevent the spread of disease.

## Incident Reports

An incident is any event that is not a part of the routine operation of the healthcare facility. An incident could be a patient or visitor falling, a healthcare worker hurting his or her back while lifting a patient, or giving a patient incorrect medication. There are also incidents that are not safety-related, such as theft or abusive language from a patient or employee. **Incident reports** (also called *quality assurance reports*) should be used to document both safety and non-safety related incidents.

If you see unsafe practices or situations, you must immediately report these incidents to a supervisor in the area. You may be asked to fill out an incident report documenting the problem (Figure 4.3). An incident report is an internal document and should not be included in a patient's medical record. Some facilities use separate reports for employee accidents versus other types of incidents.

An incident report must be filled out accurately and completely. The report form should be available to you at all times. You must use a black pen to fill in an incident report as it is a legal document. Do not use white-out on the report. Avoid being wordy in your report—simply state the

**incident reports**

*reports used in a health-care facility to document both safety and non-safety related incidents that are not part of a routine operation in the facility*

| I. OCCURRENCE: | | | (IF NO PLATE) | | STATUS | |
|---|---|---|---|---|---|---|
| DATE | TIME | LOCATION | NAME | | ❑ INPT  ❑ VISITOR  ❑ OUTPT  ❑ OTHER | |

| AGE | SEX  ❑ M  ❑ F | Diagnosis or Procedure | Witness  Yes ❑  No ❑  Name _____  Dept._____ |
|---|---|---|---|

| Condition Prior to Occurrence | Meds in last 12 hrs (falls only) |
|---|---|
| ❑ Alert  ❑ Disoriented  ❑ Asleep  ❑ Anesthetized | |

| II. MEDICATION (all that apply) | INTRAVENOUS (Note all that apply) | FALL (Complete both sides) | |
|---|---|---|---|
| ❑ Wrong medication  ❑ Wrong amount  ❑ Wrong date/time  ❑ Wrong pt  ❑ Wrong route  ❑ Transcription error  ❑ Allergic reaction  ❑ Omission  ❑ Incorrect narcotic count  ❑ Other _____  ❑ Name of Med | ❑ Wrong solution  ❑ Wrong medication  ❑ Wrong rate  ❑ Wrong time  ❑ Infiltration  ❑ Transcription error  ❑ PCA error  ❑ Blood transfusion  ❑ Hyperalimentation  ❑ Other _____ | ❑ Ambulating  ❑ In BR  ❑ Out of bed  ❑ To FRM B/R  ❑ Other | ❑ PT has fallen prev  ❑ Restrained  ❑ Side rails up  ❑ Side rails down |

| | Equipment | Surgical — Please Comment |
|---|---|---|
| **Consent:**  ❑ Name written  ❑ Mismatch  ❑ Refused to sign  ❑ Incomplete  ❑ Other _____ | ❑ Not available  ❑ Disconnected  ❑ Procedure not followed  ❑ Nonsterile  ❑ Malfunction  ❑ Other _____  ❑ Descript. of item _____ | ❑ Delay  ❑ Consent mismatch  ❑ Unplanned return  ❑ Incorrect count  ❑ Unplanned repair/removal  ❑ Arrest  ❑ Death  ❑ Anesthesis related  ❑ Other _____ |

| AMA | Pressure Sore (complete both sides) | | Other | |
|---|---|---|---|---|
| ❑ AMA signed  ❑ Not signed  ❑ AWOL  ❑ Other | ❑ On admission  ❑ Hospital acquired  ❑ Picture taken | ❑ Stage I  ❑ Stage II  ❑ Stage III  ❑ Stage IV | ❑ Security  ❑ Engineering  ❑ Combative pt  ❑ Suicide attempt  ❑ Fire  ❑ Respiratory  ❑ Pharmacy  ❑ Code blue expired  ❑ Code blue survived  ❑ Complaint | ❑ Self abuse  ❑ Lost/damaged article  ❑ Hazardous exposure  ❑ Burn  ❑ Lab  ❑ X ray  ❑ Food services  ❑ Housekeeping  ❑ Other (comment) _____ |

| III. Severity of Outcome | | | |
|---|---|---|---|
| ❑ No Injury | ❑ Inconsequential | ❑ Consequential | |

| IV. Comments & Action | V. Follow up (Director to complete) |
|---|---|
| | ❑ Communicated with _____ |

| Name of MD notified | Date | Time | Seen by MD? | ❑ Employee counseled  ❑ In-service  ❑ Policy change/new  ❑ Trend  ❑ Other _____ |
|---|---|---|---|---|
| | | | Yes ❑  No ❑ | |

| X-ray / Lab / Tests ordered | Equipment | |
|---|---|---|
| Yes ❑  No ❑  State _____ | Sent for repair ❑  Removed from Service ❑ | |

| Reported by — Date — Dept | Persons Involved     Dept | Department Director Sign — Date |
|---|---|---|

**Figure 4.3** An incident report should be filled out to document both safety and non-safety related issues that could lead to problems in the workplace.

facts. There are a variety of incident report forms that different facilities use, but the following information is included on most report forms:

- date of incident
- names of persons involved
- location and time of incident
- person to whom the incident is reported
- date and time of the reporting
- brief description of what happened
- names of any witnesses
- name of any machine or piece of equipment involved
- action to prevent recurrence
- signature of person filling out the report

### Real Life Scenario

**Reporting Accidents**

James does clerical work in a pediatrician's front office. One day he notices a 5-year-old boy running around in the reception area. Suddenly, the boy trips over his untied shoelaces and bumps his head on a chair. His mother assures James that it is no big deal, as the boy is clumsy. James doesn't notice a cut or any bleeding where the boy hit his head. Should James tell his employer about the boy's fall? Should James write up the incident even though the mother says not to bother? Have you ever had to report an incident while on the job?

## Patients' Bill of Rights

As you learned in chapter 3, patients have detailed rights stated in the Patients' Bill of Rights. These rights have been written to ensure that patients receive high-quality healthcare services, particularly regarding their safety.

## *Employee Safety*

In order for a healthcare facility to operate successfully, it must maintain employee safety. Employee illness and injury can affect patient care. An injury can also have serious professional consequences and may result in loss of a job. For example, a nurse who suffers a serious back injury can no longer perform his or her nursing duties.

### OSHA

**Occupational Safety and Health Administration (OSHA)**
*a government agency put in place to oversee employee safety in the workplace*

The *Occupational Safety and Health Act of 1970* established the **Occupational Safety and Health Administration (OSHA)**, a government agency put in place to oversee employee safety in the workplace. OSHA enacts and enforces workplace safety standards intended to prevent on-the-job injuries and illnesses among workers in the United States. Training in the OSHA standards through in-service programs at the workplace must be offered to all healthcare workers. Two important OSHA standards relevant to healthcare are the Hazard Communications Standard and the Bloodborne Pathogens Standard. The Bloodborne Pathogens Standard will be discussed in the infection control portion of this chapter.

**OSHA Hazard Communication Standard.** The **OSHA Hazard Communication Standard** directly affects healthcare workers. This standard ensures that employees are educated about chemical hazards in workplace.

Chemical injuries, such as those caused from inhaling toxic fumes or from splashing acid into the eyes, may occur in a healthcare facility. Members of the housekeeping, custodial, laboratory, and food service teams, as well as pharmacy assistants, medical assistants, and dental assistants are just a few of the employees who may be at risk of a chemical injury.

The most common chemical injury is a burn. The site of the chemical contact should be flushed with water immediately. The skin might simply turn red at the site, but proper first aid must still be applied right away. Various chemicals may also produce harmful gases, causing burns to the respiratory tract, shortness of breath, a certain type of pneumonia, or other respiratory distress. To reduce the risk of chemical injury

- wear gloves when using chemicals (eye goggles and protective safety clothing may also be required);
- do not use chemicals in unlabeled containers;
- read chemical labels carefully, double-checking before use;
- never mix unknown chemicals;
- use chemicals in a well-ventilated area;
- clean up all spills immediately using a special spill kit; and
- immediately flush the skin or eyes if they come in contact with a chemical, and continue to do so for up to 10 minutes. Your facility may have a safety shower or an eyewash station for you to use (Figure 4.4).

Contact lenses are not protective safety gear. Contact lenses must be protected by safety goggles to prevent serious injury to the eye. Some healthcare facilities prohibit contact lens wearers from handling certain chemicals. Check with your facility for guidelines.

Every chemical used in your healthcare facility should be accompanied by a **material safety data sheet (MSDS)**. Read this sheet carefully—it contains important information about the chemical's makeup, dilution and mixture concentration, and instructions for use. It also explains the possible hazards of using the chemical as well as the appropriate first aid treatment needed in case of an accident or spill.

**OSHA Hazard Communication Standard**
*a standard that ensures that employees are educated about chemical hazards in the workplace*

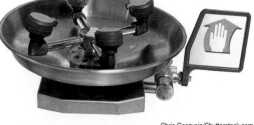
*Chris Geszvain/Shutterstock.com*

**Figure 4.4** An emergency eyewash station is used to flush the eyes when splashed with chemicals.

**material safety data sheet (MSDS)**
*a sheet that accompanies every chemical used in a hospital and which contains important information regarding that chemical*

## Extend Your Knowledge

### Burn Degrees

Burns are classified in degrees. The three degrees of burns that are most relevant to the healthcare worker include first-, second-, and third-degree burns.

First-degree: the skin is usually red and very painful, and heals in 3–5 days.

Second-degree: blisters can be present, wound will be pink or red in color, painful, and appear to be wet. These burns will take several weeks to heal.

Third-degree: All layers of the skin are destroyed, extending into tissue. Areas can be black or white, and dry. Third-degree burns may take months to heal, and could require skin grafts—the surgical transfer of healthy skin to the burned area.

## ✔ Check Your Understanding

1. Why is it important to never run in the hallway of a healthcare facility?
2. Explain the importance of hospital emergency codes.
3. What information should you include when writing an incident report?
4. What is the purpose of OSHA?
5. What is a material safety data sheet (MSDS)?

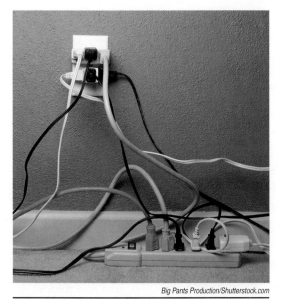

Big Pants Production/Shutterstock.com

**Figure 4.5** An overloaded electrical outlet can lead to an electrical fire.

## Electrical Safety

It is always possible to get an electrical shock when operating electrically powered equipment. Electrical shock injuries can result in moderate burns, severe skin damage, unconsciousness, or even death. Observance of safety guidelines concerning electricity can help reduce risk of such injuries. Do not overload any electrical plugs or outlets, as an overloaded plug or outlet can become a fire hazard (Figure 4.5). All equipment must have a three-prong plug, which adds further safety benefits. Equipment must be in safe, working condition with no frayed cords or loose wires.

Follow all electrical safety regulations found in a safety manual when working with electricity in a healthcare setting. It is also important to receive proper training before operating a piece of equipment. When operating electrical equipment, make sure your hands, the patient's hands, and the floor are dry. Do not perform any routine maintenance on a piece of equipment until you make sure the equipment is unplugged. Be sure to inspect equipment before use to ensure that it is safe, looking for frayed wires or other maintenance issues.

## Radiation Safety

As a healthcare worker, you must be aware of radiation safety procedures. Radiation exposure can occur when unprotected employees are near a machine that uses radiation. The degree of exposure depends on the amount of radiation, the duration of exposure, the distance from the source, and the type of shielding in place.

The radiation hazard symbol will alert you to the presence of radiation (Figure 4.6). If you are frequently exposed to radiation, you are required by law to wear a badge that records exposure. The badge should be checked periodically to make sure that you are not being exposed to damaging levels of radiation. Failure to wear a badge may result in the loss of your job.

The radiation safety principle is represented by the acronym **ALARA**, which stands for <u>A</u>s <u>L</u>ow <u>A</u>s <u>R</u>easonably <u>A</u>chievable. This principle takes into account three factors:

1. time, or duration of exposure;
2. distance from the source of radiation; and
3. shielding devices used.

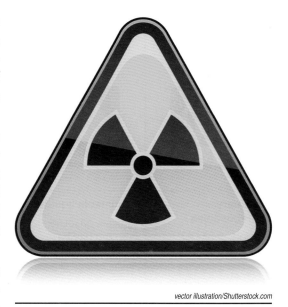

**Figure 4.6**   A radiation hazard symbol indicates that radiation is being used in the area.

## Fire Safety

Fire is one of the most feared disasters in healthcare facilities. A fire, or a threat of fire, is extremely frightening to patients, especially those who are unable to leave the facility on their own. Workers must be trained to recognize fire risks and respond in a professional manner.

The most common causes of fire include matches, heating and cooking equipment, electrical equipment and appliances, flammable liquids, and smoking (which is prohibited in all healthcare facilities). Fire can occur in any situation where three elements are present: fuel, heat, and oxygen. These three elements form what is called the **fire triangle**. If one of these elements is missing, a fire will not take place. A fire extinguisher stops the actions of a fire triangle and puts out the fire.

There are five types of fire extinguishers (Figure 4.7). Fire extinguishers must be placed around the healthcare facility and kept in working order at all times by regular, careful inspections.

**fire triangle**
*term for the three elements needed to start a fire: fuel, heat, and oxygen*

| Types of Fire Extinguishers | | | | |
|---|---|---|---|---|
| *Pressurized Water* | *Carbon Dioxide (CO$_2$)* | *Dry Chemical* | *Class D Dry Chemical* | *Multi-Purpose Dry Chemical* |
| A | B | C | D | A  B  C |
| **Ordinary combustibles** (wood, paper, or textiles) | **Flammable liquids** (grease, gasoline, oils, and paints) | **Electrical equipment** (wiring, computers, and any other energized electrical devices) | **Combustible metals** (magnesium, potassium, titanium, and sodium) | Labeled for use on ordinary combustibles, flammable liquids, and electrical equipment fires |

**Figure 4.7** Make sure the fire extinguisher you are using is appropriate for the type of fire by identifying the icons on the fire extinguisher label. Large or rapidly spreading fires should be fought by trained, professional firefighters.

## Rules for Fire Emergencies

If a fire occurs, you should stay calm. Knowing how to react will prepare you to ensure the safety of patients and yourself. It is important to familiarize yourself with your facility's evacuation routes and plans in case of a fire. Identify the location and activation methods for all fire alarms, and know the role you will play during a fire emergency. In addition to familiarizing yourself with your facility's fire emergency plan, remember the following rules to keep yourself and your patients safe during a fire:

1. Know where the fire extinguishers and the fire alarms are located (they should be in plain view) and how to use them. Make sure fire extinguishers are inspected on a routine basis.
2. Keep areas uncluttered and free of debris.
3. Evacuate ambulatory patients first (patients who are able to walk), then the patients who need wheelchairs, and finally any bedridden patients.
4. Do not prop open any fire doors.
5. Never use an elevator during a fire.
6. Don't evacuate unless instructed to do so by an authority.

### Think It Through

Does your family or do your roommates have a fire evacuation plan? Do you have fire extinguishers in the home? If so, do you know where they are located or how to use them? If your family or roommates have a fire evacuation plan, explain it. If you do not have a plan, discuss creating one with the members of your household.

7. Participate professionally during drills to ensure proper participation during a real emergency.

8. If there is no way out, close all doors between you and the fire. *Do not* open the doors without first checking to make sure they are cool to the touch.

Another way to remember how to deal with a fire is the acronym **RACE**, which stands for

1. **Rescue**: immediately stop what you are doing and remove anyone in immediate danger from the fire to a safe area.

2. **Alarm**: activate the nearest fire alarm pull stations (if applicable).

3. **Contain**: close all doors and windows that you can safely reach to contain the fire. During evacuation, close the doors behind you.

4. **Extinguish**: only attempt to extinguish the fire if it is safe to do so.

When attempting to extinguish the fire, retrieve the nearest fire extinguisher and follow the **PASS** procedure (Figure 4.8). The acronym **PASS** stands for

1. **Pull**: pull the pin to break the tamper seal.

2. **Aim**: aim low, pointing the extinguisher nozzle (also called the horn or hose) at the base of the fire. Warning: *do not* touch the plastic discharge horn on $CO_2$ extinguishers. It gets very cold and may damage your skin.

3. **Squeeze**: squeeze the handle to release the extinguishing agent.

4. **Sweep**: sweep from side to side at the base of the fire until it appears to be out. Watch the area; if the fire reignites, repeat steps 2 through 4.

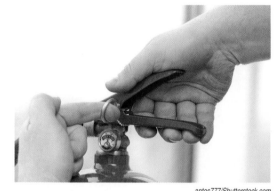

antos777/Shutterstock.com

**Figure 4.8** When using a fire extinguisher, OSHA recommends following the steps represented by the acronym PASS: pull, aim, squeeze, and sweep.

If you have the slightest doubt about your ability to fight the fire, you must evacuate immediately.

## *Body Mechanics for the Healthcare Worker*

Healthcare workers move, lift, and carry all types of supplies and equipment. They also help move or position patients. If patients are not moved properly, healthcare workers can injure themselves. Patients may struggle or twist during movement, making them more difficult to handle. Healthcare workers should educate themselves on body mechanics to ensure they do not hurt themselves.

Without the use of proper **body mechanics**, healthcare workers risk injury, particularly to their back. Back injuries can result in long periods of lost wages and even permanent disability. You can greatly reduce the possibility of a workplace injury by following simple **ergonomic** practices,

**body mechanics**
*term for the proper use of body movements to prevent injury during tasks that require lifting or moving*

**ergonomics**
*term for simple practices meant to minimize physical effort and discomfort and maximize efficiency*

which are designed to minimize physical effort and discomfort and maximize efficiency.

Practicing good body mechanics when lifting a heavy object requires you to keep your body in an upright position, with your back straight at all times. Your leg muscles should do most of the lifting work. Good body mechanics can be achieved by obeying the following principles when lifting objects:

- **Test the weight.** Before you lift, assess the weight and make sure you can lift the item safely. If not, get help or use an assistive device such as a hand truck.
- **Bend at the hips and knees.** With the lower back upright, the forces are distributed safely.
- **Maintain a wide base of support.** A solid and wide base will help reduce the possibility of slipping while lifting.
- **Hold objects as close to you as possible.** This technique reduces stress on your back.
- **Do not twist when carrying.** Always move or change directions with your feet. This decreases the stress and load on your back. Twisting often occurs when moving a patient.
- **Tighten abdominal muscles when lifting.** Your abdominal muscles help you lift while reducing strain on your lower back.
- **Think before you lift.** First, think how you will lift the object. Plan your path and make sure it is clear of any equipment or hazards.
- **Lift with your legs.** Using the large muscle groups in the legs helps reduce the forces exerted on the lower back (Figure 4.9).
- **Maintain good communication if two or more people are lifting.** Communicating with any helpers will ensure good timing when lifting, thereby reducing the likelihood of jerky or unexpected movements.

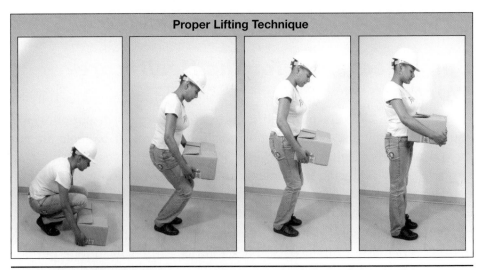

**Proper Lifting Technique**

**Figure 4.9**   In order to avoid back strain or injury when lifting, remember to always bend at the knees, lift the item smoothly, and avoid any sudden movements or twisting.

- **Push rather than pull.** It is easier to use your weight advantage when pushing.
- **Eliminate repetitive lifting duties if possible.** Store supplies that you frequently use at a reachable height to decrease lifting challenges.
- **When in doubt, get help.** Remember, some back injuries can last a lifetime.

Body mechanics are also important when you are stationary. A chair should be provided for personnel who sit for long periods of time. The height and back of the chair need to be adjustable to fit the individual. The use of a footrest may also help avoid posture problems.

When sitting for extended periods of time, you should relax periodically by standing and moving your body (Figure 4.10). At a computer station, glare should not appear on the screen. A vertical document holder, either attached to a flexible equipment arm or free standing, eases eyestrain and improves posture.

A good wrist support should be available to keep your wrists as straight as possible. The support should have rounded edges and padding, and should be about two inches high. As Figure 4.11 shows, **carpal tunnel syndrome** is a progressively painful hand and arm condition caused by a pinched nerve in the wrist. This condition can be prevented, or lessened, by maintaining a proper wrist position while operating a computer keyboard. The fingers should be lower than the wrist.

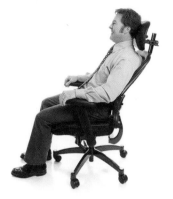

*Lisa F. Young/Shutterstock.com*

**Figure 4.10** An ergonomic chair gives the body proper support.

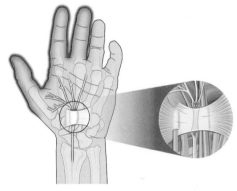

*Alexonline/Shutterstock.com*

**Figure 4.11** Carpal tunnel syndrome occurs when the median nerve becomes pinched. Surgery may be required to treat this condition.

**carpal tunnel syndrome**
*a painful, progressive hand and arm condition caused by compression of a key nerve in the wrist; can be caused when wrists are not supported during keyboard use*

# Disaster Preparedness in the Healthcare Facility

A disaster is any sudden event that brings great damage, loss, or destruction. Individuals in the healthcare profession must be prepared for unexpected events due to terrorism, catastrophic accidents, earthquakes, explosions, fires, tornadoes, hurricanes, and gun violence. In the event of a disaster, you will most likely find yourself working alongside police, firefighters, and emergency medical personnel.

Healthcare facilities are required to draw up plans for dealing with disasters. The facility in which you work will also have disaster drills. When you are hired, you will be given instructions for how to handle a disaster and what your specific role will be in those situations. These instructions may include procedures for evacuating patients, recognizing evacuation routes, and working as a team in emergency situations.

During a disaster, it is critical that you act in a professional manner, remain calm, carry out your assigned task without complaint, and obey directions given by your supervisor.

# Safety in the Science Laboratory

Throughout your education to become a healthcare worker, you may take several science courses. Science courses often have labs connected to them. There are several safety issues to keep in mind while working in the science laboratory. These considerations can also apply to any career that involves working in scientific research laboratories, hospitals, or independent laboratories.

There are significant safety risks in the science laboratory. When working in a laboratory, you must adhere to the following guidelines:

- Obey all of the rules your instructor or supervisor has posted in the laboratory. These are often also printed and given to students. There will most likely be a zero tolerance policy for disobeying safety rules.
- Clothing is an important consideration when working in a laboratory. Exposed heels and toes are vulnerable to injury, so it is best to avoid these types of shoes. Do not wear loose-sleeved blouses or shirts if fire sources are in use.
- Protective safety equipment must be worn when working with chemicals, blood, pathogens, and other items that pose a safety risk. If you are not sure when to use such equipment, ask your instructor or supervisor.
- Be aware of all safety symbols in the laboratory. For instance, a chemical's label may have a warning symbol indicating that the chemical within is flammable. Figure 4.12 illustrates some safety symbols that you should be familiar with when working in the laboratory.
- When doing a laboratory exercise, you may be tempted to read through the directions quickly in an effort to complete the exercise on time. For the sake of safety, read all directions carefully. Instructions for safely working with equipment and handling substances are most likely included in the laboratory exercise directions. If you are confused, ask your instructor or supervisor to explain.
- When working in a laboratory setting, make sure that your workspace is neat and clean during and after the procedure. You will be given instructions on how to leave your laboratory station for the next user. Imagine how you would react if the last person using your station left behind a puddle of dangerous acid.
- In the event of an accident, refer to the instructions and procedures given to avoid and treat injuries. Eyewash stations should be available if you are working with any liquid chemicals that might accidentally splash into your eyes. Protective eyewear must be worn if there is a possibility of chemicals splashing into the eyes.
- Burns, fires, and equipment failures that result in injuries are considered emergencies. Read through all emergency policies before starting any laboratory exercise. All accidents, no matter how minor, must be reported to your instructor or supervisor immediately. As in a healthcare facility, you may have to fill out an incident or accident report.

| Laboratory Safety Symbols | | | |
|---|---|---|---|
| **Safety goggles** | Safety goggles must be worn to protect the eyes while performing any task that involves chemicals, flames, heating, or glassware. | **Lab coat** | A lab coat or apron must be worn to protect the skin and clothing from harm. |
| **Gloves** | When working with harmful chemicals or microorganisms, disposable gloves must be worn at all times. Dispose of used gloves properly. | **Heat** | Do not touch hot objects with your bare hands; instead use a clamp or tongs. |
| **Flames** | Follow your instructor's or supervisor's directions when working with flames. Tie back loose hair and clothing before working with flames. | **Corrosive chemical** | When working with a corrosive chemical, avoid contact with the skin, eyes, or clothing and do not inhale the vapors. Wash your hands thoroughly after working with corrosive chemicals. |
| **Animal safety** | Avoid harming any animals or yourself when working in the lab. Wash hands thoroughly after handling any animal. | **Poison** | Avoid contact with poisonous substances and do not inhale vapors. Wash hands thoroughly after working with poisonous substances. |
| **Scissors** | Sharps, including scissors, knives, scalpels, or needles must be handled with care to avoid puncturing or cutting the skin. Always direct the sharp point of the object away from yourself and others. | **Biohazard** | Materials that are harmful and pose a threat to your health must be handled with care. Avoid contact with biohazards including used needles, toxins, infectious substances, and other medical waste. |

*Ecelop/Shutterstock.com; Max Griboedov/Shutterstock.com; andromina/Shutterstock.com; Miguel Angel Salinas Salinas/Shutterstock.com; Barry Barnes/Shutterstock.com*

**Figure 4.12** Laboratory warning symbols alert you to any specific hazards you may encounter when working in a lab.

- Familiarize yourself with the location and operation of safety equipment such as a safety shower and eyewash station(s).

Following safety guidelines in all areas of healthcare, including science training, is critical whether you are a student or an employee.

# *Infection Control*

There is a constant battle in healthcare facilities to prevent the spread of microorganisms that can cause infectious disease. These microorganisms, known as pathogens, present major problems both for patients and employees. Today, most healthcare facilities have a separate department devoted exclusively to infection control. Many facilities call this the Department of Hospital Epidemiology and Infection Control (HEIC).

# Quality Assurance

Since the 1960s, serious efforts have been made to initiate **quality assurance** policies (also called *quality control*) in hospitals. Quality assurance policies are put in place to ensure that hospitals monitor and evaluate services based on predetermined criteria. Should these criteria not be met, corrective action will be required. The establishment and monitoring of such policies has been carried out by the Joint Commission on Accreditation of Healthcare Organizations (JCAHO).

All healthcare organizations that are members of the JCAHO have a three-year accreditation cycle, meaning their membership in the JCAHO must be renewed every three years. Clinical laboratories are surveyed every two years. The JCAHO does not share all of its findings with the public. However, it does share the accreditation decision, the date that accreditation was awarded, and any standards that were cited for improvement. An organization must be in compliance with all, or most, of the standards to become accredited.

Examples of quality assurance in a healthcare facility include keeping records of incidents that occur in the facility; ensuring all machinery is monitored on a regular basis, with strict records of maintenance; and completing patient care documentation in a clear, consistent, accurate, complete, and timely manner.

There are so many tasks involved in maintaining quality assurance that most medium and large facilities have a separate department dedicated to providing the best quality of care that can be offered to patients.

# Introduction to Microorganisms

Microorganisms such as **bacteria**, **viruses**, and **fungi** are everywhere in our environment—in the air, on our skin, in food, and on everything that we touch. You cannot see bacteria without a microscope. Viruses, which are much smaller than bacteria or fungi, cannot even be seen using a standard microscope.

Many microorganisms normally do not cause illness; these are called *nonpathogenic* microorganisms. Nonpathogenic microorganisms maintain a balance in the environment and in our bodies. The bacteria in our colons are an example of nonpathogenic microorganisms. When in balance, these bacteria do not cause health problems and help to break down waste and nutrients. In some circumstances, such as surgery that perforates (punctures) the bowel, the bacteria in the colon can spill into the body cavity and cause serious infection. Persons with compromised immune systems are susceptible to infections and may become ill from microorganisms that do not usually affect individuals with healthy immune systems.

# Bacteria

Pathogenic bacteria cause many diseases. Bacteria are initially classified by their **morphology** (or form and structure) as seen under a microscope. After observing bacteria under the microscope, the clinical microbiologist then identifies the actual family of the bacteria through further testing.

The basic forms of bacteria are spherical (*coccus*) and rod-like shapes (*bacilli*). Figure 4.13 illustrates several shapes of bacteria, including those that appear as twisted cylinders (*spirochetes*), spherically-shaped cocci arranged in clusters (*Staphylococcus*), cocci forming chains (*Streptococcus*), and cocci in pairs (*Diplococcus*).

**morphology**
*term for the form and structure of an organism*

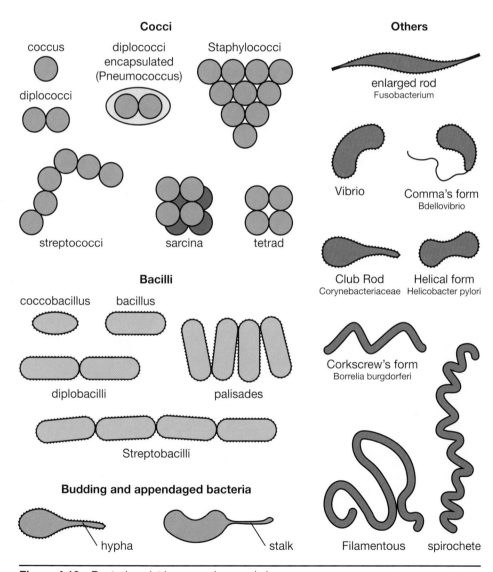

**Figure 4.13** Bacteria exist in many sizes and shapes.

Bacteria cause major illness in our bodies. Hospital stays are often prolonged caused by the bacterium called *staphylococcus aureus* (or *S. aureus*) infection. The Black Plague that killed approximately 25 million people in fourteenth century Europe was caused by the rod-shaped bacterium, *Yersinia pestis*. Today, *Yersinia pestis* is easily treated with antibiotics. Another bacterial infection, syphilis, is caused by a spiral bacterium called a *spirochete*. Bacterial infections are treated with antibiotics—drugs that kill the disease-inducing microorganism.

## Viruses

Much smaller than bacteria, viruses depend on a living cell to survive because they cannot reproduce on their own. Viruses are the cause of the common cold, smallpox, chicken pox, measles, influenza, human papillomavirus (HPV), herpes simplex, and AIDS. Many more illnesses are caused by viruses.

Antibiotics do not kill viruses. Usually, time and rest are necessary to let most of these illnesses run their course. Physicians will advise patients to stay home, take nonaspirin pain relievers, and get plenty of rest. However, vaccines have been developed against many viral diseases. A vaccine introduces small amounts of the microorganism into the system in an effort to boost the immune system against the microorganism. An increasing number of antiviral remedies are being developed. These remedies will prevent the virus from replicating, or reproducing itself.

## Fungi

Microscopic fungi include yeasts and molds. Some fungi can cause disease, especially if the immune system has already been compromised by a different disease or disorder.

Examples of fungal infections include athlete's foot, thrush (an infection of the mouth or throat), vaginitis, and certain lung diseases. Fungal infections are treated with topical, oral, or injectable medications.

**protozoa**
*microorganisms that depend on a host cell to survive and replicate; can cause serious illness*

**parasites**
*organisms that live in or on another organism*

**rickettsiae**
*parasites that normally choose fleas, lice, ticks, or mites as their host organisms; can cause severe infections*

## Protozoa

Although they are larger than viruses, protozoa also depend on a host cell to survive and replicate. **Protozoa** are found in water and soil and cause amebic dysentery, an inflammation of the colon that results in fever, abdominal pain, and severe diarrhea. They also cause amoebiasis, trichomoniasis, and malaria (a disease contracted via a mosquito bite). In a malaria patient, the protozoan lives in red blood cells. Protozoal infections are treated with oral and injectable anti-protozoal medications.

## Rickettsiae

Rickettsiae are **parasites**, or organisms that live in or on another organism. Parasites like **rickettsiae** normally choose fleas, lice, ticks, or mites as their host organism. If one of these creatures bites a human, that human's body becomes the parasite's host. Rickettsiae cause Rocky Mountain spotted fever and types of typhus, both of which are severe infections that have been known to cause serious epidemics. Rickettsiae are treated with appropriate antibiotics.

---

#### ⊣Extend Your Knowledge⊢

##### Super Bugs

In the news today you hear a great deal about antibiotic-resistant bacteria, or *super bugs*. Over the years, certain bacteria have developed a resistance to antibiotics. This resistance makes some infections difficult to treat.

Some bacteria are resistant to most antibiotics. Such resistance can develop when antibiotics are used improperly. Antibiotic resistance can develop when

- patients do not take all of their prescribed antibiotics (the bacteria may not be completely killed, which will cause further illness or even drug resistance);
- antibiotics are prescribed when not needed or indicated (antibiotics will not be effective against the flu, which is caused by a virus);
- antibacterial substances are contained in cleaning products;
- antibiotics are found in animals consumed as food; or
- genetic mutation of bacteria has occurred.

Some bacteria that have become resistant to antibiotics include *Mycobacterium tuberculosis*, *Streptococcus*, *Enterococci*, *Klebsiella*, *Acinetobacter*, *Pseudomonas*, and *Enterobacter*. One of the most highly publicized bacterium in this category is **Methicillin-resistant *Staphylococcus aureus* (MRSA)**. MRSA is responsible for a difficult-to-treat infection. MRSA is prevalent in hospitals, prisons, schools, and nursing homes, where patients with open wounds and weakened immune systems are confined in close quarters. These patients are at greater risk of infection than the general public.

Careful monitoring of antibiotic use is necessary to prevent the development of antibiotic resistance and to reduce the spread of antibiotic-resistant bacteria.

**Methicillin-resistant *Staphylococcus aureus* (MRSA)**
*an antibiotic-resistant bacterium responsible for a difficult-to-treat infection; sometimes prevalent in hospitals, prisons, schools, and nursing homes*

---

## The Chain of Infection

During a hospital stay, a patient does not expect to acquire an infection. Unfortunately, patients often do acquire new infections while in the hospital. Hospital-acquired infections are known as *nosocomial infections*, or *healthcare-associated infections*. Examples of such infection include bacterial and fungal infections. Nosocomial infections can cause pneumonia and infections of the bloodstream, the urinary tract, and other parts of the body. The reduced infection resistance of hospitalized patients contributes to the rate of nosocomial infections.

As part of a team working continually to prevent the spread of infection, you need to understand the various ways that infection can be transmitted from person to person. The **chain of infection** is used to visualize the sequence of events that allows infection to invade the human body (Figure 4.14).

**chain of infection**

*the visualization of the sequence of events allowing infection to invade the human body*

## Interrupting the Chain of Infection

There are several methods used to control the spread of infection. The infection control department of a healthcare facility focuses on interrupting the chain of infection before it spreads throughout the hospital. Once it becomes clear that an infection has developed, it is important that the clinical laboratory identifies the infectious agent as soon as possible. Appropriate treatment must be started immediately.

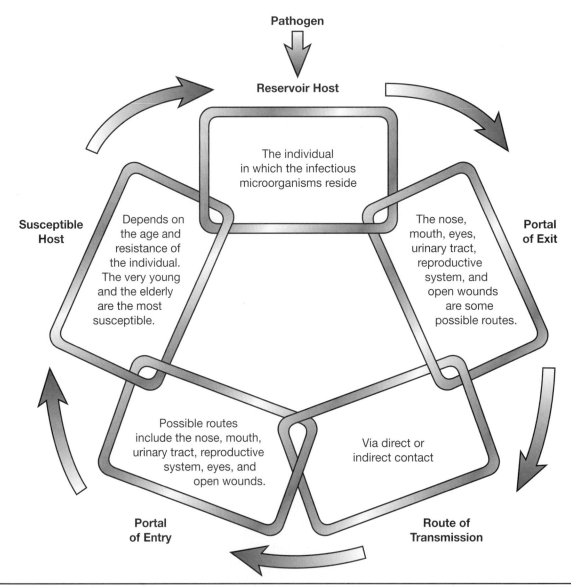

**Figure 4.14**   The chain of infection is a sequence of events allowing infection to invade the human body.

# Hand Hygiene

Employees must maintain excellent hygiene, which includes **hand hygiene**. Hand hygiene is considered the single most important way to prevent the spread of infection. It can be accomplished through hand washing with a detergent or antimicrobial soap and water, or by applying an alcohol-based hand rub. Hand sanitizers do not kill severe gastrointestinal infections such as *Clostridium difficile* (or *C. difficile*) or the norovirus. Alcohol-based hand wipes have been found to be useless against any viruses not coated in lipid envelopes.

The **Centers for Disease Control and Prevention (CDC)** is a federal agency that conducts and supports health promotion, prevention, and preparedness activities in the United States. In an effort to prevent the spread of infection, the CDC has issued guidelines for hand hygiene for healthcare workers. These guidelines state that hands should be washed

1. before eating;
2. after the restroom has been used; and
3. when dirt or body fluids such as blood, mucus, urine, and feces are visible on the hands.

The use of alcohol-based hand products is acceptable throughout the day, except under the previously stated circumstances. Alcohol-based hand rubs have become popular today because they do not dry out the skin as much as hand washing. As a result, alcohol-based hand rubs are widely used in healthcare facilities.

**hand hygiene**
*hand washing with a detergent or antimicrobial soap and water, or by applying an alcohol-based hand rub; considered the single most important way to prevent the spread of infection*

**Centers for Disease Control and Prevention (CDC)**
*federal agency in the United States responsible for protecting public health and safety by promoting awareness, control, and prevention of disease, injury, and disability*

---

**Did You Know?**

### Proper Hand Washing

It takes at least fifteen seconds to wash your hands properly, which is about how long it takes to sing "Happy Birthday to You" twice.

How to wash your hands:

- wet hands with water
- apply enough soap or hand wash to cover all hand surfaces
- rub hands palm to palm (the friction caused by rubbing is key to removing contaminants) with fingers pointing down and not touching the sink
- right palm over the other hand with interlaced fingers and vice versa
- palm to palm with fingers interlaced
- backs of fingers to opposing palms with fingers interlocked
- rotational rubbing of left thumb clasped in right palm and vice versa
- rotational rubbing backward and forward with clasped fingers of right hand in left palm and vice versa
- rinse hands with water
- dry thoroughly with towel, using the towel to turn off faucets

How seriously do you take hand hygiene in your everyday life? How many times a day do you wash your hands? How do you clean your hands? Under what daily circumstances do you practice hand hygiene?

In addition to practicing good hand hygiene, hospital workers and other healthcare employees must not come to work when sick with a contagious disease.

## Cleaning the Healthcare Facility

There are at least three levels of cleaning that take place in the healthcare environment. These include sanitization, disinfection, and sterilization.

**Sanitization** is defined as the use of antimicrobial agents on objects, surfaces, or living tissue to reduce the number of disease-causing microorganisms to nonthreatening levels. An example of sanitization is cleaning tables in a hospital cafeteria before disinfection.

**Disinfection** involves the use of antimicrobial agents on nonliving objects or surfaces to destroy or deactivate microorganisms. Disinfectants are applied and allowed to dry according to the directions of the chemical manufacturer. Disinfecting floors and walls in a hospital room is an example of disinfection. Disinfecting an object does not mean that all of the bacteria, viruses, and fungi have been removed. Some microorganisms form thick walls around themselves called *spores* that protect them from harsh environments. This makes it difficult for disinfectants to completely remove the microorganisms.

In order to kill all microorganisms on a surface, the surface must be sterilized. The most common method of **sterilization** in many healthcare facilities is the use of the **autoclave**. An autoclave is a machine that employs hot, pressurized steam. The steam's high temperature kills all microorganisms and their spores (Figure 4.15). Other methods of sterilization include dry heat, gas, ionized radiation, and specialized chemicals designed for the purpose of sterilization.

**sanitization**
*term for the use of antimicrobial agents on objects, surfaces, or living tissue to reduce the number of disease-causing microorganisms*

**disinfection**
*term for the use of antimicrobial agents on nonliving objects or surfaces to destroy or deactivate microorganisms*

**sterilization**
*the act of killing all microorganisms and their spores on a surface; methods of sterilization in a healthcare facility may include hot pressurized steam, dry heat, gas, ionized radiation, and specialized chemicals*

**autoclave**
*a machine that employs hot, pressurized steam to kill all microorganisms and their spores on a surface*

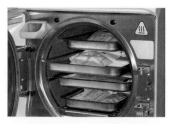

Robert A. Levy Photography, LLC/Shutterstock.com

**Figure 4.15** The autoclave, using steam under pressure, is the most common method of sterilization in many healthcare environments.

### What's the Most Hygienic?

Scientists at the University of Westminster in London performed a study to measure what was most hygienic—drying freshly washed hands with paper towels or using an electric hand dryer. Their study measured the number of bacteria on subjects' hands before washing and after drying them. Three different drying methods were used: paper towels, the warm air dryer, and a high-speed jet air dryer.

Paper towels were found to be clearly superior to the other methods, resulting in a 76% decrease in bacteria on the finger pads and 77% decrease on the palms. In contrast, warm air dryers caused bacteria counts to increase by 194% on the finger pads and up to 254% on the palms. The jet air dryers increased the bacteria on the finger pads by 42% and by 15% on the palms.

Additionally, the warm air dryers had a potential for cross contamination of other bathroom users. The jet air dryers could potentially contaminate other users up to 7 feet away. The warm air dryers had the potential of contamination range of about 10 inches.

In a hospital, the Central Services Department handles sterilization procedures. Autoclaves are widely used in physicians' offices, but many supplies used in patient care are prepackaged and sterilized by the manufacturer and are disposable. As a result, the use of an autoclave has declined somewhat in the healthcare facility.

# Preventing the Spread of Bloodborne Pathogens

In order to avoid exposure to potentially harmful substances, employees must strictly follow instructions stated by the **OSHA Bloodborne Pathogens Standard**. This standard went into effect in the United States in 1992. It was designed to reduce the risk of transmitting **bloodborne pathogens** within the healthcare facility. Bloodborne pathogens are infectious microorganisms found in human blood that can cause disease in humans. Examples of these pathogens include, but are not limited to, hepatitis B (HBV), hepatitis C (HCV), and human immunodeficiency virus (HIV).

The rules set forth by the OSHA Bloodborne Pathogens Standard apply to all patients receiving care in any healthcare facility, regardless of their diagnosis or infection status. The standard lists **potentially infectious materials (PIM)**, which include a range of body fluids. In order to protect themselves and their patients, healthcare workers should always proceed as if these body fluids are infectious. There are several body fluids that have the potential to transmit harmful pathogens:

- human blood and its components (plasma, serum, platelets, and immunoglobulin)
- semen and vaginal secretions
- body fluids such as cerebrospinal, synovial (joint), pleural (lung), pericardial (heart), peritoneal (abdominal cavity), and amniotic (surrounding unborn baby) fluids
- body fluids visibly contaminated with blood or other unidentified substances (such as saliva in dental procedures)
- human tissue such as a **biopsy** specimen
- any bodily substance from a person known to be infected with HIV

In addition to practicing good hand hygiene and cleaning contaminated surfaces, employees *must* dispose of all potentially infected materials in a proper manner.

Gloves are not always worn when giving patient care, but they *must* be worn when there is the possibility of an employee being exposed to blood and body fluids. Healthcare workers must always wash their hands before putting on gloves and again after removing their gloves between patients. Used gloves that are visibly contaminated with blood or other body fluids have to be disposed of in a biohazard receptacle.

**OSHA Bloodborne Pathogens Standard**
*a standard applied to all patients receiving care in any healthcare facility; lists potentially infectious materials and mandates that healthcare workers should always proceed as if the materials are infectious*

**bloodborne pathogens**
*infectious microorganisms in human blood that can cause disease*

**potentially infectious materials (PIM)**
*materials designated by OSHA that require healthcare workers to proceed as if they are infectious*

**biopsy**
*a small piece of tissue removed from the body for examination*

## *Patient Isolation*

The purpose of isolation is to separate patients with certain infections from other patients and prevent the transmission of pathogenic microorganisms in hospitals. Reverse isolation protects susceptible patients from contagious diseases by isolating them from others.

Guidelines for patient isolation have been identified by The Center for Disease Control and Prevention (CDC) and the Hospital Infection Control Practice Advisory Committee (HICPAC). There are two levels of isolation precautions: standard precautions and transmission-based precautions.

## Standard Precautions

Standard precautions apply to all hospitalized patients, regardless of their diagnosis. Standard precautions are used when there is the potential for exposure to blood; these apply to all body fluids, and any secretions or excretions (except perspiration), whether they contain visible blood or not. These also apply to non-intact skin and mucous membranes.

## Transmission-Based Precautions

Transmission-based precautions are designed for patients with highly transmissible infections and require additional precautions beyond standard precautions. Transmission-based precautions are divided into three categories based on how the infections are transmitted: airborne precautions, droplet precautions, and contact precautions. Transmission-based precautions may be used alone, or in combination with standard precautions. Transmission-based precautions are always used in addition to standard precautions.

**Airborne Precautions.** These precautions are used to prevent the spread of diseases transmitted by tiny, airborne droplet residue or dust particles containing the microorganisms. Airborne precautions require that the patient be placed in a private room or with another patient who has the same disease. The door to the room must be kept closed and the room must have special ventilation. Respiratory protection in the form of a N95 respirator should be worn when giving patient care. Tuberculosis is an example of a disease requiring airborne precautions.

**Droplet Precautions.** These precautions are used to prevent infection spread through large droplet transmission. In these cases, disease transmission occurs through coughing, talking, and sneezing. People within a three-foot radius or less are susceptible.

Isolation precautions include placement in a private room or with a person who has the same diagnosis. Masks should be worn within three feet of the patient. Because the droplets do not remain suspended in air, no special air handling or ventilation is required. Influenza and *Bordetella pertussis* (whooping cough) are examples of infectious diseases requiring droplet precautions.

**Contact Precautions.** Contact precautions are designed to reduce the risk of transmission of certain infectious microorganisms through direct or indirect contact. Direct contact transmission occurs when patients are touched and there is physical transfer of pathogens during direct patient care. Indirect contact transmission occurs when pathogens are transferred from a contaminated object or surface to a susceptible host. Whenever possible, patients should be placed in a private room or with another patient with the same condition. Hepatitis A and impetigo are examples of infectious diseases requiring contact precautions.

## Isolation Procedures

When employing isolation precautions, a variety of practices will be used. These practices are dependent upon the type of isolation precautions in use. Healthcare facilities often have special **isolation rooms**. Signs are placed on the door to signal the type of isolation in place. Standard precautions are always used, with great attention paid to hand hygiene. Protective gloves, masks, and face shields serve as barriers against infection. Various types of gowns are worn to prevent contamination of clothing and to protect the skin from blood and other body fluids. Impermeable gown, leg, and shoe covers are available when greater protection is required. Special handling of patient supplies and equipment is important. Disposable dishes and other items are often used. Thorough cleaning and disinfection of the room and equipment is done regularly and upon patient discharge.

Patients in isolation should be moved as little as possible. When it is necessary for an isolated patient to be transported in the hospital and airborne or droplet precautions are in place, the patient should wear a mask. Caregivers must never forget that the patient in isolation is especially in need of compassionate care and understanding so that the patient does not feel unnecessarily shut off from the world.

**isolation rooms**
*rooms in a healthcare facility used to contain contagious diseases as well as protect immune-compromised patients from disease*

**personal protective equipment (PPE)**
*equipment worn by workers to protect them from serious workplace injuries or illnesses*

## *Personal Protective Equipment*

OSHA requires that all workers wear the appropriate **personal protective equipment**, or **PPE**, for their position. PPE protects workers from serious workplace injuries or illnesses resulting from contact with hazards of a microbial, chemical, radiological, physical, electrical, or mechanical nature. This equipment can include face shields, safety glasses, goggles, gowns, gloves, and face masks (Figure 4.16).

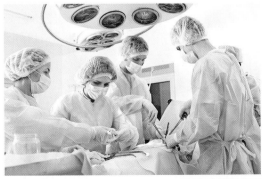

*Poznyakov/Shutterstock.com*

**Figure 4.16** Personal protective equipment includes gloves, gowns, and masks.

You should wear a face mask if your patient has a respiratory infection and is coughing and sneezing. In a doctor's office, wear a face mask if you have a cold or if you are going to be exposed to a patient with a cold.

## *Needlesticks and other Sharps*

**sharps**

*needles or any other object that could puncture or cut the skin*

**needlesticks**

*any accidental puncture of the skin by a needle; can be dangerous in a healthcare setting because the puncture can cause a potentially serious infection*

**biohazard sharps container**

*a puncture-resistant container used for disposing of waste-contaminated sharps, including needles, scalpels, glass slides, and broken glassware*

Needles and other **sharps** (any object that could puncture or cut the skin) are a risk in the healthcare environment. Injuries related to **needlesticks** (any accidental puncture of the skin) or other sharp-related injuries can be both painful and dangerous.

In the healthcare environment, all needles are considered sharps, including needles with syringes and attached tubing, or needles from vacutainers (devices that enable phlebotomists to draw several blood tubes at one time). Sharps also include blades such as razors, scalpels, and lancets. These items must be placed in a **biohazard sharps container**, whether or not they are contaminated with biohazardous waste (Figure 4.17).

*Any* object that has been contaminated with biohazardous waste and has the potential to puncture a garbage bag must be placed in the biohazard sharps container. Such items might include broken glassware, glassware with sharp edges or points, pipettes, or glass slides. If these items are *not* contaminated with biohazardous waste, they may be placed in a rigid container and marked with the words "broken glassware."

A needlestick or other sharp-related injury immediately opens the skin to the potential of infection with bloodborne disease and other pathogens. Any skin abrasion, including acne, presents an opening for pathogens to enter your body. Be sure to bandage any cuts or breaks in the skin, and keep your hands away from your eyes and face to avoid infection.

Nurses, EMTs, paramedics, phlebotomists, clinical medical assistants, housekeeping personnel, and other healthcare personnel may be at risk of exposure to bloodborne pathogens. A highly effective hepatitis B vaccine is available and is given in a series of three injections. Employers must offer this injection if their employee is at risk of being exposed to bloodborne pathogens. There is no vaccine for HIV or hepatitis C.

**Needlestick Safety and Prevention Act**

*law enacted in 2000; mandates that OSHA require employers to identify, evaluate, and introduce safe medical devices to avoid needlesticks*

**The Needlestick Safety and Prevention Act** was signed into law on November 6, 2000. Under this act, OSHA requires employers to identify, evaluate, and introduce safe medical devices. Devices are available to shield a needle as soon as it is withdrawn from the patient. A needle should never be recapped once it has been used on a patient. OSHA requires that safety-engineered needles—such as ones that have needle shields—must be used. After use, needles should be immediately placed in a puncture-resistant biohazard sharps container to prevent accidental exposure to a needlestick.

If you are stuck by a needle or another sharp object, or get blood or potentially infectious materials in your eyes, nose, mouth, or on broken skin, immediately flood the exposed area with water. Clean all wounds with soap and water or a skin antiseptic, if available. Immediately report the incident to your employer and seek medical attention. Your facility safety manual should clearly explain how to proceed after such an exposure.

The OSHA Standard requires the following:

- Sanitize your hands after direct contact with each of your patients.
- Use protective barriers such as gloves when working with blood and other potentially infectious body fluids. In addition, gowns, aprons, masks, and goggles must be used when there is a danger of being splashed or sprayed with body fluids. Remember, gloves that are worn when giving patient care are not puncture-proof.
- Collect and properly dispose of needles and other sharps in a biohazard sharps container.
- Do not recap needles.
- Cover all of your cuts and broken skin with a waterproof dressing before putting on gloves and handling blood or other potentially infectious body fluids.
- Promptly and carefully clean up spills of blood and other body fluids as directed by your facility safety manual.
- Facilities should use a safe system for healthcare waste management and disposal.

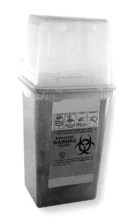

*Steve Carroll/Shutterstock.com*

**Figure 4.17** Any object that is contaminated with biohazard waste and can puncture through a garbage bag must be placed in a biohazard sharps container.

## *Real Life Scenario*

### *Needle Safety and Procedures*

Isabella just started her job as a phlebotomist at North Haven Hospital. It is her first week drawing blood, and her supervisor is very strict about procedures. Isabella already feels that her supervisor does not have much faith in her abilities.

Isabella's next patient is a male adult who admits to being afraid of needles, increasing Isabella's anxiety. Isabella's hands are shaking, and she worries that her supervisor will come into the drawing room to watch, so she hurries through the blood draw. She is able to draw the blood quickly, but in her haste to put away the needle she sticks herself with it.

Isabella immediately decides that she won't tell anyone about the needlestick for fear of getting in trouble, or possibly fired.

What could be the possible consequences of Isabella's failure to report this incident? Do you think her supervisor should fire her? What if her patient has a bloodborne disease? What would you do?

# Chapter Review and Assessment

## Summary

All healthcare workers are responsible for the safety of the patients, visitors, and their coworkers. General safety rules must be obeyed in the healthcare facility, such as never running in the halls, exercising caution when opening swinging doors, and keeping floors and hallways free of obstructions. You must continually be aware of potential safety hazards in the facility, such as liquid spills, loose rugs, and disoriented patients. When positioning patients, healthcare workers should practice proper body mechanics to avoid injuring themselves.

Read your department's safety manual to familiarize yourself with the specific safety concerns in your area. Incident reports must be filled out whenever an act occurs that compromises the safety and health of a patient, visitor, or employee. This could include any event that is not a part of the routine operation in the healthcare facility, such as a patient falling, abuse from a patient or an employee, or an accidental needlestick.

OSHA oversees employee safety in the workplace. It is important that you are aware of OSHA's Hazard Communication Standard. Additionally, you must know and practice safety regulations regarding chemical, electrical, radiation, and fire hazards. Follow instructions for disaster preparedness and participate in disaster drills.

Safety is also a serious concern for students and employees working in a science laboratory. Following safety guidelines both in school and in the workplace is critical for the healthcare student and employee.

Infection control in healthcare facilities is a constant battle to prevent the spread of disease-causing microorganisms. Special attention must be given to OSHA's Bloodborne Pathogens Standard. Employees must know how to interrupt the chain of infection using strategies such as observing proper hand hygiene, wearing appropriate attire, and proper disposal of all potentially infected materials. Employees should also follow proper procedures regarding patients in isolation areas. The employee must pay attention to special instructions for using personal protective equipment when a patient is isolated.

Needles and other sharps are prevalent in the healthcare environment. Accidental needlesticks are dangerous and must be avoided. To ensure the safety of all, used needles and other sharps should be placed in a puncture-resistant, biohazard sharps container.

Safety must be a serious concern for students and healthcare professionals working in a healthcare facility or the science laboratory. Following safety guidelines in school, the workplace, at play, and at home is critical for the healthcare student and employee.

## Review Questions

*Answer the following questions using what you have learned in this chapter.*

### Short Answer

1. What is an incident report?
2. What is a nosocomial infection?
3. Name the five types of fire extinguishers.
4. List three basic principles of body mechanics involved in safely lifting an object.
5. What is meant by the chain of infection? Name five parts of the chain.
6. Define pathogen.
7. What is meant by hand hygiene?
8. What is a biohazard sharps container and why is it used?
9. Describe two OSHA standards that apply to the healthcare facility.
10. Define quality assurance.

### True or False

11. *True or False?* Isolation rooms can be used to contain contagious diseases such as tuberculosis.
12. *True or False?* Hands do not need to be washed after you have removed your gloves.

13. *True or False?* A carpal tunnel injury is often a result of incorrect lifting.

14. *True or False? Streptococcus* and *Staphylococcus* are parasites that cause disease.

15. *True or False?* Viruses are the cause of the common cold.

16. *True or False?* The friction caused by rubbing hands and fingers together when hand washing is key to removing contaminants from the hands.

17. *True or False?* Always check the patient's identification wristband before carrying out any procedures.

18. *True or False?* Personal protective equipment is only worn by employees of the fire department.

19. *True or False?* Antibiotic-resistant bacteria are also known as *superbugs*.

20. *True or False?* Gloves do *not* need to be worn when attending to a cut on a patient's arm.

## Multiple Choice

21. Which of the following situation(s) could merit filling out an incident report at a hospital?
    A. an employee yelling at a patient
    B. a patient falling while walking to the restroom
    C. a patient experiencing a serious allergic reaction to an ingredient in their dinner
    D. All of the above.

22. To avoid back injury, which of the following should be avoided?
    A. holding objects as far away from you as possible
    B. lifting with your legs
    C. tightening stomach muscles when lifting
    D. pushing rather than pulling objects

23. Which of the following is a correct procedure for infection control?
    A. use a puncture-proof biohazard container to dispose of needles and other sharps
    B. follow proper hand hygiene procedures between contact with each patient
    C. use protective barriers when in direct contact with blood
    D. All of the above.

24. In a fire emergency, which step should *not* be followed?
    A. Follow facility evacuation plans.
    B. Keep areas uncluttered and free of debris.
    C. Run through the halls shouting "Code Blue!"
    D. Know how to operate fire extinguishers.

25. Antibiotic resistance can be caused by _____.
    A. not taking the full prescription of antibiotics
    B. overprescribing antibiotics when not needed
    C. antibacterials contained in cleaning products
    D. All of the above.

26. The acronym PASS stands for _____.
    A. pinch, aim, spray, stop
    B. pull, aim, sweep, spray
    C. pin, aim, shake, squeeze
    D. pull, aim, squeeze, sweep

## Critical Thinking Exercises

27. Do you and your family have disaster preparedness plans? Establish response plans for any natural disasters that might occur in your city or town.

28. What steps do you and your family take to avoid getting sick? vitamins? good nutrition? plenty of sleep? Do you think these steps are sufficient, or is there more you could do to stay healthy?

29. Research a specific antibiotic-resistant bacterium online. Remember to make sure you are using reputable sources. Identify the antibiotic-resistant bacteria that are emerging today as "super bugs?" How dangerous are they? Are there any measures we can take personally to prevent the development of such dangerous antibiotic-resistant bacteria?

30. What are the differences between bacterial and viral infections? What treatments are available for both infections?

31. Sanitization, disinfection, and sterilization are three levels of cleaning that take place in the healthcare environment. Explain the significance and use of each level.

# Chapter

# 5

# *Study Skills*

## Terms to Know

active listening
auditory learner
critical thinking
kinesthetic learner
learning styles

mnemonic devices
motivation
stress
time management
visual learner

## Chapter Objectives

- Identify the importance of motivation for achieving your career goals.
- Describe learning styles and their application for effective learning.
- List ways to manage your time well.
- Identify what is meant by *critical thinking*.
- Discuss how to practice active listening.
- Explain how to take effective notes while listening intently to presentations.
- Discuss ways of improving your memory.
- List effective ways to study for and take a test.
- Explain steps to take after finishing a test.
- Explain how maintaining good health helps you work toward success.
- Discuss strategies for managing stress.

Learning is a lifelong adventure. People who enjoy success in life are often those who continue to study and learn throughout their lives. When pursuing a career in healthcare, you will be faced with many challenges in your field, including technological, societal, and economic changes. To succeed in the face of such challenges, you will need to learn and practice new skills in school, at work, and in your private life.

You may be undecided about what course of study you would like to pursue. Depending on your career goal, you could be looking at anywhere from six months of coursework, to eight or more years of schooling. Regardless of your course of study, you will have opportunities for furthering your education even after you achieve your career goal.

This chapter will present a variety of approaches to mastering the skills every successful student needs. These skills include

- learning how to self-motivate;
- working to maintain good health;
- successfully handling **stress**;
- understanding your particular style of learning;
- managing your time well;
- practicing critical thinking;
- listening carefully to instructors;
- taking effective notes;
- improving your memory; and
- preparing for, and taking, tests.

If you can build and improve your study skills, you will greatly increase your chances of reaching your career goals. Learning how to study effectively can bring you closer to a dream job. Good study skills may also help you advance up the career ladder.

**stress**
*the feeling of being overwhelmed by worry and pressures in your life*

## *Assessing Your Study Habits*

Before you begin reading this section, take a moment to reflect on your study habits. Do you hit the books as soon as your teacher announces an upcoming test? Are you more successful when studying in a quiet environment, or do you prefer listening to music while studying? Some students have a hard time getting motivated to study before a test. Does that sound like you?

Analyzing your study habits now will allow you to access the study skills presented in this chapter, and decide which strategies might work best for you. Many factors influence your study habits. As you read this section, think about your level of motivation, whether or not you have trouble staying focused, and strategies for setting and meeting your goals.

### Motivation

One important factor that shapes a person's study skills is the level of his or her motivation. **Motivation** is what causes us to act, whether that

**motivation**
*a process by which one initiates, guides, and maintains goal-oriented behavior*

means baking cookies to satisfy a craving or researching new biomedical treatments to complete a homework assignment. When motivated, you are more likely to study for an important test, even though there are other things you might rather be doing. Motivation helps us reach our personal and career goals.

Staying motivated can be difficult. You might feel motivated at one moment, but you might lose that motivation when you experience a failure. Negative thoughts and concerns about the future can be distracting. At some point, everyone doubts his or her abilities. What separates the successful from the not-so-successful is the ability to stay motivated and keep moving forward despite those doubts.

Learning how to nurture motivating thoughts, ridding yourself of negative thinking, and focusing on the task you wish to complete can help you become motivated again. There are several strategies to help you stay motivated, including staying focused on your goal, being confident in your abilities, and establishing a direction as you pursue your goal.

## Focusing on Your Goal

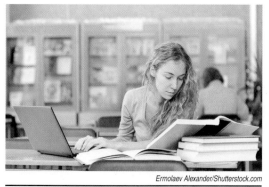

Ermolaev Alexander/Shutterstock.com

**Figure 5.1** Staying focused on your goals is critical to academic and career success.

One way to stay motivated is to establish a goal, and focus on ways to achieve that goal. Have you chosen a career goal? Let's say that you want to be a registered nurse. How can you achieve your goal? Talk to a career counselor at your school to find out about loans, grants, and scholarships for higher education. Your counselor may also know if work-study programs are available, and which nearby schools offer a nursing degree. Work with a counselor when applying for a medical course. Map out the courses you will be taking to help you move from being unfocused to focused. Keep your eye on the ball and do not let yourself be distracted from your goal (Figure 5.1). A lack of focus is the first barrier to motivation.

## Build Your Confidence

Lack of confidence can also affect your overall motivation. Past failures, bad luck, and personal inadequacies may cause you to lose confidence. You may use these things as excuses for why you cannot succeed.

The way to get out of this negative mindset is to focus on what's good in your life. Make a list of your strengths, past successes, and the positive aspects of your life. It is human nature to take our positive achievements for granted and to focus on our failures. Tell yourself that you have the ability to be successful. Positive thoughts can motivate you to pick up your textbook and study for the test you are confident you will ace.

When you truly believe that you deserve success, you will find it easy to create ways to achieve your goal. Feeling confident in your abilities will enable you to be a successful student and healthcare worker.

 *Check Your Understanding*

> Do you have trouble listing your strengths or the positive aspects of your life? If so, do the negatives interfere with this exercise? What does that tell you?

## Establishing a Direction

Once you have focused in on a goal, you need to establish a direction, or specific strategy to achieve your career aspirations. If you do not have an established direction, you may lose motivation and begin to procrastinate. Procrastinating occurs when you put off an action until a later time. You may tell yourself that studying today is unnecessary because you will have time tomorrow or the next day, but this strategy often hampers your success.

If your motivation starts to disappear, establish your direction by creating a step-by-step plan that includes small tasks to accomplish as you work toward your ultimate goal. A first task might be studying to get a good grade on an upcoming biology quiz. Your next task can focus on a long-term goal such as planning your courses for the next year.

You will have periods of low energy, bad luck, and even failure. Do not let such periods block you from your career goal. Establish a goal, identify the direction you plan to take, and stay confident in your abilities to realize your career goal. These practices will help you stay motivated as you work toward academic and career success.

## *Learning Styles*

Another way to improve your study habits is to determine how you learn best. Research shows that students can perform better on tests if they change study habits to fit their learning styles.

Just as people have different personalities, they also possess a variety of **learning styles**. There are three basic types of learning styles—visual, auditory, and kinesthetic. We rely on our senses to process the information around us. As a result, some students best remember materials they have seen, others materials that they have heard, and still others materials they have experienced firsthand. Most people possess a combination of the three learning styles, but one style is often dominant.

**learning styles**
*different ways that people learn; three basic types include visual, auditory, and kinesthetic; most people have a mixture of all three*

# Determining Your Learning Style

To determine your learning style, you may want to talk to your school's counselor. There are also learning style tests that can be found online. Just make sure the test comes from a credible source. Once you have determined your style, you must remember that there is significant variation in each style and each person. The following are descriptions of each style. See if you recognize your own traits in these descriptions. Remember that people can have more than one learning style.

## *The Visual Learner*

**visual learner**
*one who learns through seeing things; charts, color-coded notes, and videos can be helpful tools for this learner*

**Visual learners** are those who learn by seeing things (Figure 5.2). A visual learner

- may not enjoy or immediately understand a lecture;
- often enjoys colors and fashion;
- understands and appreciates charts and PowerPoint presentations;
- may spell well but could forget your name; and
  - needs quiet when he or she studies.

If you are a visual learner, the following suggestions may help you while studying:

- create outlines to help learn the material
- copy what is on the board during a lecture
- take extensive notes, using color coding if possible
- make lists
- watch videos on the subject you are studying
- use flashcards
- use highlighters to circle key words and underline important phrases
- if you study history, draw a timeline of events
- whenever possible, create an illustration to represent the topic being studied

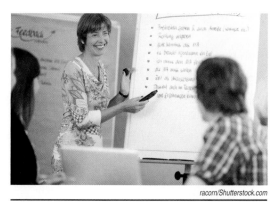
racorn/Shutterstock.com

**Figure 5.2** Visual learners often appreciate instructors who use charts while teaching.

The visual learner usually does well on tests that require reading a map, writing an essay (if the student has studied using an outline), and showing a procedure. The more challenging tests for a visual learner are "listen and respond" tests, such as listening to a piece of music and answering questions about what you have just heard.

## *The Auditory Learner*

**auditory learner**
*one who learns best by listening; lectures, discussion, and talking things through are helpful tools for this learner*

**Auditory learners** learn best by hearing things. You may be an auditory learner if you are someone who

- likes to read to yourself out loud;
- often enjoys giving speeches and presentations in class (Figure 5.3);
- does well in study groups;
- likes to teach others;
- is good at remembering names;

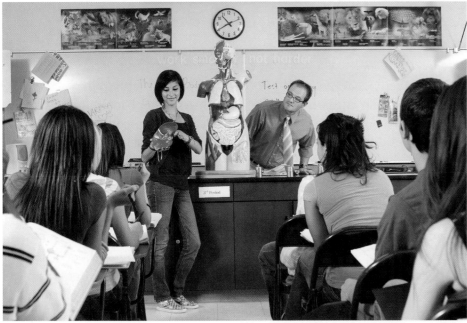
bikeriderlondon/Shutterstock.com

**Figure 5.3** Auditory learners may enjoy giving presentations in class.

- enjoys music; and
- follows spoken directions well.

Auditory learners can successfully use the following strategies when studying:

- recording lectures (provided that you get permission from your instructor)
- repeating facts
- participating in group discussions
- using tapes when learning a language

Auditory learners may find timed tests challenging if the test requires reading passages and writing answers about the material. These learners are good at writing information in response to lectures they have attended. They can also excel at oral exams, such as those given in foreign language classes.

## The Kinesthetic Learner

**Kinesthetic learners** are those who learn through hands-on experience. These learners are also called *tactile learners.* You may be a kinesthetic learner if you are someone who

- needs to move around in his or her seat after a short period of listening to an instructor;
- may have some trouble with spelling;
- may have less than perfect handwriting;
- loves active learning situations, such as conducting experiments in the lab (Figure 5.4);

**kinesthetic learner**
*one who learns through experiencing and doing things; labs, field trips, and study breaks can be helpful for this learner*

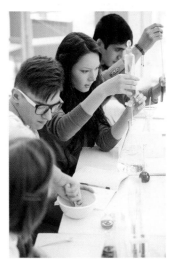
Hasloo Group Production Studio/Shutterstock.com

**Figure 5.4** Lab activities are especially useful for kinesthetic learners.

- can study while listening to loud music;
- enjoys participating in sports;
- likes action movies; and
- needs to take breaks while studying.

Kinesthetic learners may do well studying with others. Memory games and flash cards may be helpful instructional tools for the kinesthetic learner. Some kinesthetic learners also appreciate when an instructor moves around while lecturing. In general, kinesthetic learners do better on tests with short definition, fill-in, and multiple choice questions; they may have a harder time with a long, essay-heavy exam.

Sometimes an instructor's teaching style does not satisfactorily address a student's learning style. Understanding the differences between learning styles will help you to deal with an instructor whose teaching methods favor a learning style that you do not possess. You might benefit from a conference with the instructor to explain how your style differs from his or her teaching methods. This will allow the two of you an opportunity to brainstorm ways you can succeed in her classroom.

 *Check Your Understanding*

Review the learning styles. Did you recognize yourself in any of these descriptions? Which learning style do you think best fits you? Could you have more than one style? How can this information help you study more effectively?

# *Time Management*

**time management**

*the process of planning and controlling the amount of time spent on specific activities to increase efficiency and productivity*

Effective **time management** is an important skill for every student to learn, as it allows you to schedule time for studying. Successful, effective studying requires that you review material while you are alert and motivated. To study well, you must manage your time wisely. Most of us do not have the luxury of unlimited time, so we must make the most of the time we have for studying. Here are some tips for scheduling study time to effectively review your material:

- **Determine the best time of day to study.** Many people feel refreshed and clearheaded early in the morning. Others do their best studying after midnight.
- **Study the hardest or least interesting subject first.** Focusing on this information first will ensure that you have the energy to get through it. Save your favorite subjects for later. The fact that you enjoy those subjects should motivate you even if you have been studying for a while.
- **Get rid of distractions.** Try to eliminate or minimize distractions such as TV, music, the Internet, and your cell phone. Let others know that

you need to study, and will respond to them when you are done. If you have to leave your study area, write a note to yourself detailing what you were studying when you were interrupted.

- **Take advantage of downtime.** If you have to wait 20 minutes for a doctor's appointment or have an hour between classes, use this time to study. Always be prepared to sneak in short study periods that will allow you to accomplish small tasks. For example, write formulas or vocabulary terms that you have to memorize on an index card and carry that with you. iPads and other mobile devices are convenient study tools, and some educational programs offer mobile sites that you can visit using your smartphone.

- **Find the ideal study area.** Finding an area where you can study allows you to focus more quickly (Figure 5.5). You might do well studying in a well-lit, quiet library or even in a classroom environment. A desk with a comfortable, supportive chair can be helpful. Make sure you have all of the necessary supplies nearby, including a computer or tablet, pens, pencils, paper, and your textbook.

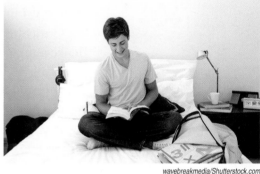

*wavebreakmedia/Shutterstock.com*

**Figure 5.5**  Some students might prefer to study at a quiet table in the library, while others are more comfortable studying in their room.

- **Join a study group.** Study groups could be unhelpful for students who are easily distracted by others. However, fellow students in a study group may be able to explain something that you do not understand. Such groups can be encouraging and give you energy that you did not have when studying alone.

## Extend Your Knowledge

### Cultural Attitudes toward Time

There are many different approaches to managing time; these can vary among cultures. For example, in countries such as the United States, Great Britain, Norway, and Sweden, meetings usually start on time. However, in some South American countries, meetings may start at least half an hour late. In some cultures, arriving on time to an event may even be considered rude.

When studying with people of different cultural backgrounds, be aware of differences in their concept of time. Others may not consider showing up late to a group study session to be rude or careless behavior. However, to maximize the time your study group has together, you should make sure all members know the planned start time for each study session.

**Think It Through**

Where do you study most effectively? What are the main distractions that you face while studying? How can you minimize these distractions?

It's important to occasionally evaluate your use of time to identify any potential time management issues. Take note of a study session in which you did not make any real progress. Ask yourself what you did that wasted time. Being aware of the specific ways in which you managed your time poorly will help you improve in the future.

# *Critical Thinking Skills*

**critical thinking**
*a process of actively and skillfully analyzing and evaluating information to draw a conclusion*

**Critical thinking** and problem-solving skills often mark the difference between average and exceptional healthcare workers. Critical thinking is a process that involves examining and evaluating information. This process involves an attitude—a need to explore, question, and search for answers. Critical thinking helps a person analyze a situation, identify the important aspects of the situation, and reach intelligent conclusions.

Qualities of a critical thinker include the ability to ask relevant questions, and to examine statements and arguments. Critical thinkers should not be judgmental or jump to conclusions, but should analyze the facts without emotion. To be a critical thinker, you must have an open mind and an interest in finding new solutions for problems.

Critical thinking can be used in every aspect of your life. What evidence supports an article online that claims you can cure the common cold by eating 10 bananas a day? Where did the author of this article get his or her information? Which candidate will you support in the next presidential election? Will you simply follow your parents' political beliefs?

If you are a critical thinker, you can see the whole picture and reach reasonable conclusions based on the facts. However, some common errors can derail effective critical thinking, such as making generalizations and false assumptions; rushing to judgment; and stereotyping:

- **Generalizations.** A generalization occurs when we conclude that something is true about a person or group without examining the facts. An example of this is, "all children play video games and do not read." Perhaps your neighbor's children constantly play video games rather than read, but that does not mean that *all* children do the same.
- **Rushing to judgment.** Sometimes we make up our minds about something before we have all of the necessary information or facts. Perhaps you instantly dislike the new medical assistant, even though you don't really know him. Later on, you realize that he reminded you of someone who once let you down, and find that he is actually a great person. You rushed to judgment and your initial impression was wrong.
- **Making false assumptions.** A false assumption is a belief and/or idea that you do not question. Imagine that a coworker tells you that the medical clerical supervisor in your new office is unfair and mean. When you first meet this supervisor, you are very wary. Then you find out that she is quite warm and approachable. You based your assumption on another person's opinion, not your own experience.
- **Stereotyping.** A stereotype is a judgment held by a person or group about members of another group. An example of a stereotype is, "all old people are cranky." Learn to see individual differences among groups of people. Following stereotypes is lazy thinking.

You will need to think critically and problem solve throughout your life. As the world of healthcare—healthcare technology in particular—continues to evolve, you will have an ever-increasing need to obtain, analyze, understand, and share information. Becoming a skilled critical thinker will set you up for success in your personal and professional life.

 *Check Your Understanding*

Do you think of yourself as a critical thinker? If not, which error or errors in critical thinking do you believe you have made? What have been the results? How can you become better at critical thinking?

### Real Life Scenario

*Using Critical Thinking at Work*

Two weeks ago, Mei's supervisor spoke to her about being late for work. Mei was on time last week, but this week had many problems that prevented her from arriving at work on time. One morning, Mei's car wouldn't start, making her 15 minutes late. Another day this week Mei's babysitter ran late, preventing her from getting to work on time yet again. Today, she made it to work on time, but was 20 minutes late getting back to work after running errands at lunch. Mei's supervisor has requested a meeting with her to discuss this problem again.

Think about this scenario from the perspectives of both Mei and her supervisor. What are some ways to resolve this issue?

## Reading to Learn

Reading is a critical element when perfecting your study skills. Being an effective reader will not only allow you to absorb the material in your textbook, it will also make you a better note-taker. In school, you will take notes from reading material as well as during lectures. Reading is the foundation of successful studying. You will learn more about developing effective reading skills in chapter 6.

## Active Listening

Information presented in class frequently contains the core concepts of the course and the material most likely to be included on exams. Yet, students frequently do not realize the importance of listening and taking notes. Lecture notes can be a critical tool for test preparation, and to take useful lecture notes, you must practice **active listening**.

Listening is a skill that must be developed—people do not always instinctively listen well. Listening requires focus. Your instructor may not be the most entertaining or interesting speaker, but you are responsible for

**active listening**
*the act of listening intently to not only hear the words being spoken, but to understand the complete message being sent*

receiving the information he or she is presenting. Information presented during a lecture is critical for studying. The following suggestions may be helpful when listening to a lecture in school or when learning a new procedure at work:

- Listen for the main ideas of the lecture or presentation. If you have trouble distinguishing between unimportant details and information worth writing down, ask the instructor after the lecture.
- If you have trouble hearing the speaker, sit somewhere that allows you to hear. Move away from anything or anyone that might be distracting.
- Do not let your mind wander. You can increase your attention span by making a conscious effort to do so.
- Be an active listener. Even if you are not interested in what the speaker is saying, listen and absorb the information he or she is presenting (Figure 5.6).

## Taking Notes

There are many reasons to take careful lecture notes. Taking notes forces you to listen carefully and test your understanding of the material. When you are studying, your notes provide a list of important topics to remember for the test. Personal notes that you write down are usually easier to remember than what you read in a textbook. The action of writing down ideas helps reinforce the material (Figure 5.7).

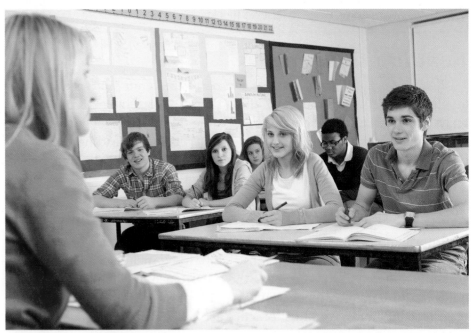

Monkey Business Images/Shutterstock.com

**Figure 5.6**   It's important to focus on what the speaker is saying, especially when you are in class.

Instructors will typically give you clues as to what information is most important and might be on a quiz or test. Important material may be found in

- the information the instructor writes on the board;
- any material that is repeated and emphasized;
- word signals that indicate the number of important points in a chapter or covered by a subject;
- summaries given at the end of the lecture; or
- reviews that the instructor gives before quizzes and tests.

Once you are familiar with the instructor's lecturing methods, and can identify the important topics of his or her lecture, you can perfect your note-taking skills. The following suggestions may be helpful for taking notes:

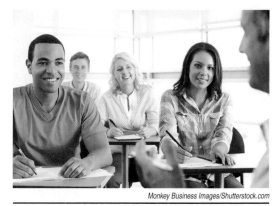

*Monkey Business Images/Shutterstock.com*

**Figure 5.7** Well-written and organized notes can be one of your best study tools.

1. **Get organized.** It's important to have the materials you need for note taking on hand during class. This might include bringing a separate notebook to each class. If you use your tablet or laptop computer for note taking, create a separate document for each class's notes, and save these documents with an easily-identifiable file name. You may want to create a folder for each semester or class.

2. **Be brief.** Use phrases and words instead of long sentences when taking notes. If you write down everything the instructor says, you will fall behind quickly and possibly miss important material.

3. **Notes should be neat.** Make sure that your handwriting is neat and legible. Unreadable handwriting will present a challenge when you are studying your notes. You may not remember what your notes mean when reviewing them for a test.

4. **Notes do not have to be exact.** Your job is not to write down exactly what the instructor is saying. However, formulas, definitions, and specific facts should be recorded exactly as they are presented. Review specific details in your textbook as well, if you have one for the class.

5. **Outlining can be helpful.** Outlines allow important points to stand out in your notes.

6. **Do not stop taking notes if you miss a point.** Leave space on the page or in the document and come back to it later. Your instructor or classmates can help you fill in this information after the presentation.

7. **Color coding your notes can be very helpful.** Using several different colored pens might help you better understand your notes when it comes time to study. One color could be used for points the instructor stresses, another for information what will be on the test, and a third color for points you do not understand. Highlighters can be very useful as well, especially for visual learners.

8. **Rewrite or type your notes after lecture.** The repetition of rewriting or typing notes helps some students retain the material.

9. **Identify new vocabulary in your notes.** Consider using an equal sign (=) between a new term and its definition. For example, "procrastination = putting things off." You may want to underline new words with two lines as well.

As you take notes, do not write down everything you hear. Be alert and attentive to the main points. It is important to stay focused and resist distractions. Notes should consist of key words or very short sentences. Keep notes in order and in one place, like a notebook with plenty of pages. After taking your notes, reread them and add extra points, spelling out unclear items. You may quickly forget the details of the lecture, so review the notes as soon as you can. Look over notes regularly before tests—these are an essential study tool.

## *Memorization*

Before you study for your next exam, you might want to learn a few strategies for boosting your ability to remember important information. There are a number of excellent techniques you can use to improve your memory. These strategies help you recall information and increase your retention of material presented in class, at work, or in your textbook.

## Mnemonic Devices

**mnemonic devices**
*learning techniques such as rhymes, catchphrases, and acronyms used to help remember and retain information*

**Mnemonic devices** are techniques students often use to help memorize material. Using mnemonic devices helps translate information that may be hard to remember into a more memorable form, such as a song or funny saying. There are several types of mnemonics:

1. **Rhymes.** Turning a spelling rule or date in history into a rhyme will help you remember and employ that rule. For example, "i before e, except after c" is a rhyme used to help spell words such as *receive*.

2. **Spelling catchphrase.** To spell *potassium* correctly, you can remember that there is, "one tea, two sugars" in the word. This should help you recall the proper numbers of the letters *t* and *s* in the term.

3. **Expression acronyms.** Many subjects will require you to memorize a specific order or number of things. For example, many biology students must memorize the classification of organisms. The phrase "Kids Prefer Cheese Over Fried Green Spinach" can be used to remember the order of Kingdom, Phylum, Class, Order, Family, Genus, Species.

You can invent your own mnemonic device to help remember a specific piece of information that you have to memorize. Get creative—sometimes the most amusing mnemonic devices are the easiest to remember!

*Focusing on the Essence of a Chapter*

Studies have found that, when reading a textbook, people have an easier time learning material that comes at the beginning or end of the chapter. Recalling the information that comes in between can be difficult. Dedicate extra time to study this information in the middle of the chapter. Remember that difficult material should be studied at the beginning of a study session, when you are most alert.

## Making Connections between Topics

Information is often organized into related groups in your memory. Grouping similar concepts and terms together may increase your chances of retaining this information. Make an outline of your notes and textbook readings to help recognize related concepts. For example, when studying the history of healthcare, you might first study cultures that made significant impacts on ancient medicine and then study individuals who made exciting medical discoveries.

When you are learning unfamiliar material, take time to think about how this new material relates to things you already know. If you establish relationships between new ideas and existing knowledge, you can dramatically increase the likelihood of recalling the new information.

## Reading Out Loud

Reading materials out loud can significantly improve your recall of the material. This can be especially helpful to auditory learners. Teaching the material to others also enhances understanding and recall. Having a study partner who is focusing on the same materials can be very helpful when using this strategy (Figure 5.8).

Repeatedly reading information out loud will help you commit it to your long-term memory. To recall information, you need to store it in your long-term memory. It may be helpful to read the definition of a key term, study the definition, and then read the definition again. After repeating this process a few times, you should recall the term more easily.

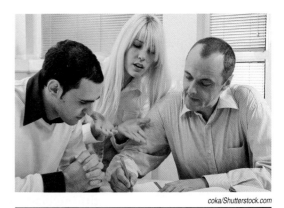

*coka/Shutterstock.com*

**Figure 5.8**   Study partners can help you with memorization as well as explaining topics you do not understand.

## Visualizing Information

Many people, especially visual learners, benefit from visualizing the information they are studying. Focus on photographs, charts, and other graphics in your textbooks. If you do not have visual cues, create your own. Draw charts or figures in the margins of your notes, or use highlighters or pens in different colors to group related ideas in your study notes.

**Did You Know?**

### Cramming and Pulling All-Nighters

Cramming and pulling all-nighters are not effective study methods. Reviewing materials over several study sessions gives you time to adequately absorb the information. Students who study regularly remember the material far better than those who did all of their studying in one last-minute session. Remember that being well-rested makes learning much easier.

## Alternating your Study Routine

It may be helpful to occasionally change your study routine. If you often study in a specific location, try moving to a different spot during your next study session. If you study best in the evening, try spending a few minutes each morning reviewing material you looked at the previous evening. Occasionally changing your study routine will increase the effectiveness of your efforts, and improve your long-term recall of the information.

How well you remember information depends on your attitude, interest level, awareness, mental alertness, distractibility, observation skills, memory devices, and the willingness to practice remembering the material.

## *Test Taking*

Have you ever said to yourself or heard someone say, "I'm just not a good test taker"? Everyone can improve their test-taking skills by thinking about taking a test in three parts:

1. test preparation
2. the test itself
3. after the test

## Preparing to Take a Test

Preparing to take a test should start on the first day of class. The syllabus provided for the course will include the quizzes and exams you will be expected to complete. From the first day, you should be paying attention during class, taking good notes, and studying regularly.

### *Managing Your Schedule*

Assess the amount of time you think a course will require of you. If possible, examine the syllabus and determine how much of your time will be required to complete the projects, papers, and exam prep for this course. Is the final a take-home test or an in-class examination? Is this a subject that you love, or is it a required course that you are not excited to be taking? Take all these facts into consideration as you budget your time, considering other classes and your personal and professional responsibilities.

**Think It Through**

What techniques do you use to memorize information before an exam? Do you use any of the methods listed in this chapter? Are there any methods not mentioned in the text that you have found useful? What is the most effective memorization technique that you use?

### Attending Review Sessions

Review sessions present a wonderful opportunity to prepare for an upcoming exam. Listen carefully to hints that the instructor may give about the test. This is the time to ask questions about any concepts you find confusing. You can also make an appointment with the instructor during his or her office hours to get extra help with material you do not understand. Ask the instructor about areas that will be emphasized on the test.

### The Day of the Test

Review any material that will be on the test well before the examination, rather than the night before. Many students do not do well after staying up all night before the test to cram. You will most likely perform best when you are well rested. Go over practice tests, homework, sample problems, review material, the related textbook chapters, and class notes. Allow plenty of time to study all of these sources.

Eat before the test. Having nutritious food in your stomach gives you energy. Avoid heavy, sugary food that might make you groggy. Also be sure to visit the bathroom before going to your classroom. You do not want to be uncomfortable during the test.

On the day of the test, you should arrive at class early (Figure 5.9). Being late can cause you to feel stressed before the examination starts, instead of feeling relaxed and ready to go. Arriving a bit early may also give you a chance to look over your notes one more time. Be sure to set your alarm (and maybe a backup alarm as well) if your test is scheduled in the morning.

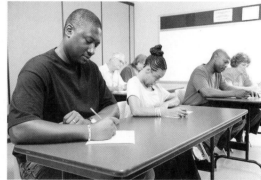

*Lisa F. Young/Shutterstock.com*

**Figure 5.9** On the day of an exam, show up to class at least five minutes early to ensure you are relaxed and ready to go when the exam begins.

## Taking the Test

There are many strategies you can employ to more successfully take tests. A few of these strategies follow:

- First, make sure you put your name on the test.
- Be sure to bring proper writing instruments (pen or pencil—whichever your instructor tells you to use) with good erasers, if needed. If you are to use a calculator, be sure to bring it and any other approved resources (consider packing all of your test-taking resources the night before).
- If a clock is not available in the classroom, bring a watch so that you can pace yourself.
- Try to stay relaxed. If you find yourself tensing up, take several deep breaths and then continue.
- Keep your eyes on your own test. Do not ask for trouble by appearing to cheat (Figure 5.10).

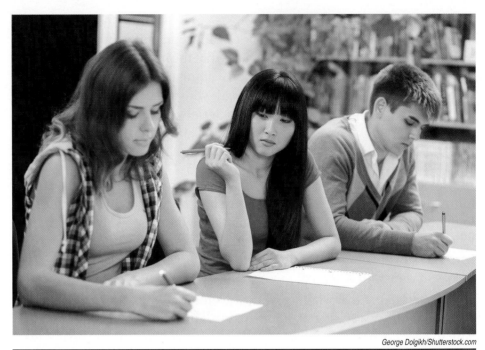

George Dolgikh/Shutterstock.com

**Figure 5.10** Keep your eyes on your own exam—even if you are not guilty of cheating, your teacher may interpret the situation as cheating.

- When you receive the test, scan it to figure out how to budget your time.
- Pace yourself and do not rush. Read the entire question before you begin to answer it. Read everything carefully and pay attention to details.
- Answer the questions that have been assigned the largest point value first.
- When you do not understand what a question is asking or what the instructions of the test say, ask your instructor for an explanation.
- Write legibly when answering all questions (especially essay questions). You do not want a question to be marked wrong because of poor handwriting.
- If you do not know an answer, skip the question and come back to it later. Other parts of the test may have information that will help you with the skipped question.
- Do not panic if everyone seems to be finished and you are not. Focus on your test and ignore everyone else.

## After the Test

After your instructor passes back the examination, you should look it over to make sure there are no grading mistakes. Make sure you understand why your answers were marked wrong. If the instructor does not go over the test, make time to ask him why a question may have been marked wrong.

If the instructor does go over the test in class, make notes on what he wanted to see in the answer for questions or problems that you got wrong. If you are not satisfied with your grade, ask if it is possible to retake the test, or if there is extra credit available. In college, extra credit is probably not offered, so it is best to study harder and analyze how you might improve on the next exam.

If a test is returned to you, save it and use it as study material for future tests and quizzes in the class.

## *Managing Your Health*

Now that you are familiar with study skills and habits that will help you succeed, let's look at habits to keep you healthy. There are several ways to improve your personal practices in an effort to become a healthy, productive student and worker. Working toward your career goal will require that you develop effective methods of maintaining your health. You will be dealing with the demands of school—studying for exams, writing papers, meeting deadlines, and preparing presentations—while also juggling family responsibilities and planning for the future. Such demands will create stress on your body and mind.

### Eating Healthful Foods

Eating healthful foods gives your body the energy it needs. Taking in the proper nutrition can reduce depression, headaches, fatigue, and insomnia. The United States Department of Agriculture (USDA) helps educate people on healthful eating by publishing a nutrition guide called *MyPlate* (Figure 5.11). MyPlate helps consumers adopt healthful eating habits by encouraging them to build a healthier plate.

The USDA's dietary guidelines include

- an emphasis on eating fruits, vegetables, whole grains, and fat-free or low-fat milk and milk products;
- consuming proteins from sources such as lean meats, poultry, fish, beans, eggs, and nuts; and
- limiting intake of saturated fats, trans fats, cholesterol, salt (sodium), and added sugars.

### Maintaining a Healthy Weight

You will have more energy and enjoy better health if you maintain a reasonable weight for your height, body frame, and age. Eat only when you are hungry, not because you are depressed, bored, or worried. Also, avoid skipping meals—you need to eat regularly to supply your body with fuel for your busy life. Eat slowly and try not to eat on the run.

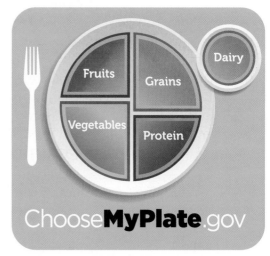

**Figure 5.11**   MyPlate guidelines presented by the United States Department of Agriculture (USDA).

If you are overweight, talk to your physician about losing weight without trying fad diets or fasting. You should also speak to your doctor if you find yourself exhibiting signs of disordered eating. Disordered eating habits include severely restricting your calorie intake, extreme exercise sessions that are too long or frequent, binge eating, or purging.

## Getting Plenty of Rest

The amount of sleep you need varies from person to person. Most adults need six to nine hours of sleep per night. Your mind works much better when you have had plenty of rest and sleep.

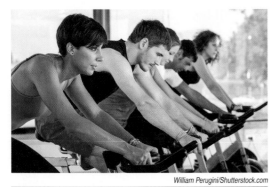

William Perugini/Shutterstock.com

**Figure 5.12**  Exercise is essential for maintaining both your physical and mental health.

## Exercise

The health benefits of aerobic exercise are numerous. Regular aerobic exercise involves raising your heart rate above its normal level for at least 20 minutes a day, three or four days a week. Aerobic exercise reduces stress; strengthens the immune system and heart; reduces excess fat; and increases stamina (Figure 5.12). The key is to start slowly, building up gradually until you are capable of maintaining a consistent exercise schedule. If you have any physical problems, talk with your physician about a safe exercise routine before starting any exercise program.

## Establishing Healthy Relationships

Enjoying successful relationships with others not only contributes to your happiness, but also increases your energy and improves your overall health (Figure 5.13). If you spend all your time studying, you will miss the satisfaction of a pleasant evening with friends and family.

Friends and family can help us think through problems; brainstorm ideas; overcome boredom; and bring us joy and laughter. Establishing healthy relationships with others will also create a support system of people who will provide encouragement when you have a bad day at work, or become overwhelmed at school. Neglecting your family and friends because you are busy at school and work can create barriers to healthy relationships.

## Managing Stress

Everyone experiences daily stress throughout life (Figure 5.14). Sometimes, situations can introduce multiple sources of stress to a person. High levels of stress can impact your physical and mental health. An overwhelmed student may lose focus and even give up on educational and careers goals because the stress of school is too much to handle. Learning to manage and prevent stress can help reduce the impact of stress on your overall health and personal goals.

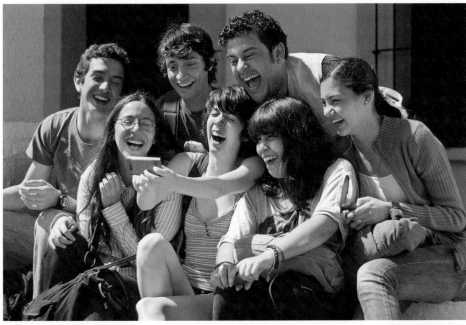

photomatz/Shutterstock.com

**Figure 5.13** It is important to find time in your busy schedule to enjoy the company of your family and friends.

| Common Stressors | |
|---|---|
| *Life-Altering Events* | *Daily Challenges* |
| Death of a family member or friend | Misplacing or losing items |
| Divorce or separation | Concern about physical appearance |
| Personal injury or change in health | Arguments in the household |
| Change in health of family member | Difficulties with friends or significant other |
| Loss of job | Decision making |
| New baby in the household | School/job responsibilities |
| Pregnancy | Change in sleeping habits |
| Moving | Loneliness |
| Starting classes at a new school | Peer pressure |
| | Uncertainty of the future |
| | Money concerns |

**Figure 5.14** How many of these common stressors have you experienced?

Each person responds differently to stress. What may be stressful to one person may not be to another. One student might think the world is ending after earning a C in a course, while another is happy with a C. A third student might be motivated to turn the C into a B by studying harder.

## Personality Types

Reactions to stress often depend on personality types. Some people (sometimes known as *type A personalities*) are ambitious, organized, impatient, and sometimes take on more than they can handle. Others (often called *type B personalities*) are generally patient, relaxed, easygoing, and are not plagued by a sense of urgency. A third personality type (*type C personalities*) is described as suppressing emotional expression, denying strong emotional reactions, having trouble coping with stress, and feeling hopeless or helpless.

Most people have some qualities belonging to each personality type. Depending on a person's personality, he or she will react to stress in various ways, too.

## Attitude

When considering how a person may cope with stress, attitude may be a more important factor than personality. Those who approach problems as challenges to overcome are more likely to react positively when faced with stressful situations. Research has found that positive outcomes are more related to your reaction to stress than to the types of stressors in your life.

## Strategies for Stress Management

It is important to recognize the signs of too much stress. Frustration, irritability, and depression are common emotional reactions to stress. Headaches, upset stomachs, and fatigue are indications that you have too much stress in your life. After identifying the source of these symptoms, take a deep breath, relax, and sort out what is causing your stress.

You cannot avoid stress and, in fact, some stress in your life can motivate you to perform well and achieve your goals. Adopting some of the following strategies will help you work through stress and achieve a positive outcome.

- **Stay healthy by eating a nutritious diet, staying physically fit, and getting plenty of sleep.** A balanced diet will give you energy to complete tasks required for effective studying. Physical exercise produces endorphins (substances secreted during exercise that can give the person a feeling of well-being), and exercise can also help to control weight. As discussed before, a well- rested person can be more productive than someone who has not gotten enough sleep.
- **Avoid substance abuse.** Many people feel that alcohol and other drugs will relieve stress. However, such substances only mask stress

symptoms. Eventually, substance abuse will add new stressors to your life, creating physical and mental health problems. Substance abuse can also ruin healthy relationships and may lead to fights, accidents, and even arrests.

- **Learn how to relax.** Set aside time for enjoying leisure activities. Everyone has different ways of relaxing. You might like to listen to music, read a good novel, or exercise. Some people may find relaxation techniques such as yoga, deep breathing, and meditation to be helpful (Figure 5.15).
- **Adopt positive strategies for effective time management**. Maximize the time you have set aside for studying. Having a good balance of work, school, and life will make you happier, healthier, and a more effective student.
- **Reach out to your support system.** Family members, friends, school counselors, social workers, religious leaders, instructors, and psychologists can all help you deal with stressful situations. In return, you can support them when they are in need.
- **Be positive about your abilities.** Remember your strengths and have a positive attitude. Avoid dwelling on failures or negative qualities; doing so will only leave you feeling discouraged and more stressed. If you are confident in yourself, you will find it easier to work through a stressful situation.

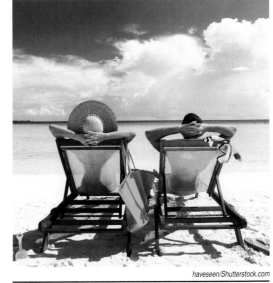

*haveseen/Shutterstock.com*

**Figure 5.15** Visualizing your favorite spot or taking a vacation can be a great way to relax and decompress.

## *Real Life Scenario*

### *One Student's Stress*

Inez is stressed! She is working part-time to pay for her college tuition, and her biology instructor has just announced that there will be a test in two days. Inez has not read any of the five chapters that will be covered on the test. She also has not been sleeping well lately. On top of everything, she and her fiancé have been fighting recently. He feels Inez is too busy studying to pay any attention to their relationship.

How might Inez deal with these stressful situations? Discuss some strategies Inez might use. Have you ever felt stressed and overwhelmed? How did you alleviate your stress?

Review Figure 5.14 and ask yourself: how many of these stressors have you experienced? How do you deal with stress in your daily life? Are you successful at reducing stress?

# Chapter Review and Assessment

## Summary

In this chapter you learned study skills every serious student needs to succeed. Successfully handling stress, maintaining motivation, staying healthy, and discovering your particular learning style are important factors when developing effective study habits.

Critical thinking is a skill that can be used in your personal life, at school, and at work. The critical thinking process involves analyzing and evaluating information to reach an intelligent conclusion. Critical thinking is especially helpful when taking tests and writing essays.

One way to ensure your studying is effective is to develop your memory. Mnemonic devices, reading out loud, and making connections are all strategies for improving your recall. It is much easier to remember facts you have studied over time than what you reviewed when cramming the night before an exam. Taking effective notes and actively listening in class will also improve your retention and recall of important information.

Mastering all of these study skills is important, but you must also know strategies for test taking to truly excel. Begin preparing for your tests as soon as possible. On the day of the test, arrive early, and be prepared both mentally and physically for the exam period. When your graded test is returned, review the incorrect answers and make sure you understand why these answers are wrong.

Eating well, getting enough rest, and managing your stress will make you a stronger student and healthcare worker. Effective studying involves maintaining your mind and body.

Following the study tips, test-taking strategies, and health guidelines presented in this chapter will help prepare you for the rigorous demands of school and a career in healthcare.

## Review Questions

### Short Answer

1. Explain motivation as it relates to studying.

2. List three strategies you can adopt to maintain your health.

3. Describe the differences between visual, auditory, and kinesthetic learners.

4. What is a mnemonic device?

5. Describe the differences between type A, B, and C personalities.

6. How might creating outlines contribute to effectively committing material to long-term memory?

7. What is time management and why is it important when studying?

### True/False

8. *True or False?* The USDA symbol for nutritional balance is a plate.

9. *True or False?* Kinesthetic learners can sit for long periods of time.

10. *True or False?* Critical thinking involves reaching reasonable conclusions based on important facts.

11. *True or False?* Using stereotypes can be helpful when analyzing people.

12. *True or False?* Mnemonic devices are helpful when memorizing material.

13. *True or False?* Visual learners appreciate charts and PowerPoint presentations.

14. *True or False?* Type B personalities are characterized by their ambition, extreme organization, and occasionally taking on more than they can handle.

15. *True or False?* A diet rich in lean protein from eggs, nuts, and fish is beneficial for your health.

### Multiple Choice

16. To be _____ is to feel overwhelmed by worry and life pressures.
    A. motivated
    B. fatigued
    C. stressed
    D. irritated

17. A(n) _____ is a specific strategy implemented to help you achieve your goals.
    A. outline
    B. direction
    C. goal
    D. motivation

18. Which of the following should be done when preparing for a test?
    A. pay attention during a lecture
    B. take clear notes
    C. budget your time to allow for ample studying
    D. All of the above.

19. People with type A personalities tend to be _____.
    A. patient
    B. relaxed
    C. unorganized
    D. ambitious

20. When taking a test you should _____.
    A. rush through the questions
    B. look around to see how your classmates are doing
    C. ignore the clock to avoid feeling rushed
    D. answer the questions with the highest point values first

21. Which of the following should *not* be done before taking a test?
    A. Eat a heavy meal before the test.
    B. Arrive to class at least five minutes early to take a test.
    C. Visit the bathroom before taking a test.
    D. Bring a watch so you can pace yourself.

22. All of the following concepts affect critical thinking negatively *except* _____.
    A. generalization
    B. rushing to judgment
    C. evaluating information
    D. stereotyping

23. A healthful diet is one that includes _____.
    A. lean proteins such as poultry, fish, beans, and nuts
    B. an emphasis on fruits and vegetables
    C. limiting your intake of saturated fats, sodium, and sugar
    D. All of the above.

24. After receiving your graded test, you should _____.
    A. immediately recycle the old test
    B. ask your classmates what grade they received
    C. check for grading errors
    D. look only at your score, disregarding the questions you answered incorrectly

25. Which of the following is *incorrect* when talking about the importance of motivation?
    A. Motivation is a process that guides a person toward a goal.
    B. Motivation is something that causes us to act.
    C. Motivation helps us reach our career goal.
    D. Motivation is always easy to maintain.

## Critical Thinking Exercises

26. Most schools offer extensive resources to help students achieve their academic and professional goals. What resources are available to you at your school? Have you used any of these resources in the past? If not, do you plan on using these resources in the future?

27. Do you have any problems with motivation? If so, which motivation barriers do you experience? Will these motivation issues affect your ability to achieve your career goals?

28. Do you have short- and long-term goals for becoming a healthcare professional? List and explain how you plan to accomplish them.

29. What steps do you take to remain healthy? Are there things you could do better?

30. How do you handle stress? What do you do to reduce stress?

31. Make a list of all the things that keep you from listening well in each of your classes. How can you overcome these distractions?

32. In your experience, what is the best advice you could give someone who is about to take a very important test?

33. Critical thinking is not used only for academic purposes. Think about a situation or problem in your daily life that required critical thinking. Explain how critical thinking was used in this scenario.

# Chapter

# Reading Competence

## Chapter Objectives

- Discuss the benefits gained from daily reading.
- Identify techniques for improving your vocabulary.
- Explain some possible advantages of e-readers.
- Discuss what is meant by *active reading*.
- Explain the SQ3R reading system and how it is used to improve your reading skills.
- Identify some strategies for taking effective notes while reading textbooks.
- Explain different reading approaches to use in a variety of courses.
- Discuss why it can be helpful to highlight your textbooks and notes.
- Identify some strategies to use when reading difficult and dense material.
- Explain what a decoding problem is and how this relates to dyslexia.
- Discuss some ways to increase your reading speed.
- Explain ways to decrease eye strain when reading or using the computer.

Reading is a skill that is essential to understanding school and work assignments. Effective studying relies on excellent reading skills. Reading a variety of materials is very important for developing different reading strategies. Such reading materials might include textbooks, newspapers, novels, magazines, blog posts, or poetry.

## Benefits of Reading

Experts recommend that people attempting to improve their reading skills should spend 20 minutes reading for pleasure each day (Figure 6.1). Why would experts recommend reading every day? What are the actual benefits of reading?

- Keeping your brain active and stimulated through reading sharpens brain function.
- Knowledge is gained by reading. This new knowledge may help you handle challenges you face in school, at work, or in your personal life.
- Memory is enhanced by remembering concepts you have read.
- The growth of your vocabulary and exposure to different authors' writing styles through reading helps improve your writing skills.

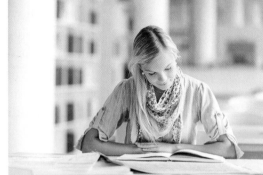

*lightpoet/Shutterstock.com*

**Figure 6.1** Make it a habit to read a variety of materials.

- Enjoying a good book and getting lost in an interesting story can distract you from daily stresses, allowing you to relax.
- Reading promotes focus when you dedicate your attention to a story.
- Reading is free entertainment if you take advantage of local libraries.

As you learned in chapter 5, strong reading skills provide the basis for effective studying. By becoming a better reader, you will find it easier to take effective notes during lectures, and outline and review your textbook and notes.

## Vocabulary Building

It can be an overwhelming challenge to read and understand a chapter in any book if you have a limited **vocabulary**. To read, write, and study well you must have an adequate vocabulary.

When you embark on a career in healthcare, your vocabulary will expand as you learn medical terminology (see Chapter 8, *Medical Terminology and Disease*). A certain amount of memorization will take place when you are introduced to medical terms, but learning basic word elements will help you understand new medical terms. To progress in your healthcare education and career, it is critical that you become fluent in medical terminology.

Do not be frustrated by a limited vocabulary—there are simple solutions to this problem. One solution is to keep a dictionary or **thesaurus**

**vocabulary**
*a set of words known and used by a person*

**thesaurus**
*a resource that identifies words with the same meaning*

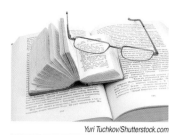

**Figure 6.2** Having a dictionary at hand while reading makes it easy to quickly look up new vocabulary words.

with you at all times (Figure 6.2). A traditional, printed dictionary or thesaurus is a useful resource to add to your personal library. If you prefer an electronic version, many online dictionaries and thesauruses are available. Reliable dictionaries often have an app that can be downloaded on your smartphone or tablet to look up words when you are on the go.

As you work to build your vocabulary, many instructors recommend you keep a list of new words you have learned. You can record new words, along with their definitions, in a notebook, on flashcards, or in an electronic list saved on your smartphone or computer. Keeping a word list is particularly important in vocabulary-heavy courses such as medical terminology. Review your word list each day and set a goal for how many new words you would like to learn every day or every week.

In addition to building a word list and using references like dictionaries and thesauruses, there are many simple ways to improve your vocabulary:

- **Read every chance you get**. Look up the definition of any word you do not understand, and add the term to your word list.
- **Break down the word elements**. Medical terms are composed of basic word elements—prefixes, word roots, combining vowels, combining forms, and suffixes—that can be used to decipher the term's definition. Identifying these word elements can help you understand the term as a whole. You will learn more about breaking down word elements in chapter 8.

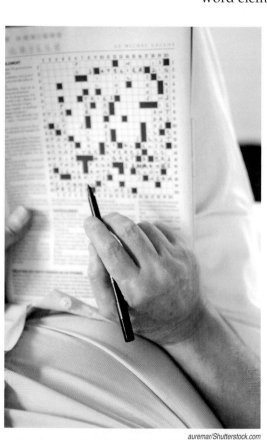

**Figure 6.3** Working on crossword puzzles is an easy way to improve your vocabulary.

- **Challenge yourself with word games**. Word games such as crossword puzzles, word jumbles, Boggle®, Scrabble®, or Bananagrams® are a fun way to learn and practice vocabulary (Figure 6.3). Many of these games are also available online.
- **Listen to your friends, family, instructors, and coworkers for words you do not know**. Do not be afraid to ask others to define words you are unfamiliar with, or to look up the words later.
- **Highlight new words in lecture notes**. Later, you can write the definition above the highlighted word and add it to your word list.
- **Learn at least one word (or more) every day**. Buy a word-of-the-day desk calendar and you will learn a new word every day for a year. Many online dictionaries offer you the option to subscribe to their word-of-the-day emails.
- **Use the new words you have learned**. Incorporating the terms on your word list into your daily vocabulary will help you remember the terms and expand your vocabulary.

# Tablets and E-Readers

Today, many people choose to do their pleasure reading on e-readers such as the iPad, Kindle, or other tablets (Figure 6.4). Increasingly, classrooms around the nation are providing or requiring tablets for their students. There is a growing trend for textbooks to be available as e-books. There are advantages to using tablets and e-readers, either for pleasure or in the classroom:

1. E-readers are portable, many fitting easily into purses and backpacks.
2. Hundreds of books can often be stored on an e-reader or through cloud (online) storage.
3. You can often insert digital highlighting, underlining, and notes in an e-book.
4. The e-book bookmarks your page for you.
5. Many local libraries offer e-books for rent through their digital library system.
6. Most e-readers have high resolution screens with options to reduce or increase the print size.

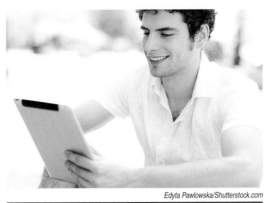
*Edyta Pawlowska/Shutterstock.com*

**Figure 6.4** Many printed textbooks are also offered in an electronic format that can be accessed using a tablet or e-reader.

# Active Reading

College courses demand that you read much more than you were expected to in high school. How will you find the time to read through all the assignments given to you each week? Many studies show that students do not read with any strategy in mind. Adopting a reading strategy such as active reading will improve your level of **retention**.

Whether you are reading a novel on vacation, studying material for a test, or reading for a work assignment, you must become actively involved with the material you are reading. If you are not interested in the subject you are assigned to read, you will have a hard time retaining information you have read.

**retention**
*the ability to preserve information in the mind*

 *Check Your Understanding*

What did you already know about reading competence when you began this chapter? Are you satisfied with your reading speed and comprehension? If not, what can you do to improve your reading abilities?

**Active reading** involves your level of concentration while reading. Have you ever had the experience of finding yourself halfway through a chapter in a textbook, but unable to remember what you had read? Your

**active reading**
*reading with extreme concentration and focus to ensure you are fully present and aware of what you are reading; note taking and reading out loud are sometimes part of active reading*

eyes moved across the page, but your brain did not process the information. Perhaps you were tired, distracted, or just bored by the topic. This is an example of passive reading—not being involved in processing the information.

There are several strategies to help students become active participants while reading. The strategy highlighted in this chapter is called the *SQ3R reading system.*

## SQ3R Reading System

**SQ3R reading system**
*study strategy used to increase comprehension while reading; stands for Survey, Question, Read, Recite, and Review*

**comprehension**
*an understanding of what you have read or heard*

The **SQ3R reading system** is a study strategy designed to help students comprehend a text by teaching them to think a certain way. SQ3R stands for Survey, Question, Read, Recite, and Review (Figure 6.5).

This system was first introduced by Professor Francis Robinson in his 1946 book, *Effective Study.* Originally designed for college students to improve their reading **comprehension**, this five-step method has also been used in elementary schools and high schools for decades. The five steps of this method should be applied when a student approaches a textbook chapter:

1. **Survey**. Before you begin reading the chapter, survey or examine some of the basic parts to assess key points of the material. Read the chapter title, introduction, and summary. Determine how the chapter is organized by reading the headings and subheadings. Notice the use of italic and bold fonts; the objectives; and the review questions. After you gather this information, assess the author's purpose for writing this chapter.

2. **Question**. As you begin each section of the chapter, write down some questions you think will be answered in the section. As you actively look for answers to these questions, your mind will become truly engaged in the text. Questions you might ask include, "What is the main idea of this section?" "What examples support this idea?" "What key events will be discussed?"

3. **Read**. As you actively read the material, search for answers to the questions you posed as part of step 2. Continue to ask questions as you read.

4. **Recite**. After you read a section, stop and review your questions for the section. Can you answer each question? Saying the answers out loud or writing them down promotes concentration and creates understanding of the material.

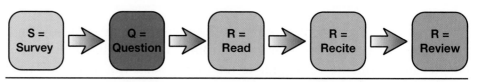

**Figure 6.5**    The SQ3R reading system can be used to improve your reading comprehension.

5. **Review**. Once you have finished reading the chapter and completed the preceding steps, go over your questions. See if you can still answer the questions; if you cannot, refresh your memory and then continue. It might also be helpful to write a summary of the chapter. This summary can be read out loud to increase retention. Study groups may provide an opportunity to explain concepts to others, and creating note cards provides a review opportunity and study tool.

There are other proven reading systems that can also be explored to help you improve your reading comprehension. Some alternative systems include

- the five-part reading system;
- the Wilson Reading System®; and
- the adult learning cycle.

If you are serious about improving your active reading skills, many resources are available to you.

 *Check Your Understanding*

Read a chapter in another textbook you are studying using the SQ3R method. Did this method help you to learn and retain more information? Why or why not?

## *Real Life Scenario*

*Last-Minute Cramming*

Ian always puts off studying until the night before a test. He has over 200 pages of reading to do for a test tomorrow in his Intro to Health Sciences class. Ian enjoys staying up late and feels that he does his best studying at night. Unfortunately, on the night before his test, Ian is especially tired and stressed after a busy day. He finds himself feeling sleepy after only an hour of reading.

What reading strategies should Ian employ to remain focused on the material? What might he have done differently to prepare for the test? Have you found yourself in a similar situation?

## Reading for Different Courses

You may want to use some different reading strategies when you read for specific course material. The subject matter presented by various courses may require you to analyze the material in different ways.

### *Reading a Math Textbook*

As you read your math textbook, take notes in the margins of the book after figuring out each problem. Include reminders and tips that will help you solve similar problems in the future. Spend an ample amount of time studying tables, formulas, and any other visuals used to explain complex

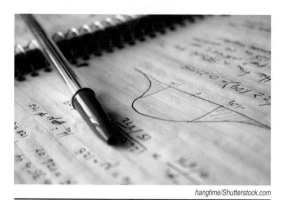

hangtime/Shutterstock.com

**Figure 6.6** Taking notes while reading complicated material such as your math textbook can help you retain information and serves as a valuable study tool.

concepts. Ask as many questions as you need to until you understand the concepts and how to apply them to questions and problems. To help you memorize important formulas, write them down on note cards or take notes describing the use of each as you read (Figure 6.6).

## Reading for Science Classes

Reading a science textbook may be more challenging for students than other types of reading. Science vocabulary can be difficult to understand, making it hard for many students to comprehend what they are reading. Reading about detailed scientific concepts (such as the laws of physics) requires concentration and focus for readers at all levels.

Reading strategies become essential to retaining information in a science textbook. Writing down vocabulary words as you read may help increase your focus and concentration on the subject. Study skills such as the mnemonic devices discussed in chapter 5 may be particularly helpful when reading dense, challenging material for your science classes.

## Understanding Your History Textbook

Filled with facts, dates, and important people, history textbooks can be overwhelming. When you are studying history, it's important to look for common themes or trends. Closely observing the textbook's visuals can help put the details into perspective. For example, you might review a map to see where two countries at war are located.

Creating an outline is a useful practice for keeping material clear in your mind. A timeline with important dates and events will put such details in a form that makes the information easier to understand. A timeline can connect important people to key events as well.

## Reading the Social Sciences

Social science courses study the nature of society, and human relationships and behavior. Courses such as psychology, sociology, or anthropology will discuss major theories about human behavior. As you read the textbooks for such courses, write down the theories presented and explain them in your own words. Study how psychological research led to various conclusions. Social science textbooks often present many key terms for you to learn. Flash cards can be a helpful review tool for remembering these terms and their definitions.

## Literature

Reading novels, plays, short stories, or poetry in your literature course is much different than any other reading you will do in school. These materials require particular attention to detail.

To answer broad questions such as, "what is the purpose of this piece?" you must first study smaller elements of the literary work. When you are studying the characters in a story, make a list of the important people and describe their personalities, actions, and motives. Doing so will help you determine what the author is saying through the characters in the story.

Take care to examine the plot points, themes, and any literary devices employed by the author including foreshadowing (suggestions of what is to come), symbolism (the use of symbols to express ideas), or metaphor (a way of connecting two things). Visualize each scene in your mind as you are reading. Use your imagination to further enhance your reading experience.

## Taking Notes While Reading

A very effective way to retain information presented in a textbook, especially for technical subjects, is to take notes while you are reading. If you read and take notes in the process, you are taking an extra step to reinforce what you have just read. This extra step will help you retain and recall information faster and with less effort.

## Highlighting

In high school, writing or highlighting in your textbook is greatly discouraged. However, most college courses require that you purchase the textbook. If you own the textbook, you can indulge yourself by highlighting the text and underlining information with a pencil or pen (Figure 6.7). Using different colored highlighters can help a visual learner quickly absorb and retain material.

However, it's important that you don't get too carried away with underlining and highlighting. Doing so will defeat the purpose of making the most important material stand out when you review the text. Highlight sparingly, usually less than 10 percent of the text.

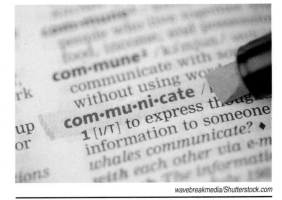

wavebreakmedia/Shutterstock.com

**Figure 6.7** Highlighting can make the most important material stand out when reviewing a text or your lecture notes.

> ### Think It Through
>
> Do you have a favorite subject matter to read? Is reading about psychology more appealing to you than reading formulas for math class? Do you have any courses with particularly challenging reading assignments? If so, what do you think makes this subject matter so difficult for you to read? Are you disinterested in the material? What strategies can you use to improve reading for a course that is hard for you?

## Adding to Your Notes and Textbook

To get even more creative, you can mark your text using the following techniques:

- Put an exclamation point (!) or an asterisk (*) after a particularly important sentence or term.
- Put a **T** in the margin when you think the material might appear on a test.
- Put a **Q** next to a concept you do not understand so that you remember to ask your instructor for an explanation.
- Circle terms that you cannot define. Look these terms up immediately and write the definition in the margin next to the term.

- If you notice your instructor has emphasized certain material, write comments in the margin where that information can be found.

These techniques can also be used with your lecture notes. Have the necessary writing utensils—pens, highlighters, pencils—handy at the time of the lecture to use these notation strategies. It's important to emphasize and add detail to the points the instructor has made before you forget the importance of the information.

**Did You Know?**

**Note Taking**

Did you know that using different highlighting colors could improve your note taking? What strategies do you use when taking or reviewing your notes? How could you improve your note taking?

## *Reading Difficult Material*

Sometimes the strategies you use while reading easy and interesting material do not help when you are faced with a particularly challenging text. Perhaps the material is very dense and technical. Maybe the text itself is hard to read because the print is small, there are double columns on each page, little white space, and no illustrations. What can you do in such situations to improve your reading experience and retain the material for a test?

When approaching difficult material, several techniques can be used to help you master the text:

1. Preview the reading assignment by scanning for key words, emphasized sections, headings, and end-of-chapter summaries. These will provide a foundation on which you can build an understanding as you read through the text.

2. After previewing the assignment, skim the chapter again, spending more time looking for key phrases and ideas.

3. After previewing and then skimming the chapter again, you are ready to read the assignment in more detail.

4. If you find you are still having a hard time understanding the chapter after completing steps 1–3, put the material down and take a break. Go for a walk, watch a television program, or tackle the material the next day when you are well rested after a good night's sleep.

5. Summarize each section that you read by writing down, or reading out loud, what you think you have just read in your own words.

6. If you continue to have problems or questions, talk to your instructor. Take advantage of any study groups that exist for the course (Figure 6.8). Sometimes other people can explain a concept in a way that will help you understand.

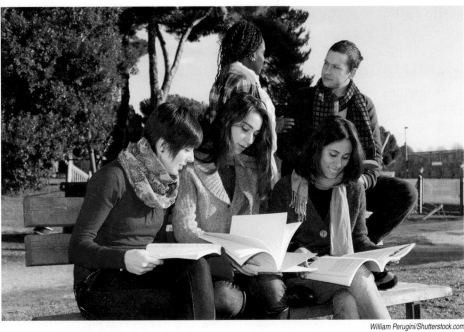

William Perugini/Shutterstock.com

**Figure 6.8**  Explaining concepts you understand to the other members of your study group will help you reinforce the material you have learned.

7. When you are studying and come to something you do not understand, physically change positions. Walk around, stand while you read out loud, or find a different chair. Perhaps your body needs to stretch and find a more comfortable position that will help your concentration.

8. Sometimes it is necessary to move ahead to the next section of the assignment. The next main point may help you better understand what you previously read.

9. Explore the library to find a similar textbook that may be written in a way that is easier for you to understand.

10. Explain the concept you are studying to another person to make sure that you are clear about what you have read.

## *Overcoming Reading Challenges*

Some students may find reading to be a particularly challenging task. The good news is that you can improve your reading abilities by taking many of the steps included in this chapter. Some challenges to successful reading may be easy to overcome, like reducing eye strain. Other challenges, such as the reading disability dyslexia or reading too slowly, may require dedication and time to overcome. Many resources are available to help you, including professionals at your school's learning center and other community resources. Above all, it is important that you have a

**Think It Through**

Have you ever been part of a study group? If so, was it a positive or negative experience? Can you think of any disadvantages of studying with others? How might such problems be resolved? If you have never worked with a study group, how could you join or create such a group?

positive attitude as you work to overcome any challenge you might face in school, work, or your personal life.

## Maintaining a Positive Attitude

Sometimes improving your reading skills can feel like an impossible task—especially when it seems easier to watch the movie version of a

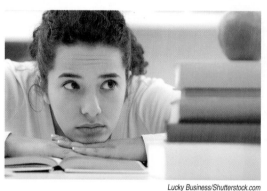

novel, or listen to the news instead of reading about what's happening in the world. To have a positive attitude about reading, you have to get rid of any negative thoughts you associate with reading. Negative impressions such as, "I read too slowly to finish the long reading assignment for this course," will set you up for failure (Figure 6.9). It takes time and patience to become good at any task that is worthwhile. Did you learn to drive in a day?

Work on improving your attitude over time. The more you read, the more your reading skills will improve. Work to reverse any negative reading habits you have developed. This will allow your reading to improve, making reading a much more positive experience.

*Lucky Business/Shutterstock.com*

**Figure 6.9**   Reading problems can be frustrating, but it's important to overcoming those feelings of frustration.

## Decoding the Text

**decoding**
*the process used to break down words into recognizable units as part of a word*

**Decoding** is the process that people use to break down words into units that are recognizable as part of a word. The process of decoding can present a serious challenge to some readers, hurting their ability to comprehend, or understand the material. Signs of decoding problems include

- having trouble sounding out words;
- an inability to recognize words out of context;
- confusing the sounds that letters make;
- reading out loud at a slow pace;
- reading with little or no expression; and
- skipping over punctuation while reading.

Professional intervention is available for such problems, which are usually identified early in a student's life.

**dyslexia**
*a learning disorder characterized by problems processing words; often causes difficulties when learning to read*

**Dyslexia** is a learning disorder that causes reading problems in the areas of decoding, comprehension, and retention of information. People with dyslexia may see words or letters in reverse order, have difficulty seeing similarities between words, or find it hard to remember sequences.

Dyslexia is a genetic (inherited) disorder that affects how the brain processes information. Although this disorder does not go away, people with dyslexia can learn strategies to become successful readers. Diagnosing dyslexia early in life may help a person develop the skills needed to read at the appropriate grade level. To learn more about strategies for treating dyslexia, talk to your school's counselor or an expert in the field.

Experts estimate that dyslexia affects as many as 15 percent of all Americans. Noteworthy individuals who have overcome dyslexia include Whoopi Goldberg, George Washington, Albert Einstein, and Thomas Edison (Figure 6.10).

## Improving Your Reading Speed

Many college freshmen express a concern about their reading speed. Students can become overwhelmed by the volume of reading expected of them, and slow readers often fear that they cannot complete all the reading assignments on time.

Although this number varies greatly, the average adult reads about 250 to 300 words per minute. Many people believe that if you read rapidly, you will not comprehend as much as if you read at a slower pace; this is a myth. Research finds that there is little connection between rate of reading and comprehension of what you read. Identifying main ideas before you begin to read the chapter and following the steps outlined in the SQ3R strategy will increase your attention span and understanding of the material.

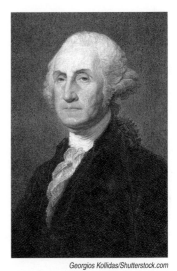

*Georgios Kollidas/Shutterstock.com*

**Figure 6.10** Historians believe George Washington was dyslexic.

If you are serious about improving your reading rate, other strategies to increase your speed and understanding of what you read include:

- **Relaxing**. It is easier to read faster when you are relaxed. Feeling relaxed also helps you to concentrate on your subject. Stress interferes with your ability to focus and concentrate.
- **Sitting up at a desk or table**. Reclining on a couch or bed may prevent successful reading.
- **Overcoming bad habits**. There are many habits that you may have fallen into that can slow down your reading. Avoid reading every letter in a word, instead absorbing whole words and phrases at a glance. Do not carelessly choose your reading environment—is it too noisy, cold, or warm?
- **Skimming for main ideas**. If you are running out of time and are overwhelmed by the amount of reading you need to cover, skimming the text can be a good option. Read headings, subheadings, the first sentence of paragraphs, lists, graphs, and the summary at the end of the chapter. Notice italicized or bold words. Search for phrases such as "The four most important factors in…" and lists set off by numbers or bullets. Skimming can also be a good pre-reading tool to improve your comprehension when you have time to read the chapter in its entirety.
- **Timing yourself**. Assess your reading ability and determine reachable goals after timing yourself while reading. If you find you can easily read 35 pages in an hour, attempt to read the same amount in 50 minutes. Do you still understand the material when you read a bit faster? Push yourself to increase your reading speed while still retaining comprehension.

- **Being flexible**. Speed reading is not always useful. You may want to slow down when reading dense material and important subjects, such as your advanced calculus textbook. Vary your speed according to the type of material you are reading.

---

### Extend Your Knowledge

*Reading Resources*

If your reading comprehension and speed need improvement, you might want to explore what help is available in your community. Courses or workshops on speed reading strategies may be offered. Your school may also have resources to help you increase your reading speed.

---

## Avoiding Eye Strain

In today's digital world, eye strain has become a major job-related complaint. Many students and healthcare workers spend a great deal of time in front of a computer screen while working on projects, researching online, and keeping up with social media. Stress and studying late into the night can also cause eye strain. Some people also suffer from dry eyes, which can worsen eye strain. Spending long periods of time reading your textbook can cause serious eye strain as well.

If you find that your eyes tire easily, the following steps can help you to reduce eye strain:

- **Make sure your eyes are healthy and properly corrected, if necessary**. Annual eye examinations are recommended to make sure you do not have any underlying eye problems (Figure 6.11). Eye examinations will ensure that you have proper vision and that your glasses or contact lens prescription is accurate and adequate for the work you are doing.

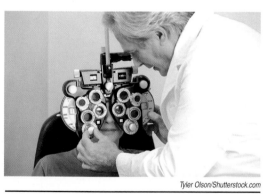

Tyler Olson/Shutterstock.com

**Figure 6.11** Regular eye examinations will ensure your eyes are healthy.

- **Reduce glare**. Glare can cause your eyes to tire quickly. If you are reading near a sun-filled window, close the blinds or curtains. The computer screen is the source of the most glare (Figure 6.12). Installing an anti-glare screen on your monitor, or adjusting the monitor's brightness can help reduce glare. Also, if you wear glasses, lenses can be treated with anti-reflective coating. This coating reduces the amount of light reflecting off your lenses.

- **Treat dry eyes**. Dry eyes can become a problem when reading for long periods of time. Remember to blink often or use artificial tears to moisten your eyes. Many work environments have especially dry air, which can increase dry eye problems. Staying hydrated at all times also helps. If your dry eyes persist, see your eye doctor for further help.

- **Invest in computer glasses**. These glasses do not have a prescription lens, but do help your eyes focus on the computer, rather than the glare on your screen. Computer glasses are designed to optimize your vision, reduce eye strain, and prevent fatigued eyes and headaches.
- **Take time to exercise your eyes**. Focusing may become difficult after reading or looking at a computer screen for an extended period of time. Look away from your book or computer every 15 to 20 minutes and focus on a distant object for at least 30 seconds. Looking away relaxes your eye muscles and reduces eye fatigue. You can also shut your eyes and relax for a short time. Rolling your eyes and closing them tightly several times can also relax tired eyes.
- **Take frequent breaks during long reading sessions**. Walk around your house for five minutes; get something to drink; stretch your arms, legs, back, neck, and shoulders. You might even want to develop a series of exercises to reduce tension and refresh your body before continuing to read.

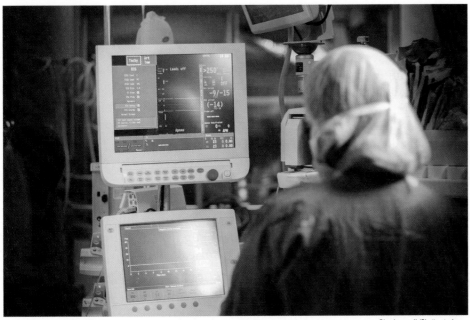

*Oleg Ivanov IL/Shutterstock.com*

**Figure 6.12**   The glare on a monitor, such as the bottom monitor in this operating room, can make the screen hard to read, often resulting in eye strain.

# Chapter Review and Assessment

## Summary

Many of the skills you will master by using this textbook overlap. For example, effective studying depends on excellent reading skills. To read, write, and study well, an adequate vocabulary is necessary. Increasing your vocabulary requires discipline and will help improve your reading skills.

Active reading means concentrating while reading. Strategies like the SQ3R reading system will help you become an active participant in your reading. These strategies are also designed to increase your reading comprehension.

You will be required to take a variety of courses throughout your education. Different courses may require that you adapt certain strategies to read the materials specific to that subject matter. Improving your retention of information can be achieved by highlighting passages of importance, as well as underlining, writing in the margins of the text, and defining new words.

Reading dense, difficult material for a class or for your job can be made easier by strategies such as skimming, summarizing, and working with study groups. You can overcome reading problems by maintaining a positive attitude.

Dyslexia is a genetic learning disorder that can be managed, but will present a challenge throughout a person's life. To learn more about dyslexia, you can find information online or by consulting your school counselor.

Some students may have a desire to increase their reading speed—a goal that can be accomplished by relaxing, timing yourself, and being flexible in your reading speed and habits. Finally, eye strain can present a challenge to reading. Adopting the practices presented in this chapter can help alleviate this problem.

## Review Questions

### Short Answer

1. Identify three benefits of reading.
2. Name four ways to improve your vocabulary.
3. What is active reading?
4. What are some advantages to using an e-reader?
5. What does SQ3R stand for?
6. Identify three strategies that will help you read difficult material.
7. How might reading for a social science course be different from reading for a literature course?
8. Describe dyslexia.
9. How might highlighting and note taking improve your reading skills?
10. Name three ways to decrease eye strain while studying.

### True/False

11. *True or False?* Dyslexia is easily cured.
12. *True or False?* Never write in your textbooks, even if you own them.
13. *True or False?* Expanding vocabulary is an important goal for the student and the healthcare worker.
14. *True or False?* You can read rapidly and still understand what you are reading.
15. *True or False?* Retention means being able to retrieve information you read from your memory.
16. *True or False?* Active reading occurs when you have skimmed a passage but recall nothing of what you just read.
17. *True or False?* When reading your history textbook, all you need to remember are the dates of historical events.
18. *True or False?* Before you begin reading a challenging chapter, it is helpful to skim the material for key phrases and terms.

### Multiple Choice

19. The SQ3R reading system includes each of the following steps, *except* _____.
    A. survey
    B. quantify
    C. read
    D. recite

20. Which of the following statements about eye strain is false?
    A. Eye strain problems have increased as workers spend many hours in front of a computer screen.
    B. Eye strain cannot be prevented.
    C. Eye strain is particularly problematic when the air is dry.
    D. Eye strain can be helped by using eye drops to add moisture to the eye.

21. What is a good method for identifying important or hard-to-understand material in your textbook?
    A. Put a Q next to material you don't understand.
    B. Mark particularly important concepts with an asterisk (*).
    C. Circle or underline terms you do not understand.
    D. All of the above.

22. When reading difficult material, it may be helpful to _____.
    A. summarize what you have read
    B. scan the document for key words and headings
    C. physically change positions
    D. All of the above.

23. When highlighting your notes or textbook, try to highlight less than _____ of the material.
    A. 50%
    B. 5%
    C. 15%
    D. 10%

24. Identifying common themes to help put dates and facts in order is helpul when reading a _____ textbook.
    A. social science
    B. math
    C. science
    D. history

25. _____ is the process used to break down words into recognizable units.
    A. Comprehending
    B. Deciphering
    C. Decoding
    D. Articulating

26. To improve your reading speed, it is helpful to _____.
    A. skim for main ideas
    B. time yourself
    C. relax
    D. All of the above.

27. When reading for a _____ course, it is important to explain theories in your own words.
    A. literature
    B. social science
    C. math
    D. history

28. _____ indicates a possible decoding problem.
    A. Reading with great expression
    B. Reading out loud at a slow pace
    C. An inability to recognize words out of context
    D. B and C only.

## Critical Thinking Exercises

29. Take a minute to think about your personal vocabulary. How would you rate your vocabulary? Does it need improvement? Does texting affect how you express yourself? Do you find yourself using excessive amounts of slang or swear words when trying to get your point across? Do you think people who use big words are pretentious?

30. What challenges have you faced when completing reading assignments? Would any of the strategies presented in this chapter make you a more efficient reader? Explain your answer.

31. How much reading do you do every week? Track your reading time and create a chart listing how long you read, what material you read, and if you experienced any challenges while reading.

32. What is your favorite material to read? Do you enjoy fiction or nonfiction? Would you prefer reading magazines or novels? Have you used e-books downloaded on your computer or tablet? After considering your reading preferences, review the chart you created for question 31. Did you read mostly for pleasure, school, or work in the past week?

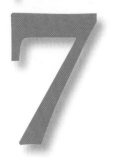
# Verbal and Written Communications

## Terms to Know

adjective
adverb
capitalization
complex sentence
compound sentence
conjunction
consonants
contraction
grammar
interjection
nonverbal communication

noun
paragraph
parts of speech
preposition
pronoun
proxemics
punctuation
simple sentence
verbal communication
verb
vowels

## Chapter Objectives

- Describe the role that verbal communication skills play in the workplace.
- Identify potential communication barriers and challenges.
- Describe how to take a complete telephone message.
- Describe strategies for giving a successful presentation.
- Discuss some general rules for attending and holding a meeting.
- Discuss the significance of nonverbal communication.
- Define *proxemics* and discuss the types and significance of personal territory.
- Explain the importance of active listening and the barriers that can occur.
- Explain and demonstrate the importance of mastering the elements of effective writing, including recognizing the parts of speech, and the use of proper grammar, spelling, and punctuation.

Reinforce your learning with additional online resources
- **Practice** vocabulary with flashcards and interactive games
- **Assess** with posttests and image labeling
- **Expand** with activities and animations

Companion
*G-W Learning*

www.g-wlearning.com/healthsciences

**Study on the Go**

Use a mobile device to practice vocabulary terms and review with self-assessment quizzes.

Mobile
*G-W Learning*

www.m.g-wlearning.com

If you chart your daily activities, you will find that much of your time is spent communicating in some way, be it verbal, nonverbal, or written communication. Communication skills affect your ability to be understood and to understand others, establish positive relationships, and perform your job well. For some people, communicating with others is one of the biggest challenges they face in their jobs. This chapter will provide you with tips and tools for improving your communication skills.

Being a good communicator is important in both personal and professional aspects of life. Being able to communicate clearly with patients and coworkers is vital in the healthcare industry. Miscommunication can lead to serious physical, and even legal, consequences. When you become a healthcare worker, you *must* be able to communicate precisely and effectively. One tip to remember is that a simple smile can improve your ability to communicate. A smile can reassure an anxious patient or welcome a new coworker on their first day (Figure 7.1).

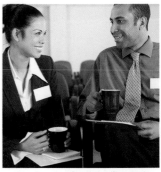
*Blend Images/Shutterstock.com*

**Figure 7.1** A smile enhances communication.

# Verbal Communication

**Verbal communication**, also known as *speaking*, is an important form of communication in a healthcare facility. During the course of a work day most healthcare workers spend time talking with coworkers, supervisors, managers, or patients. Planning and organizing your thoughts is a critical part of verbal communication. This involves thinking about who will receive the message and what you want to convey. Making notes before a phone call, having an agenda for a meeting, or researching information you wish to give to someone in advance are all methods you can use to ensure clear communication.

**verbal communication**
*expressing your thoughts out loud; speaking*

According to motivational speaker and entrepreneur Pat Croce, effective communication involves much more than choosing the right words. Mr. Croce recommends five rules to incorporate while conveying a message, known as the *5 Cs of Communication*:

1. **Clear.** Speak in black-and-white terms to clearly state your message. Allow questions from the recipient of your communication to ensure you are understood.
2. **Concise.** Do not ramble. Your important message can be lost in the nonessential information you include—get to the point.
3. **Consistent.** Make the message consistent at all times. If you are telling your supervisor about an incident that you have observed, do not change your story to make it more dramatic. Report your findings in a consistent, accurate manner. Do not tell one person what you saw and later change your observations as you retell the story to another person.
4. **Credible.** People can tell if your words are insincere—make sure your message is real. Do not heap praise on someone just because you want to win their favor. It is important that you mean what you say.

5. **Courteous.** Words and phrases such as "hello," "thank you," "please," "excuse me," and "I'm sorry" are easy, effective ways to demonstrate respect. Being courteous when you communicate sets the right tone and attitude. Courtesy is mandatory in the workplace, even if you are interacting with someone you dislike. Keep your personal feelings out of your work interactions.

Having an open mind during verbal communication is also very important. Making assumptions about what someone is going to say before he or she speaks might cause you to miss the essence of the message. If you have had disagreements with the speaker, you might negatively translate a message into your assumption about what you are hearing. Keeping an open mind and listening respectfully without emotion is critical to open, clear communication.

**Did You Know?**

**Listening and Attention**

Several studies have shown that 20 minutes is about the maximum amount of time listeners can stay attentive (Figure 7.2). After 20 minutes, listeners' attention levels begin to drop. Speaking is more stimulating than listening, so although it may be exciting to talk for long periods of time, chances are your listeners may be having a hard time staying focused.

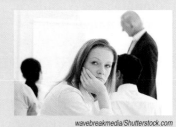

*wavebreakmedia/Shutterstock.com*

**Figure 7.2** When a speaker sees that the audience is being inattentive, he may call for a break.

The most successful communicators in the healthcare profession form positive relationships with coworkers and patients through mutual respect and professionalism (Figure 7.3). Having a bad day is no excuse for using an irritated tone when speaking with a patient or coworker. Personal problems should not be brought into the workplace.

It is also important to be cognizant of how patients wish to be addressed. Some patients, especially the elderly, may feel disrespected if you call them by their first names. To be safe, use the titles Mrs., Mr., or Ms. and their last name when speaking to adult patients. They may ask you to call them by their first name, which is acceptable with permission. Pet names like "Honey" or "Sweetie" could offend many patients who feel you are talking down to them.

When addressing your patient, speak clearly and use a tone that can be easily heard. Shouting or mumbling will not help get your point across. Careless slang expressions, especially vulgarities, are also unacceptable when dealing with patients.

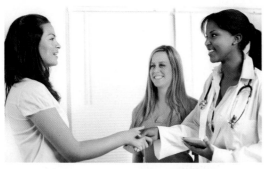

*Pablo Calvog/Shutterstock.com*

**Figure 7.3** A medical professional can put a patient at ease with a warm greeting.

☑ *Check Your Understanding*

In order to comply with HIPAA regulations, you should not call patients by their full names in the reception area. In the interest of confidentiality, use their first or last name only. For example, when addressing a patient in front of other patients, use Mr. Mercer rather than John Mercer.

Some people have a tendency to be sarcastic, or use words that mean the opposite of what you feel, to express frustration or in an attempt to be funny. Sarcasm must be avoided with patients and coworkers. Sarcasm adds a biting edge to words and can be hurtful or misunderstood.

# Verbal Communication Challenges

Anything that interferes with communication can lead to a misinterpretation of your message. However, various factors can interfere specifically with your ability to communicate verbally with your patients. Patients such as the hearing impaired, some intellectually disabled individuals, or a patient who does not speak your language pose challenges for verbal communication, possibly requiring the use of a translator. Speaking may be difficult for a patient who has suffered a stroke or stutters badly.

In addition to these considerations, communication must be geared toward a patient's ability to understand. This often means substituting basic terms for challenging medical terms that could confuse some people. Even if a coworker is translating for you, you can't assume that a fellow employee unfamiliar with your specific field will understand your use of technical terms. You may want to simplify your language for both the translator and the patient.

## Hearing Impaired Patients

Communicating with someone who is hearing impaired presents special challenges. If you have the opportunity, learning American Sign Language (ASL) would be valuable as a healthcare facility employee (Figure 7.4). However, many deaf people can read lips. If this is the case with your hearing-impaired patient, speak slowly and face the patient in a well-lighted area.

When a hearing-impaired patient is accompanied by an ASL interpreter, your conversation is still with the patient, not the interpreter. Face your patient and speak directly with him or her. Speak in a normal tone of voice, slowly, and clearly. People often speak loudly when talking to a deaf person, but this tendency is unhelpful and should be avoided.

## Think It Through

Have you had an experience communicating with a hearing-impaired individual? If so, what methods have worked for you to ensure the hearing-impaired person understands what you are saying?

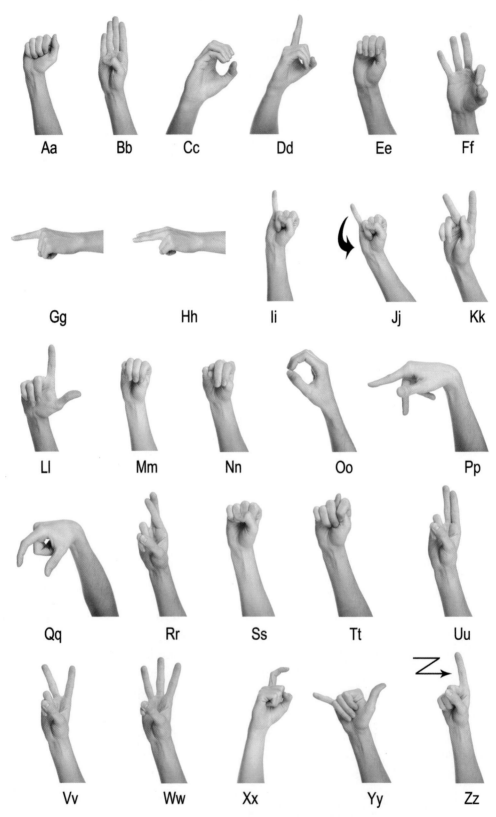

**Figure 7.4**   The ASL alphabet

## Visually Impaired Patients

Patients with visual impairments present unique communication challenges. Verbal communication is one of the main ways a visually challenged person communicates with the outside world. When working with a visually impaired person, you must hone your verbal skills so you are able to communicate successfully with your patient.

Many blind patients will be accompanied by someone who will help them adjust to the environment. However, the patient may be left with you temporarily, perhaps in a treatment room. Introduce yourself and address the patient by name, so he or she knows you are addressing them and not another person in the room. If the patient is standing, guide the patient to a chair by placing his or her hand on the chair. Remember to ask the patient what assistance is needed instead of assuming what is needed.

Ensure that the patient is included in discussions about procedures and medical plans. Visually impaired individuals can still hear and understand what is being said. Be sure to inform the patient what you are doing throughout each step of the procedure. For instance, you do not want the patient to be startled when you apply a blood pressure cuff. Let the patient know what you are about to do by saying, "Now I'm going to place the cuff around your arm."

Visually impaired patients may have a service animal (Figure 7.5). The animal must stay with the patient throughout the entire visit, including when the patient visits other facilities. Remember that the service animal is working and should not be petted or otherwise distracted.

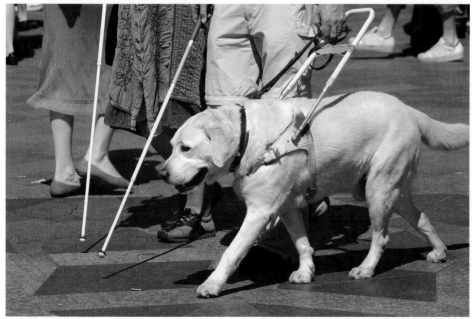

*Lars Christensen/Shutterstock.com*

**Figure 7.5**  Do not distract a service dog who is accompanying a visually impaired patient.

## Mentally Ill or Incompetent Patients

Mental illness may affect a person's judgment, making them incompetent, or unqualified to make decisions on their own. Most patients who have a mental illness that interferes with their judgment will be accompanied by a legal guardian. When communicating with someone who is mentally ill or incompetent, you should speak to the patient first and then to the guardian. Repeat any instructions you may give the patient, making sure that the guardian understands as well. You might also want to demonstrate to the guardian any task that the patient has been shown.

## Distressed Patients

Patients can become nervous, confused, scared, sick, and angry when they enter the unfamiliar environment of a healthcare facility. Becoming angry or frustrated with an unsettled patient will only make the situation worse. Remain calm and speak in a steady, confident voice.

Be sympathetic when you see the patient's distress. Sentiments such as "I am so sorry you are upset," and "let's see if we can make things easier for you" can be very helpful and calming to the patient. Put yourself in the patient's place and respond with compassion. Hopefully, the distressed patient has brought someone to help him or her understand what you are trying to communicate. If not, proceed slowly and carefully as you work with distressed, unaccompanied patients.

## Communicating with Young Patients

When treating children, you must remember that the child is the patient, but the parent is also important in such interactions. Serious illness in children is overwhelming for all parents, but even minor illness can be frightening. The following points are important to remember when you work with children, especially in a healthcare facility environment:

- Find out where the child is most comfortable—on a parent's lap or on the floor playing with toys.
- Pay attention to the distance between you and the child—many children like you to physically be at their level.
- Work with the child using an unstructured, open approach, perhaps even incorporating play during your time with a small child.
- Take the child seriously and do not talk down to him or her.
- Offer the child support and praise.
- A child may be more relaxed during a procedure if you first demonstrate the procedure on a stuffed animal so the child will know what to expect (Figure 7.6).

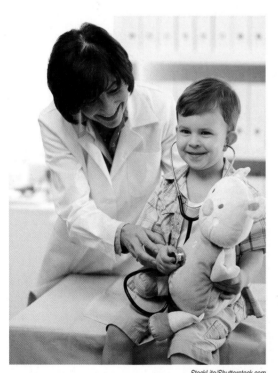

StockLite/Shutterstock.com

**Figure 7.6** Toys can make a child more comfortable during a medical examination.

**Children and the Truth**

Part of treating a child with respect is being honest with him or her. Telling a child that a shot or a blood test is not going to hurt may cause lasting distrust of healthcare professionals. Telling a child, "you may feel a little pinch" might be more appropriate.

# Language Barriers to Communication

Some patients will not be able to communicate with you because they speak another language. Most hospitals have a policy in place to deal with this situation. Additionally, many facilities have a list of employees who speak other languages in addition to English. Be particularly careful to avoid slang expressions as these can be especially confusing to non-English speakers.

Most importantly, make sure that the patient can understand the information being communicated. You should also make sure you understand any questions that the patient wants to communicate.

# Telephone Etiquette

Regardless of where you will work in a healthcare facility, sooner or later you will be answering the telephone. The following steps are an introduction to proper telephone etiquette.

- Answer a ringing phone promptly! If you need to put someone on hold, get their permission before doing so. For example, you might say, "May I put you on hold, please?" Do not leave the caller on hold for more than a minute or two without returning to see if they wish to continue to hold.
- When answering the phone, identify the facility or department in which you work, and give your name and title. For example, "Laboratory, this is Jean Smith, laboratory secretary. May I help you?"
- Before making a call, plan what you are going to say.
- When you leave a telephone number, speak slowly and repeat the number twice.
- Speak clearly with a pleasant, professional tone (Figure 7.7).
- Take a clear, concise message. Ask the caller to repeat the message if you are not sure whether you have heard or recorded it properly.
- A proper message must include the date and time of the call, the caller's name spelled correctly, and the telephone number (including the area code). You should also include your name as the person who took the call. Always repeat all numbers, including telephone numbers, addresses, numerical results, and

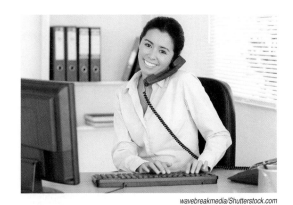

wavebreakmedia/Shutterstock.com

**Figure 7.7** You sound friendlier on the telephone when smiling.

times. Be sure to double-check that you have taken the message down correctly.

- If the message is for someone else, be sure you deliver the message to the correct person. If you are the recipient of a message, return the call as soon as possible.
- Pay special attention to the spelling of the caller's name. Ask for a full name in case the caller has a common name.
- Use "please" and "thank you" and avoid using slang expressions.
- Hold the receiver an inch or an inch and a half from your mouth and speak directly into the receiver.
- Make sure you have confirmed all aspects of the message before you hang up.
- When a doctor calls, answer questions promptly, or transfer the call as soon as possible.
- Remember that you are not authorized to give medical information to a family member or friend of a patient unless the patient has given written permission to do so.
- Do not allow any conversation that identifies a patient or contains personal information to be overheard by other patients or visitors.

## Public Speaking

You may be called upon to give a presentation in class or in your role as a healthcare worker. Whether you are giving a short talk to fellow classmates or explaining a procedure to fellow workers, there are several public speaking strategies to keep in mind.

- Be prepared. Practice your presentation several times. Know more about your material than you include in your speech. Use humor, personal stories, and conversational language if relevant.
- Look at the audience and establish direct eye contact. Smile, develop rapport, and notice if your audience looks like they are following what you are saying or if they look puzzled or confused (Figure 7.8).
- Relax and slowly count to three before beginning to allow yourself time to calm down. Don't apologize for being nervous. Realize that people want you to succeed.
- Know your room. Arrive early to the venue and walk around the speaking area. Practice using the microphone if possible, and make sure any visual aids you may have are present and in working order.
- Remember to be concise and avoid a long, repetitive presentation. Be aware of signs of lagging attention in your audience.

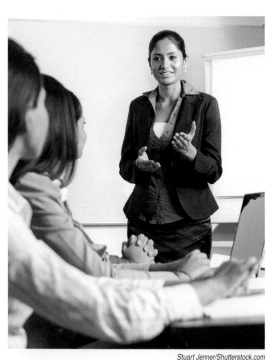

Stuart Jenner/Shutterstock.com

**Figure 7.8** Direct eye contact is critical when giving a presentation.

- Develop visuals if appropriate. You may use projected visuals, hand-outs, PowerPoint® presentations, or demonstrations. Visuals can effectively reinforce your speech. Make sure any technology you might need to use for your visuals is working before the presentation begins.
- Be well-acquainted with your topic. Reading continually from note cards loses your audience's attention. Write down key phrases, quotes, and stories in large letters on note cards to jog your memory as you are talking. Show enthusiasm for your topic.
- Practice, practice, practice! Speak slowly and calmly, but louder than your usual speaking voice (unless you are using a microphone).

# *Meetings*

When you become a healthcare worker, you will be asked to attend many meetings. As you take on more responsibility in your job, you may be asked to hold meetings as well.

## Attending a Meeting

Meetings vary in importance. Some will be brief, others will be lengthy. Whatever type of meeting you are asked to attend, there are some general rules that need to be followed:

- **Know the details of the meeting.** Where will it be? What time does it start? What topics will be discussed? Reconfirm these details before the meeting starts to make sure the location and time have not changed.
- **Be on time!** Arrive a few minutes early so that you can get organized before the meeting begins.
- **Come prepared.** You may need paper and pen to take notes. What you will need to bring with you will depend on the type of meeting you're attending.
- **Dress respectfully, yet comfortably.** Your appearance will vary depending on what type of meeting you're attending. If you wear a uniform, make sure it is clean and free from stains. If the meeting is more formal, make sure you wear nicer clothing. Check ahead of time to make sure you won't be underdressed or overdressed.
- **Pay close attention and listen carefully.** Turn your cell phone off and resist the temptation to bring other electronic devices that could divert your attention. The organizer of the meeting will expect you to understand what is being said. If you do not, ask questions at an appropriate time to make sure you understand. Try not to yawn.
- **If your participation is needed or expected, make sure you take part in the meeting.** Participation shows that you are listening and are engaged in the conversation. Make sure you show respect for everyone attending.

## Holding a Meeting

Meetings can be very productive, but they can also be a waste of time. Ineffective meetings not only stop normal workflow with little gain, but they also affect employee morale. You need to know how to run a meeting that will produce productive results. Here are some techniques to follow:

1. **Send out a meeting request.** Make sure key players can attend at the requested time. Set up another time if the people you want to attend cannot come due to scheduling conflicts. In your request, state the purpose of the meeting. Also, prepare an agenda after thinking through and preparing each topic of discussion. Your meeting request should be accompanied with meeting material, such as an agenda, at least two days before the meeting.

2. **Make copies of relevant materials for everyone attending the meeting. It is important to supply each attendee with the documents to be discussed during the meeting.**

3. **Start the meeting on time.** Wait no more than five minutes for latecomers.

4. **Set up ground rules for the meeting.** Make it clear that you will need attendees' full attention, and ask them to turn off all electronic devices.

5. **Get to the point!** Allow a minute or two of pleasantries; make it clear when it is time to get down to business.

6. **Prioritize meeting subjects.** If you have ten topics to discuss, start with the most important items.

7. **Follow your agenda.** Do not allow anyone to get off topic. Be firm when it is time to move on.

8. **Take notes.** This will assure participants that you are listening to their points. If the meeting is complex with many topics, try to have someone else take minutes, or notes, for you.

9. **Know when to end the meeting.** If you have set a time to end the meeting, do not go over your time limit. If topics are not discussed, you may have to hold a follow-up meeting. Watch for signs from your audience that you have talked long enough. If the group starts to fidget, look at their watches, or seem inattentive, it is time to stop. Go over action items that may have been discussed during the meeting and ask for questions.

10. **Send out an overview after the meeting.** The overview should contain a record of who attended, what was discussed, any agreements that were reached, and action items that were assigned. The overview should be completed soon after the meeting is over.

When done correctly, meetings are a good way to make employees feel valued and in the loop.

# Nonverbal Communication

**Nonverbal communication**, or *body language*, is a critical form of communication. This natural, unconscious language reveals your true feelings and intentions in any given moment.

When you interact with others, you continuously give and receive wordless signals. All of your nonverbal behaviors—the gestures you make, the way you sit, how fast or loud you talk, how close you stand to others, whether or not you make eye contact—send strong messages. These messages do not stop when you stop speaking. Even when you are quiet, you're still communicating your thoughts and feelings (Figure 7.9).

Some nonverbal messages are subtle, such as posture. What message does the posture of the students in Figure 7.10 give to their instructor during a lecture?

Frequently, what we say and what we communicate through body language are two different things. When faced with these mixed signals, the listener has to choose whether to believe your verbal or nonverbal message. Often, a listener will be more influenced by nonverbal signals because these tend to be more reliable than words.

**nonverbal communication**
*any form of communication that does not involve speech, including gestures, the way one sits, eye contact (or lack of), and facial expressions; body language*

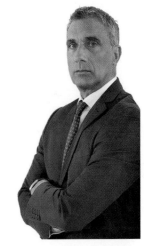

*auremar/Shutterstock.com*

**Figure 7.9** What does this man's body language suggest? Does he seem welcoming?

## *Real Life Scenario*

### *Inattention*

Rusty is quite anxious to discuss an upcoming exam, so he makes an appointment with his instructor. The instructor greets Rusty and asks him to sit down. However, as Rusty begins to ask questions, the instructor continues to look at his e-mail. What message does the instructor's inattention send to Rusty?

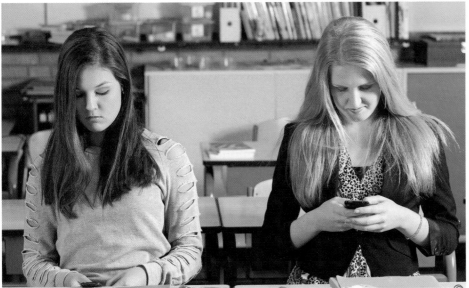

*Simone van den Berg/Shutterstock.com*

**Figure 7.10** Do these students look like they are listening to the instructor?

# Gender Differences in Nonverbal Communication

Studies have shown that men and women differ in their use of nonverbal communication. Women use facial expressions to express emotion more often than men. Women are more likely to smile and use facial and body expressions to show friendliness. Men do not smile as much. Women may demonstrate more friendly nonverbal cues, but their posture tends to be tenser than men's. Men seem more relaxed and will use more gestures, whereas women tend to rely more on verbal communication.

Women tend not to stare, while men use staring to challenge a powerful person. Men will often wait for the other person to turn away from an initial gaze, whereas women are more likely to avert their eyes. The differences in nonverbal signals between men and women further add to the complexity of communication.

# Cultural Differences in Nonverbal Communication

Hand and arm gestures, touch, and eye contact (or lack of eye contact) are some aspects of nonverbal communication that can vary significantly depending on a person's cultural background. Of course, it is important to remember that, within cultures, there is great variation in communication. This discussion can be used to guide you in your communication so that you do not needlessly offend someone.

## Gestures

Some gestures commonly used in the United States may be offensive to someone from another culture. An example of this is the use of a finger or hand to indicate for someone to "come here". In some cultures, this gesture may be used to call dogs. Pointing with one finger is not done in some Asian cultures and may be considered rude. Some cultures use the entire hand to point to something.

## Touch

In the United States, it is common for someone to pat a child's head as an affectionate gesture. However, in some Asian cultures, this might be considered inappropriate because they believe the head to be a sacred part of the body. In many Muslim cultures, touch between persons of the opposite sex who are not related is inappropriate.

## Eye Contact

In Western culture, direct eye contact is understood as being attentive and honest. In many cultures (Hispanic, Asian, and Middle Eastern for example), eye contact may seem disrespectful and rude. Women in some cultures may especially avoid eye contact with men as it could be taken as a sign of sexual interest.

## Proxemics

**Proxemics** is the study of our use of space. Proxemics can be divided into two categories: physical territory (rooms and furniture arrangements) and personal territory (the distance you keep between yourself and others).

Personal territory is the area surrounding a person that they psychologically regard as their own. Most people value their personal territory and feel uncomfortable, angry, or anxious when another person enters, or "invades," their personal territory (Figure 7.11). How much you permit another person to enter into your personal territory, or to what degree you enter somebody else's personal territory, can reveal your relationship with another person. Understanding the concept of personal territory when working with patients, staff, and visitors increases your ability to provide the best possible care.

There are four types of personal territory. These include intimate space, personal space, social space, and public space (Figure 7.12).

The size of an individual's personal territory can vary by locale. People living in a densely populated area tend to have a smaller personal territory, whereas people living in less crowded areas may have a much larger personal territory. What is considered intimate space in one culture may fit another culture's description of social space.

Men and women may also differ in their personal territory requirements. Women tend to stand close to others, while men seek more personal territory. However, men may be more likely to invade another's personal territory if necessary when asserting themselves during disagreements or emergencies.

**proxemics**
*the study of humans' use of space; includes physical territory and personal territory*

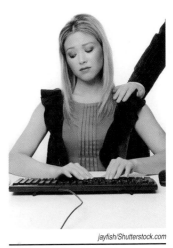

*jayfish/Shutterstock.com*

**Figure 7.11**  Has this woman's space been violated? Does she seem comfortable with his touch?

| Proxemics | | |
|---|---|---|
| *Personal Territory* | *Reserved For* | *Distance* |
| intimate space | significant others, children, close family | 18 inches or less |
| personal space | friends, work associates | 1.5–4 feet |
| social space | new acquaintances, strangers | 4–12 feet |
| public space | speeches, lectures, and theater | Greater than 12 feet |

**Figure 7.12**  Distances of personal territory can vary among cultures as well as individuals.

## Personal Territory and Touch

There are various types of touch, and each type can be received in many ways. Touch can be comforting—such as a pat on the back—or it can be offensive, possibly leading to a sexual harassment lawsuit. People who have experienced sexual abuse or other traumatic experiences may not want to be touched at all. You must be extremely careful when using touch as a communication tool.

In today's society lawsuits flourish, and any touching without a person's consent could be mistaken for something unwanted. Touch should be used with great caution. While providing care, many healthcare workers have to enter a patient's intimate space and should be sensitive to the patient's reaction.

Although a common method of greeting is the handshake, it is not appropriate in many situations in the healthcare facility. Handshakes are typically avoided to help reduce the spread of infection among the patients and healthcare workers.

The type and amount of touching that is appropriate varies with culture, age, gender, and family background. Some families hug every time they part, while others rarely hug. In some cultures and in many of the healing arts, touch is used to promote healing.

If you want to communicate more successfully in all areas of your life, you should strive to become more sensitive to body language and other nonverbal cues. This sensitivity will help you be more in tune with the thoughts and feelings of others. You also need to be aware of the signals you are sending, to ensure that the messages you are sending match what you really want to communicate.

# *Active Listening Skills*

When you think of communication, listening skills may not immediately come to mind. However, listening is a key element in all communication. If you do not receive the message that is being sent, communication has not taken place. If you understand how to be a good listener, you will be a far better healthcare worker, spouse, friend, and communicator.

As you learned in chapter 5, active listening is not the same as simply hearing what has been said. Active listening is the decision to be fully attentive and to understand the intent of the speaker. It requires physical and mental attention, energy, concentration, and discipline. As part of your career in healthcare, you will be attending meetings, following directions from your supervisor, working with patients, and giving and receiving feedback.

## Strategies for Active Listening

Applying the following active listening strategies can help you build effective relationships in school, in the healthcare environment, and in life.

1. **Desire to be a good listener.** You must want to be a better listener. Is your intention to learn about and understand the other person? Or do you feel restless until the speaker stops talking because you want to prove your intelligence and have a chance to shine?

2. **Be open and willing to learn.** When listening to someone giving you instruction, are you resistant to learning new information? Be open to different points of view, different styles of lecturing, and new ideas.

3. **Show interest.** When speaking one-on-one with a patient, it is important to show interest in the other person. Good eye contact, a gentle touch if appropriate, and other body language shows that you are interested in what the patient has to say. If you tune out the message due to disinterest, communication will not take place. Pay attention to the speaker.

4. **Resist judgment.** If the speaker is wearing strange clothing, has a reputation for being troublesome, speaks in an annoying voice, or displays other distracting features, focus on the message the person is conveying. Try not to be distracted by these less important aspects of the person.

5. **Do not interrupt.** Have you ever been continually interrupted when trying to get a point across to a friend? Recall how frustrating you found the interruptions. Allow the speaker to give you his entire message without interrupting him. If you need to ask a question, wait until the speaker finishes his general message.

6. **Show empathy and respect.** Focus on understanding the message and viewpoint of the speaker. Look for common views and ways in which you are alike. Listen with the intent to understand.

7. **Look as if you are listening.** Active listening requires high energy—sit up and uncross your legs. Maintain eye contact with the speaker and lean slightly forward.

8. **Give feedback.** Repeat what you think the speaker meant. For example: "If I understand you correctly…," "Please correct me if my understanding is wrong…," "What I believe you are saying is…"

 *Check Your Understanding*

Ethel is an 84-year-old woman who is a bit confused and in pain. You are a nurse assigned to assess this patient's problems. Ethel speaks slowly, has many concerns, and is desperate to tell you about her situation. You are very busy and have many tasks ahead of you. How do you handle this interaction?

# Barriers to Active Listening

There are many situations in which active listening is challenging. It is important to listen closely to your patients and coworkers, particularly in a healthcare facility where the well-being of your patients may be concerned. People often fail to listen when they face the following situations:

- You are interrupted by someone coming into the room, a ringing telephone, or other people talking loudly nearby.
- You move ahead in the listening process when you think you have heard what the person is saying, thinking to yourself, "I've heard all this before."
- You do not agree with what is being said and, therefore, refuse to listen (Figure 7.13).
- You cannot hear what the patient is saying because of the speaker's soft voice.
- You do not understand what the patient is saying because of a speech problem, the speaker uses challenging vocabulary, or has a thick accent.
- Your mind starts wandering, interfering with your concentration.

To be a good listener, you must concentrate on what is being said, showing a sincere interest in what the speaker is saying. To avoid being distracted, block out everything except the speaker's voice. Do not interrupt the speaker unless you cannot understand what is being said. Ask the speaker to explain what he or she is saying in greater detail. Remember that active listening can be improved with practice. Being a good listener makes you a much better employee.

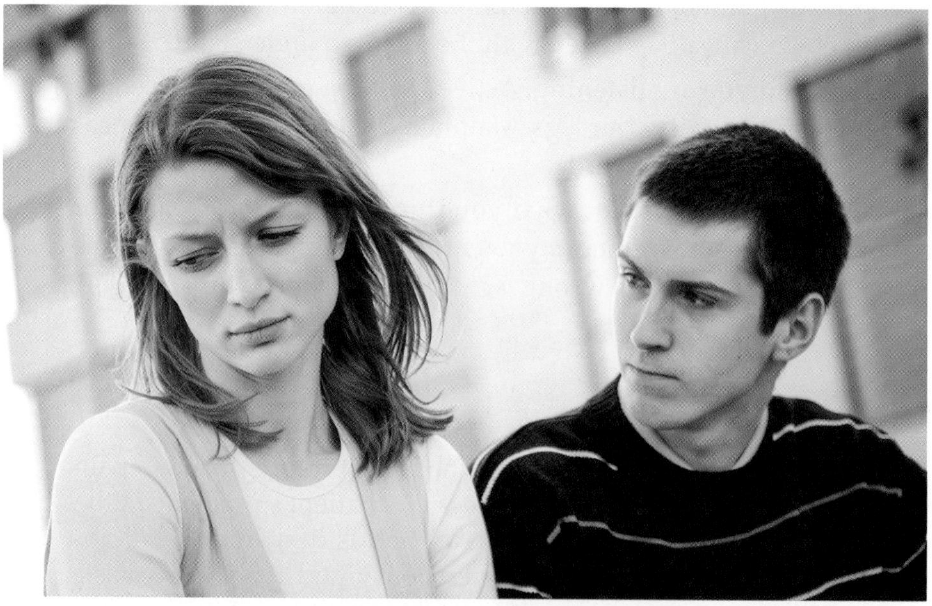

**Think It Through**

Can you remember times when you have felt that someone was not listening to you? How did it make you feel? How did you make yourself heard, if at all? How can you be a better listener?

Martin Novak/Shutterstock.com

**Figure 7.13**    Are these two people demonstrating active listening?

# Written Communication Skills

Many employers consider written communication skills to be one of the most important job skills an employee can have. Studies have indicated that the ability to write well seems to be diminishing among students. Therefore, if you can write a message clearly and accurately, that skill will benefit you in the working world. As you study to become a healthcare worker, you must practice using clear, concise writing in your assignments.

Composing written communications can be done effectively if you possess good writing skills. Written communication requires the presentation of clear, logical thoughts. Today, few written communications are actually written by hand, except quick notes like telephone messages. The vast majority of written communications are prepared electronically. As a result, keyboard skills are essential in today's healthcare world. We will learn more about computer skills in Chapter 11, *Heathcare Technology*.

Patients entering a healthcare facility may find the experience complicated, and many people struggle with understanding medications, instructions, and follow-up plans. The way the healthcare worker communicates with patients through written instructions helps to minimize confusion and lead to better patient care.

Written communications offer an excellent opportunity to make a good impression on others, but developing these skills takes time and effort. Writing requires thought, preparation, skill, and confidence. Throughout your healthcare career, you might be asked to write a variety of communications such as original letters, memos, responses to information requests, telephone messages, e-mails, patient instructions, and supply orders. You will also fill out a variety of forms on a regular basis.

Of course, to obtain a job you may be asked to present a cover letter, job application, and a résumé, all of which will require you to possess good writing skills. Job seeking information is covered in-depth in Chapter 12, *Employability Skills*.

Good writing means using several key elements to get your point across. Those elements include using grammar correctly, recognizing and correctly using the parts of speech, spelling and punctuating properly, and using clear, concise words.

# Writing an Effective E-mail

When you are writing a business e-mail—to an instructor, a fellow employee, or supervisor about a work-related subject—keep the following guidelines in mind:

- **Include a specific subject line.** If you do not put anything in the subject line, chances are your e-mail will not be a top priority. Instead of a subject line that says "Quiz," a better effort would be "Question concerning 12/8 quiz for Anatomy Class, Section 4."

- **Keep your message focused.** E-mails are meant to be short and to the point. Long, rambling messages may be only partially read or ignored.
- **Identify yourself.** When e-mailing an instructor, be sure to include the following: your name; the course name and its section number (if it has one); the days on which the course is offered; and your brief, focused message. Do not assume that the instructor knows immediately who you are by your name.
- **Do not e-mail an angry message.** If you find yourself e-mailing in anger, resist the urge. Ask the intended recipient (maybe it is your instructor or supervisor) politely if you may have a meeting with them concerning the topic you wish to discuss. By the time you have the meeting, you may have calmed down and will be able to speak rationally.
- **Proofread your e-mail.** Your point will be taken more seriously if you express yourself intelligently with excellent spelling and grammar.
- **Be courteous.** When asking for assistance and requesting a response, thank the sender by saying something like, "thank you for your quick response," or "I appreciate your assistance in this matter."
- **Do not assume that your e-mail is private.** Your message can be easily intercepted. Do not include any private information about a patient. Be professional in your communications and refrain from gossiping.
- **Avoid any fancy fonts.** Keep your message clear by using a standard font such as Times New Roman or Helvetica.

## *Grammar Review*

**grammar**

*the study of how words and their components combine to form sentences*

When speaking or writing, using correct grammar helps you send a clear message that is easily understood. **Grammar** is the study of how words and their components combine to form sentences. Writing that contains grammatical errors makes the writer appear uneducated. As harsh as this seems, there are many times when individuals are judged simply on the basis of poor writing skills and grammatical mistakes. Poor grammar can cause setbacks in certain situations, including your education and career.

It is important that you proofread, or review, your writing for grammatical errors. However, proofreading your own work is not effective if you do not know grammar rules or the correct spelling of words. You will present an unprofessional image to potential employers, patients, and coworkers if your writing has grammatical errors, misused words, and spelling mistakes. Instead of relying on a friend to review your work, use an online grammar check program, read a grammar reference book, and edit your writing once more.

## *Real Life Scenario*

### *Is Grammar an Advantage?*

Jenny and Drew are applying for the same job. They have each put together a résumé and filled out an application for the position. Drew took a considerable amount of time to craft his résumé and to fill out the application, paying close attention to grammar and spelling. Jenny has a very busy schedule. She didn't take the time to carefully review her résumé and application for grammar and spelling mistakes, but felt that her qualifications would be enough to get the job. Who is at an advantage if their qualifications are similar?

## Vowels and Consonants

When formulating words in the English language, the most basic building blocks are **vowels** and **consonants**. Written English has five vowel letters—a, e, i, o, and u (y may substitute for i). Consonants in the English language are the remaining letters of the alphabet—b, c, d, f, g, h, j, k, l, m, n, p, q, r, s, t, v, w, x, y, and z. Together, vowels and consonants form words. There are distinct sounds for each letter, depending on where it appears in the word.

## Parts of Speech

Words in the English language are divided into eight different **parts of speech**. Parts of speech can be combined to form a complete thought, or *sentence*. A sentence can combine any or even all of the parts of speech listed in Figure 7.14.

**vowels**
*five letters in the English language: a, e, i, o, and u (sometimes y is substituted for i)*

**consonants**
*all letters of the English alphabet except a, e, i, o, and u*

**parts of speech**
*collective term for eight classifications of words that denote each word's function; in English these include noun, pronoun, verb, adjective, adverb, conjunction, preposition, and interjection*

| Parts of Speech | | |
|---|---|---|
| *Part* | *Definition* | *Examples* |
| noun | a word naming a person, place, or thing | patient, clinic, medication |
| pronoun | a word taking the place of a noun | he, it, they |
| verb | a word showing action or state of being | help, run, is |
| adjective | a word describing a noun or pronoun | healthy, young, happy |
| adverb | a word describing a verb, adjective, or another adverb | rapidly, very, nearby |
| conjunction | a word connecting words, phrases, or sentences | and, or, but |
| preposition | a word relating nouns or pronouns to other words in a sentence | above, to, for |
| interjection | a word expressing strong emotion | STAT! |

**Figure 7.14**   All English words can be categorized as one of the eight parts of speech.

## Nouns

**noun**

*a word representing a person, place, or thing*

A **noun** is a type of word that represents a person, place, or thing, like *doctor, heart,* and *ambulance.* Nouns can be singular or plural (Figure 7.15).

**Proper Nouns.** Nouns can be classified as *proper* or *common.* A proper noun begins with a capital letter no matter where it occurs in a sentence. Proper nouns name a specific item. A common noun is not capitalized and does not name a specific person, thing, or place.

> **Example** (common noun): writer
> **Example** (proper noun): Ernest Hemingway
> **Example** (common noun): city
> **Example** (proper noun): Chicago

**Possessive Nouns.** A possessive noun indicates ownership by the noun or a characteristic of the noun. The possessive form of a noun is created by adding an apostrophe and an "s."

In most cases, plural nouns that end with an "s" are made possessive

| Making Singular Nouns Plural | | |
|---|---|---|
| **Guidelines** | **Singular** | **Plural** |
| **For most nouns, add *s* to the singular form to create the plural form.** | doctor | doctors |
| | X-ray | X-rays |
| | glove | gloves |
| **For nouns that end in *sh, ch, s, x, z,* or similar sounds, add *es* to the singular form. In the case of z, the z is often doubled.** | crutch | crutches |
| | box | boxes |
| | class | classes |
| | quiz | quizzes |
| **For nouns that end in a consonant and a *y,* change the *y* to *i* and add *es.*** | pharmacy | pharmacies |
| | nursery | nurseries |
| **For nouns that end in *o* preceded by a vowel, add *s* to the singular form. For most nouns that end in *o* preceded by a consonant, add *s* to form the plural. For some exceptions, add *es.*** | albino | albinos |
| | radio | radios |
| | memo | memos |
| | placebo | placeboes |
| **For many nouns that end in *f* or *fe,* change the *f* sound to a *v* and add *s* or *es* to the singular form. For others, keep the *f* and add an *s.*** | life | lives |
| | knife | knives |
| | strife | strives |

**Figure 7.15**   Singular nouns can be made plural by following these guidelines.

by adding an apostrophe after the "s".

> **Example**: The brothers' names all began with an M.

Plural nouns that do not end in "s" are usually made possessive by adding an apostrophe "s".

> **Examples**: *toys of children* would read: children's toys
> The nurse's smile made me feel welcome.

## Pronouns

A **pronoun** is a substitute for a noun. Common pronouns include *I, me, she, hers, he, him, it, you, they,* and *them*. Pronouns allow writing to flow smoothly without repeating nouns over and over.

> **Example**: Jason didn't get the job, and *he* was very upset.

**pronoun**
*a substitute word for a noun*

## Verbs

A **verb** is a type of word that describes an action or a state of being, such as *waddle, walk, run, jump, have,* or *think*.

> **Example**: Doctor Martin *diagnosed* his patient with strep throat.

Verbs such as *be, is, are, was, were,* and *am* can also show a state of being.

> **Example**: I *am* hungry.

**verb**
*any word describing an action or a state of being*

**Helping Verbs.** There are verbs that work with the main verb to show action. These are called *helping verbs*. These verbs have little meaning on their own, but they help make the main verb clearer. Helping verbs include *be, been, am, is, are, was, were, has, had, have, do, does, did, can, could, may, might, will, would, should, shall,* and *must*.

> **Examples**: I *have* interviewed for that position.
> I *should* study for the science examination.

**Voice.** Verbs also have different properties, including voice, mood, tense, person, and number. Voice can be either active or passive. Sentences using an active voice verb are considered to be more direct and easier to understand than those using passive voice. Passive voice is appropriate in some cases, such as in scientific papers to make conclusions sound more objective.

> **Example** (passive voice): The lecture *was given* by Dr. Brown.
> **Example** (active voice): Dr. Brown *gave* the lecture.

## Extend Your Knowledge

### Passive Voice

To become more aware of the use of passive voice, scan a newspaper article and underline every example you can find of passive voice verbs.

**Mood.** The mood of a verb is the way in which the writer wants the sentence to be understood. Mood can be used to ask a question or express a fact or opinion.

> **Example**: The patient in pain *raged* at the doctor.

A mood can also be a command or request.

> **Example**: Please *assist* the doctor with the procedure.

A mood can also express an idea or suggestion.

> **Example**: I *recommend* that you read the examination carefully before you start.

**Verb Tense.** Verb tense will tell you if the action takes place in the present, past, or future.

> **Example**: Jerry *arrived* at the hospital last night. His doctors *are reviewing* his test results now, but he *will have* more lab work done tomorrow.

**Did You Know?**

### Speaking and Verb Tense

Many speakers are inconsistent when expressing verb tense. Some languages do not have verb tenses, so non-native English speakers sometimes find this very challenging. When in doubt, consult a grammar text.

**Verb Person.** The person of a verb determines to whom the action or state of being refers. Verbs can refer to one of three persons: the person who is speaking (first person); the person being addressed (second person); or a person, or group of people being discussed (third person).

A first person verb is an action of the person who is speaking or writing.

> **Example**: I *am deciding* which career to pursue.

A second person verb refers to an action of someone who is being addressed.

> **Example**: You *are going* to be a wonderful nurse.

A third person verb refers to an action of someone being discussed.

> **Example**: They *are going* to become physical therapists.

**Verb Number.** Verbs should agree in number with related nouns and pronouns. Verbs connected with "I" should always be singular.

> **Example**: I *am* studying.

Verbs related to "you" are always plural.

> **Example**: You *are* studying.

Verbs in the third person should agree in number with the nouns or pronouns.

> **Example**: John and Laura *study* every day.

## Adjectives

An **adjective** is a word that modifies or describes a noun or pronoun. Examples of adjectives include *big*, *cold*, *blue*, and *silly*. Adjectives provide details about the noun or pronoun that give you a better understanding of the person, place, or thing. Adjectives can come before or after the words they modify.

**adjective**
*a word that modifies or describes a noun or pronoun*

> **Examples**: *Two* students failed the science test.
> After studying all night, Denise is *tired*.

## Adverbs

An **adverb** is a word that tells "how," "when," "where," or "how much." Some examples of adverbs include *easily*, *carefully*, *slowly*, *mainly*, *freely*, *often*, and *unfortunately*.

**adverb**
*any word that tells how, when, where, or how much*

> **Examples**: *Finally*, I finished my project.
> Jennifer will have an interview *tomorrow*.
> Sarah *quickly* finished the multiple choice section of her exam.

## Conjunctions

A **conjunction** is a word that joins other words, phrases (two or more words acting as a unit in a sentence), clauses (a group of words that contains a noun and a verb), or sentences. Examples of common conjunctions are *and*, *as*, *because*, *but*, *or*, *since*, *so*, *until*, and *while*.

**conjunction**
*a word that joins other words, phrases, clauses, or sentences*

> **Example**: *While* I could become a nurse, I might also want to be a physical therapist *or* an occupational therapist.

## Prepositions

A **preposition** is a word that connects or relates its object to the rest of the sentence. Examples include *to*, *at*, *by*, *of*, *under*, *beside*, *over*, and *during*.

**preposition**
*a word that connects or relates its object to the rest of the sentence*

> **Example**: *During* an internship, you will be working *beside* an experienced medical professional.

**Prepositional Phrases.** A prepositional phrase consists of a preposition, its object, and related adjectives and adverbs.

> **Example**: The patient is *in the examination room*.

## Interjections

An **interjection** is a word, phrase, or clause that expresses emotion. An interjection often starts a sentence, but it can be contained within a sentence

**interjection**
*a word, phrase, or clause that expresses emotion*

or stand alone. Some interjections are *oh*, *wow*, *ugh*, *hurray*, *eh*, and *ah*. Interjections should be used infrequently in workplace communications.

Interjections can appear at the beginning of a sentence that expresses strong emotion. Depending on how much emotion is expressed, a sentence containing an interjection can end with a period or an exclamation point. Interjections can also appear alone with an exclamation point.

> **Examples**: *No*, don't let the patient walk without help!
> *Oh*, you surprised me.
> *Ouch*!

## Sentences

A sentence is a grammatical unit of one or more words that expresses an independent statement, question, request, command, or exclamation. A sentence typically has a noun (called the *subject*) as well as a verb (called the *predicate*). Sentences begin with a capital letter and end with the appropriate punctuation.

In this age of abbreviated messages in e-mails, text messages, and tweets, complete sentences are not often used to communicate (Figure 7.16). However, in the workplace, complete sentences must be used in order to present professional communication skills and communicate a complete thought.

There are three types of sentences—simple, compound, and complex. The type of sentence you should use depends on how simple or complex an idea you wish to express.

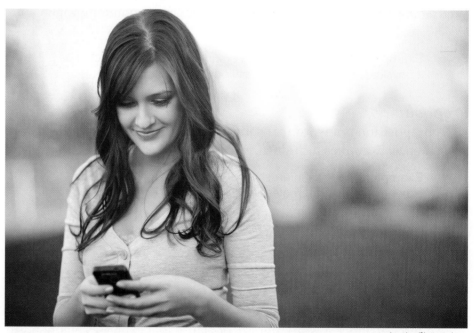

arek_malang/Shutterstock.com

**Figure 7.16** Slang used in texting is not appropriate for workplace communication.

*Check Your Understanding*

Consider the examples below. Are these sentences? Or are they sentence fragments that do not constitute a complete sentence?

1. Below the knee.
2. The calf is located below the knee.
3. The fact that Janice did not pass the anatomy test when she studied.
4. Janice studied a long time for the anatomy test and failed.
5. Because Larry is not comfortable with children, and he is assigned to work on the pediatric floor.
6. Larry worries that he will not be able to work on the pediatric floor because of his dislike for children.

## Simple Sentences

A **simple sentence**, also called an *independent clause*, contains a subject and a verb and expresses a complete thought. A noun or pronoun is always used as the subject of the sentence. In the following simple sentences, subjects are in green, and verbs are in blue.

> **Examples**: The nurse worked all weekend.
> The patient began to cough loudly.
> The phone rang at the nurse's desk.

**simple sentence**
*sentence that contains a subject and a verb, and which expresses a complete thought; independent clause*

## Compound Sentences

A **compound sentence** contains two independent clauses joined by a conjunction. Except for very short sentences, conjunctions are always preceded by a comma. In the following compound sentences, subjects are in green, verbs are in blue, and the conjunctions and preceding commas are in red.

> **Examples**: I tried to speak French, and my friend tried to speak English.
> Darryl played basketball, so Maria went shopping.
> James wants to be a physical therapist, but his mother wants him to be a doctor.

**compound sentence**
*sentence containing two independent clauses joined by a conjunction*

## Complex Sentences

A **complex sentence** has an independent clause (a group of words that can stand alone) joined by one or more dependent clauses. The dependent clause is in blue.

> **Examples**: When he handed in his homework, the instructor smiled.
> The instructor handed back the homework after she noticed an error.
> The students are nervous because they have a test tomorrow.

**complex sentence**
*sentence with an independent clause joined by one or more dependent clauses*

# The Paragraph

**paragraph**
*part of a written composition, which consists of a collection of sentences related to one topic*

A **paragraph** is a part of a written composition, which consists of a collection of sentences all related to one topic. Paragraphs express one idea or present the words of a single individual. Each paragraph can begin with an indented line. An indent is signified by hitting the Tab key, or inserting five spaces.

**Example**:

In our office, Tony is always the first one at work each morning. He was elected Employee of the Month three times because of how hard he works. Tony sets a good example for others.

I first met Tony when I was hired last year. He always has made me feel welcome in the office.

When writing a business letter, paragraphs are often not indented. Instead, the single-spaced paragraphs are separated by an extra line, or return, in between to clearly mark each paragraph.

**Example**:

Today there are many styles of writing paragraphs. Some styles include indenting paragraphs, and others do not.

Whichever style you choose, be consistent. Also, remember that a paragraph with more than six or seven sentences may be too long and will need to be broken up into a second paragraph. Chances are that there is more than one idea represented in that long paragraph.

Today, many instructors will tell you that they prefer you have at least two sentences in a paragraph. Be mindful of the length of your paragraphs. Paragraphs should be neither too short nor too long.

# Punctuation

**punctuation**
*the practice or system of using certain conventional marks or characters such as commas, question marks, and periods in writing*

**Punctuation** is defined as the practice or system of using certain conventional marks or characters in writing. Proper punctuation guides the readers and helps them understand the meaning of sentences.

### End Punctuation

There are only three ways to end a sentence: a period (.), a question mark (?), and an exclamation point (!). The period is by far the most used mark of punctuation.

**Periods.** Paragraphs can contain several sentences, and the period is used to provide structure and separate thoughts by marking the end of each sentence. Periods are also used to divide parts of an abbreviation (p.m.) or signal the end of an abbreviation. An abbreviation is a shortened form of a word or letters used to represent a word or term. Figure 7.17 provides a list of commonly used abbreviations in healthcare.

| Healthcare Abbreviations with Periods ||
| *Term* | *Abbreviations* |
| --- | --- |
| three times a day | t.i.d. |
| doctor | Dr. |
| company | co. |
| association | assoc. |
| orthopedics | ortho. |

**Figure 7.17** Some medical abbreviations are created using periods.

Many abbreviations formerly followed by a period have now dropped that punctuation. Examples of this include academic degrees (BA, MA, AA) and two-letter state abbreviations (CA, TX, SC).

**Question Marks.** The question mark is used after a word or sentence that asks a question.

> **Example**: What? Are you kidding?

**Exclamation Points.** Another form of end punctuation is the exclamation point. Exclamation points are used to express strong emotions.

> **Example**: I passed my exam!

## *Internal Punctuation*

Punctuation marks within a sentence are called *internal punctuation*. Internal punctuation marks include commas, dashes, parentheses, semicolons, colons, hyphens, apostrophes, and quotation marks.

**Commas.** Punctuation marks used to separate elements in a sentence are called *commas*. Commas provide breaks or pauses in a sentence, helping readers to more easily understand sentences. Commas are also used to separate items in a series.

> **Examples**: Doctors, nurses, and physical therapists will be at the career fair.
> Dorothy got the job by having an excellent résumé, an impressive application, and a great attitude.
> Louis enjoyed his internship in Dr. Martin's office, but he was sorry he didn't choose an internship in a hospital setting.

Some styles (preferred by newspapers and written communication in England) eliminate the last comma when separating items in a series. For example: *I prefer to wear a lab coat, a name badge and comfortable shoes*. Here, the comma is eliminated after *name badge*. However, the *Chicago Manual of Style* and most other style manuals dictate that a final comma appear before the conjunction, as shown in the examples above.

**Dashes.** Also called *em dashes*, these punctuation marks separate elements in a sentence or signal an abrupt change of thought. The dash provides a stronger break than a comma.

> **Example**: I need my anatomy book—I lost it again—before the quiz.

There are also *en dashes*, which are shorter than an em dash, but longer than a hyphen. The *en dash* is used to indicate a range of values, such as a span of time or a range of numbers.

> **Examples**: 8 a.m.–4 p.m.
> Monday–Friday
> ages 5–9

**Parentheses.** Parentheses are used to enclose words or phrases that clarify meaning or give more information. When the entire sentence is enclosed by parentheses, the period should appear inside the closing parenthesis. If the parenthetical notation falls at the end of the sentence but only encloses a portion of it, the period should *follow* the closing parenthesis.

**Examples**: I'll see you at the meeting at noon (3rd floor lounge).
Please review the medical terminology abbreviations. (They are in Appendix A.)

Parentheses are also used to enclose numbers or letters in a list that is part of a sentence.

**Example**: Your essay has errors in (1) spelling, (2) punctuation, and (3) capitalization.

**Semicolons.** When a sentence requires a stronger break than a comma, a semicolon may be used. Semicolons are used to separate clauses or some items in a series. The two clauses separated must be independent, meaning they are stand-alone clauses.

**Example**: Our entire math class took the exam; everyone passed.

A semicolon can be used to separate a series when at least one item in the series already contains commas.

**Example**: I applied for an internship in Los Angeles, California; Seattle, Washington; and Las Vegas, Nevada.

**Colons.** When introducing elements in a sentence or paragraph, a colon may be used. The elements can be words, phrases, clauses, or sentences. The colon is a stronger break than a comma.

**Example**: We need to study three things for the medical terminology quiz: abbreviations, prefixes, and suffixes.

**Hyphens.** Hyphens are used to separate parts of a compound word. Hyphens are also used when spelling out numbers.

**Examples**: My mother-in-law is a nurse.
twenty-four

**Apostrophes.** When forming possessive words and contractions, an apostrophe should be used. Possessive words show ownership. An apostrophe and a letter "s" are added to many nouns to create the possessive form. If the possessive noun is plural, the apostrophe is placed after the pluralized noun.

**Examples**: Jennifer's test score was excellent.
The nurses' cars were parked in the hospital parking lot.

| Using Hyphens | |
|---|---|
| *Rules for Use* | *Examples* |
| Fractions shown in words | one-third, one-fourth |
| Numbers less than 100 with two words | thirty-one, fifty-three |
| Telephone numbers, Social Security numbers | 1-888-2346, 558-34-1678 |
| Between letters when a word is spelled out | Awkward is spelled a-w-k-w-a-r-d. |

**Figure 7.18** Follow these guidelines when using hyphens in written communications.

A **contraction** is a shortened form of a word or term. To form a contraction, one or more words are omitted and replaced with an apostrophe. This creates a single word.

> **Example**: Rock 'n' roll became popular in the '50s.
> Dr. Hartman didn't know the patient had high blood pressure until the patient's test results were returned.

**contraction**
*a shortened form of a word or term; one or more letters are omitted and replaced with an apostrophe to create one word*

**Quotation Marks.** Quotation marks enclose short, direct quotes and some titles (such as chapter titles or article titles). A direct quote is a restatement of someone's exact words. A quote does not have to be a complete sentence. Rather, it can be a word or phrase *within* a sentence that was said or written by another person. If you have a long quote (several sentences in length or greater), it should be set apart from the paragraph. Long quotes that are set apart should not be enclosed in quotation marks.

> **Examples**: "Why do you think you would be a good choice for this job?" asked the interviewer.
> What did the administrator mean by "charitable giving"?

**capitalization**
*the use of an uppercase letter for the first letter of a word, and lowercase for the remaining letters; used for proper nouns*

# Capitalization Rules

The following rules relate to **capitalization**. Capitalization is the use of an uppercase letter for the first letter of a word and lowercase for the remaining letters.

- A sentence always begins with a capital letter.
- Capital letters are used for headings in reports, articles, newsletters, and other documents. Capital letters are used for titles of books, magazines, and movies.

  > **Examples**: The Adventures of Huckleberry Finn, National Geographic

- Capitalize the first word, and all other important words in a heading or title (conjunctions and prepositions are normally not capitalized).

  > **Example**: The Lion, the Witch, and the Wardrobe

- Proper nouns must always be capitalized.

  > **Examples**: Dr. Lang is my physician. I love Japanese food.

- Capitalize the name of months, days, cities, states, and countries (Figure 7.19).

  > **Examples**: January, Monday, New York, Great Britain

- Some abbreviations use capital letters (Figure 7.20).

  > **Examples**: HIPAA, UCLA, HTML, WI

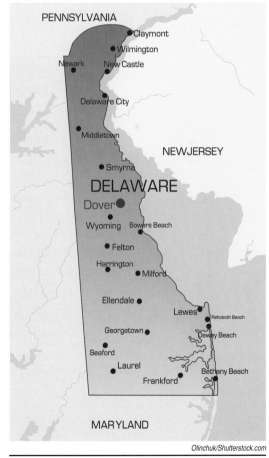

*Olinchuk/Shutterstock.com*

**Figure 7.19** The names of states and cities are proper nouns and must be capitalized.

| State Abbreviations | | | | | | | | | | | |
|---|---|---|---|---|---|---|---|---|---|---|---|
| Alabama | AL | Hawaii | HI | Massachusetts | MA | New Mexico | NM | South Dakota | SD |
| Alaska | AK | Idaho | ID | Michigan | MI | New York | NY | Tennessee | TN |
| Arizona | AZ | Illinois | IL | Minnesota | MN | North Carolina | NC | Texas | TX |
| Arkansas | AR | Indiana | IN | Mississippi | MS | North Dakota | ND | Utah | UT |
| California | CA | Iowa | IA | Missouri | MO | Ohio | OH | Vermont | VT |
| Colorado | CO | Kansas | KS | Montana | MT | Oklahoma | OK | Virginia | VA |
| Connecticut | CT | Kentucky | KY | Nebraska | NE | Oregon | OR | Washington | WA |
| Delaware | DE | Louisiana | LA | Nevada | NV | Pennsylvania | PA | West Virginia | WV |
| Florida | FL | Maine | ME | New Hampshire | NH | Rhode Island | RI | Wisconsin | WI |
| Georgia | GA | Maryland | MD | New Jersey | NJ | South Carolina | SC | Wyoming | WY |

**Figure 7.20**   State abbreviations are composed of two capital letters without periods.

- Capitalize titles that come before personal names.

    **Examples**: Ms., Dr., Officer Johnson

- Capitalize abbreviations for academic degrees and other professional designations that follow names.

    **Examples**: Jacob White, LPN; Jessie Parks, RN, BSN, MSN

- Do not capitalize seasons.

    **Examples**: fall, winter, spring, summer

## Writing Numbers

As in all aspects of grammar, there are rules for expressing numbers as figures or words. Number guidelines are not as widely agreed upon as rules for punctuation and capitalization. The guidelines listed below should be used for general writing. If you are writing a research paper or an article for publication, find out if there are written number guidelines you must follow.

General guidelines for writing numbers include

- Numbers one through nine should be spelled out with words. Numerals should be used for the number ten and anything greater.

    **Examples**: One supervisor and three workers were needed to solve the problem.
    The health unit coordinator ordered 25 black ink pens.

- Use words for numbers that are indefinite or approximate.

    **Examples**: About twenty people applied for the job.
    There were approximately ten thousand new cases of tuberculosis last year.

- When a number begins a sentence, it should be spelled out.

    **Example**: Thirty copies of the report should be made.

- When two numbers come together in a sentence, use words for one of the numbers.

    **Example**: There are 11 twenty-year-old students in my class.

- Use words to express fractions. A hyphen comes between each word.

    **Example**: The patient is to receive one-half of the dosage she previously had taken.

- When expressing time, use numerals followed by a.m. and p.m. designations. Always spell out the number that appears before the term "o'clock". A colon is used between numerals expressing hours and minutes, but is omitted when using military time (a 24-hour system).

    **Examples**: 2:30 p.m.; eight o'clock; 16:00 hrs.; 1345

- Use numerals for days and years in dates. Do not write "th", "nd", "rd", or "st" after a number.

    **Examples**: I started my job on February 10, 2014.
    I handed in my resignation at my last job on January 2, 2014.

## Common Grammatical Mistakes

The purpose of using proper grammar is to ensure that what you write is easy to read and comprehend. Many employers are immediately put off when they receive a poorly written cover letter. Such cover letters will often cause the entire application to be tossed into the wastebasket without the employer even looking at the rest of the application.

Following grammar rules when you speak conveys to others that you are an intelligent and educated person, and someone who recognizes that clear and concise language is easily understood.

### Extend Your Knowledge

*Referencing Grammar*

Because the correct use of grammar is so important, there are many reference books and multiple sites on the Internet that focus on the correct use of grammar. It may be helpful to have a grammar reference book at hand when you are composing a letter, a school assignment, or putting together an oral presentation.

The following list includes common grammar errors in the English language. Do you frequently make any of the errors listed below?

1. **don't vs doesn't**

    **Incorrect**: She *don't* answer questions in class.
    **Rule**: *Doesn't, does not,* or *does* are used for the third person singular (words like *he, she,* and *it* are third person singular words).
    **Correct**: She *doesn't* answer questions in class.

## 2. double negatives

**Incorrect**: She *does not* dislike *no one* in her class.
**Rule**: Double negatives can confuse the meaning of a sentence. Since *not* is negative, you cannot use *no one* in this sentence.
**Correct**: She *does not* dislike *anyone* in her class.

**Incorrect**: She *don't* do *nothing* right.
**Correct**: She *doesn't* do *anything* right.

## 3. gone vs went

**Incorrect**: I should have *went* to the lecture.
**Rule**: *Gone* should be used with a helping verb.
**Correct**: I should *have gone* to the lecture.

**Incorrect**: I *gone* to the game.
**Rule**: *Went* is used without a helping verb.
**Correct**: I *went* to the game.

## 4. pronoun abuse

**Incorrect**: *Me* and *my lab partner* did a great job on the assignment.
**Correction**: Rephrase the sentence without one of the subjects. Does it still make sense? Would you say "*Me* did a great job on the assignment"?
**Correct**: My lab partner and *I* did a great job on the assignment.

## 5. its vs it's

**Incorrect**: *Its* going to be hard to study with the beautiful weather today.
**Rule**: The contraction *it's* is used here because it stands for *it is*.
**Correct**: *It's* going to be hard to study with the beautiful weather today.

## 6. good vs well

**Incorrect**: You really spell *good*.
**Rule**: When an activity is being described, use *well*. When it is a condition or a state being described, use *good*.
**Correct**: You really spell *well*.

**Another example**: Lisa spelled *well* at the spelling bee; she looked *good* on stage wearing her new purple outfit.

## 7. anxious vs eager

**Incorrect**: Jenny was *anxious* to go to the graduation party in her honor.
**Rule**: In this case, Jenny was looking forward to her party but was not worried or uneasy, as the word *anxious* suggests.
**Correct**: Jenny was *eager* to go to the graduation party in her honor.

**Another example**: Jenny is *eager* to go to medical school after graduation, but her parents are *anxious* about the expense.

8. **affect vs effect**

> **Incorrect**: Leonard's terrible cold *effected* his performance on the science test.
>
> **Rule**: When you are referring to a thing (noun), you mean *effect* in almost all cases. When you are meaning an action (verb), you use *affect.*
>
> **Correct**: Leonard's terrible cold *affected* his performance on the science test.
>
> **Another example**: The *effect* of Leonard's terrible cold was that his grade on the test was negatively *affected.*

9. **lay vs lie**

> **Incorrect**: I asked the patient to lay down on the bed.
>
> **Rule**: To *lay* is to place something (there always is a noun or a "something" that is being placed). To *lie* is to recline.
>
> **Correct**: I asked the patient to *lie* down on the bed.
>
> **Another example**: *Lay* your book on the table and *lie* down on the couch.

10. **lose vs loose**

> **Incorrect**: I always *loose* my car keys.
>
> **Rule**: *Loose* and *lose* are spelled similarly, but have very different definitions. *Loose* means something is not fastened, tied up, or confined; able to move freely. To *lose* something means you no longer have it or cannot find it.
>
> **Correct**: I always *lose* my car keys.
>
> **Another example**: I *lose* my lecture notes when they are *loose* in my binder.

11. **among vs between**

> **Incorrect**: *Among* the two of us, I don't like to work with people.
>
> **Rule**: *Among* refers to three or more individuals. *Between* refers to two individuals.
>
> **Correct**: *Between* the two of us, I don't like to work with people.
>
> **Another example**: *Among* the four of us, three want to be nurses.

12. **is vs are**

> **Incorrect**: *Is* those two going to interview for the same job?
>
> **Rule**: *Is* must be used with a singular noun. *Are* is used with a plural noun.
>
> **Correct**: Are those two going to interview for the same job.
>
> **Another example**: She *is* going to the interview, but Paul and Don *are* not going to interview for that job.

---

**||Extend Your Knowledge||**

*Media Mistakes*

What grammar mistakes do you often hear in the media? Of the examples listed previously, which mistakes do you commonly make? How can you avoid them in the future? Is it important to you that you use good grammar?

---

# Spelling

In the classroom as well as in the workplace, writing containing spelling mistakes will detract from the message being delivered. Errors can take away from the sentence's meaning. If combined with a limited vocabulary and poor sentence structure, these mistakes will most likely earn you a poor grade, or you may be asked to redo your assignment.

Today, poor spellers may rely on the spell-check programs built into their word processors, but the automatic spell-check does not catch every misspelling. Your spell-check program may not recognize many medical terms which may have complicated spellings. Additionally, the program cannot help you if you substitute the wrong word, spelled correctly, for a word you intended to use.

The following are some basic English language spelling rules that should be followed closely:

- The letter *q* is followed by the letter *u*, with few exceptions.
- The letter *s* never follows *x*.
- The letter *y*, not *i*, is used at the end of English words.

    **Examples**: *my, by, why,* and *shy*

- In spelling a short vowel sound, only one letter is needed.

    **Examples**: *bed, it, lot,* and *up*

- If a word ends with a silent and final *e*, drop the *e* when adding an ending that begins with a vowel.

    **Example**: *rope* becomes *roping*; *come* becomes *coming*

- One of the most common spelling rules taught to elementary school children is: *i* before *e*, except after *c*, unless it says *a* (pronounced with a long *a*) as in *neighbor* and *weigh*.

    **Examples**: receipt, brief, or thief

- When adding an ending to a word that ends with *y*, simply change the *y* to *i* if it is preceded by a consonant.

    **Example**: *try* becomes *tries*; *fly* becomes *flies*

One of the most frustrating aspects of the English language is the number of exceptions to spelling rules. Memorization of spellings may be necessary, especially in the case of medical terminology when you may have never before encountered the terms. Chapter 8 reviews many rules for learning to spell medical terms. Of course, when in doubt, look up the word in a standard or a medical dictionary.

Figures 7.21 and 7.22 contain some of the most commonly misspelled and misused words in the English language. Do you have trouble spelling any of these words? Add your own problem words to this list.

# Putting It All Together

Now that you understand how to use all the elements of grammar effectively, keep in mind these additional tips to ensure your written communications are as clear as possible.

1. **Use precise language**. Resist the urge to use vague words like "stuff" and "thing" in your writing. Do not use jargon, or specialized language that your listener may not know.

2. **Keep your sentences short**. A very important rule to remember is that the longer the sentence, the more likely it will be for the reader to lose interest. Instead, use short, to-the-point sentences.

| Commonly Misused Words | | |
| --- | --- | --- |
| *Word* | *Definition* | *Example* |
| your | a possessive form | Your new scrubs are cute. |
| you're | a contraction form of *you are* | You're going to like the new doctor. |
| their | a possessive form | Their positive attitude made the patients more at ease. |
| they're | a contraction form of *they are* | They're going to take a small sample of blood. |
| there | a place or idea | I want to go there someday. |
| it's | a contraction form for *it is* or *it has* | It's almost time for Mr. Warner's medication. |
| its | indicates possession | The hospital room could not be used because its call button was broken. |
| then | expresses time | First we must distribute medication and then we will give the patient a bath. |
| than | used for comparison | Science is easier than English. |
| ensure | to make sure or certain | Safety education will help ensure safety in the workplace. |
| insure | refers to the provision of insurance; coverage against a specified loss | My new car is not yet insured. |

**Figure 7.21**   Use this guide to check your written communications.

| Commonly Misspelled Words | | | | | |
|---|---|---|---|---|---|
| absence | cemetery | familiar | mysterious | precedence | ridiculous |
| accommodate | changeable | February | necessary | preference | sacrifice |
| accumulate | committee | fiery | ninety | preferred | schedule |
| achievement | conceivable | foreign | noticeable | prejudice | seize |
| acquaintance | conscience | forty | occasionally | prevalent | separate |
| acquire | criticize | fourth | occurred | principal | separation |
| advice | definitely | government | occurrence | principle | severely |
| advise | desperate | grammar | omitted | privilege | similar |
| amateur | dictionary | height | opportunity | probably | sophomore |
| analysis | disappearance | immediately | parallel | procedure | specifically |
| analyze | disappoint | independence | paralysis | proceed | specimen |
| apparatus | disastrous | inevitable | paralyze | profession | studying |
| apparent | discipline | intellectual | particular | professor | succeed |
| arctic | dissatisfied | intelligence | pastime | prominent | succession |
| arithmetic | effect | knowledge | performance | pronunciation | technique |
| ascend | eligible | laboratory | permissible | pursue | temperamental |
| athletic | encouragement | laid | personnel | quantity | tragedy |
| belief | environment | led | perspiration | quizzes | unanimous |
| believe | equipped | lightning | physical | recede | undoubtedly |
| boundaries | especially | loneliness | possession | receive | unnecessary |
| business | exaggerate | lose | possibility | recommend | villain |
| candidate | excellence | maintenance | practically | rhyme | weird |
| category | experience | mathematics | precede | rhythm | writing |

**Figure 7.22**   This reference guide can be used to double-check spellings in your written communications.

3. **Reread what you have written**. Spell-check is not perfect. It is helpful to read what you have written out loud to do your own spell-check. You may hear certain words repeated, or something that seemed fine when written may sound unclear when read out loud.

4. **Seek feedback**. Your writing may not be as clear you think. Ask someone to review your writing for clarity and grammatical errors (Figure 7.23).

The ability to write clearly is becoming increasingly important. Excellent written communication skills will give you a significant advantage both when applying for a position, and in your chosen profession.

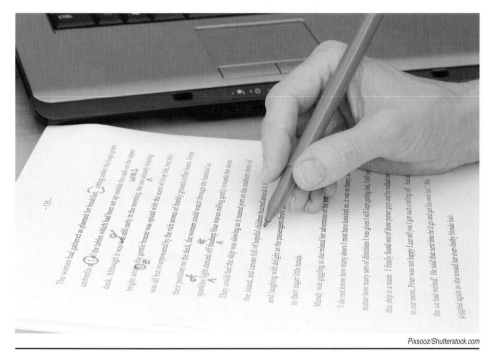

Pixsooz/Shutterstock.com

**Figure 7.23**   A good proofreader will identify spelling mistakes, grammatical errors, and passages needing clarification.

## *Real Life Scenario*

### *Testing Communication Skills in Interviews*

Jason is a 23-year-old college graduate. Since graduating a year ago, he has not been able to find a job related to his field of study and has taken several low-paying jobs to make ends meet. Jason is delighted when a friend tells him about a perfect position open in a well-paying company that offers benefits. After reading the job posting and description, Jason feels he is a great fit for this job.

Jason is surprised when he is scheduled for a lengthy interview. The process includes a writing exercise as well as a verbal interview. He feels confident after the verbal interview, and he sails through the writing portion. Jason is told he will hear about the job in two weeks.

Three weeks go by, and Jason has not heard anything. Jason decides to call the human resources representative at the company to ask if he got the job. Jason is told that his spelling and grammar are not up to the standard required for the position.

How could Jason improve his writing skills? Why do you think correct spelling and grammar usage are important to a healthcare worker?

# Chapter Review and Assessment

## Summary

To be a competent communicator, you must understand and practice English language usage rules. Your ability to communicate successfully is dependent upon your understanding of language. This is true in speaking and listening, as well as written communication through letters, reports, essays, and e-mails. Communicating clearly while giving a presentation and holding a meeting is critical for succeeding in both endeavors. If you use incorrect English in your written and verbal communications, you may be misunderstood.

Another way to communicate is through the use of body language. Reading others' body language and being aware of your own body language does much to enhance your communication skills. If you are unaware of the message your body language is sending, you may be sending a message to a patient, a coworker, supervisor, or visitors that is not what you intended at all. You must also be aware of cultural differences regarding gestures, touch, and proxemics.

Unfortunately, when you speak or write poorly, you may be judged as unprofessional or uneducated. Correct spelling, sentence structure, grammar, and punctuation are essential to your success as an employee. It is critical when working within the healthcare world that you learn and use proper English.

## Review Questions

*Answer the following questions using what you have learned in this chapter.*

### Short Answer

1. List three barriers to communication that you might encounter while working in healthcare.
2. Explain the term *proxemics*.
3. Describe three errors you could make while holding a meeting.
4. Explain what is meant by *active listening*.
5. Discuss your responsibilities as a good employee when attending a meeting.

### True or False

6. *True or False?* Meetings should start and end promptly.
7. *True or False?* It is important to read your presentation to the audience.
8. *True or False?* A healthcare worker must be respectful of a patient's personal territory.
9. *True or False?* If you are a new employee, you should not speak up in meetings.
10. *True or False?* It is permissible to leave a caller on hold for up to 5 minutes.
11. *True or False?* HIPPA stands for Health Insurance Portability and Accountability Act.
12. *True or False?* Pet names for patients make them feel welcome.
13. *True or False?* You should never tell a child that a procedure could be painful.
14. *True or False?* Personal space requirements are universal in all cultures.
15. *True or False?* In general, men seek more personal space than women.

### Multiple Choice

16. Semicolons are used in which of the following ways?
    A. They are the same as colons.
    B. They are used to separate clauses or some items in a series.
    C. Semicolons come before dashes.
    D. They are seldom used in formal writing.
17. Which of the following words is correctly capitalized?
    A. Summer
    B. wednesday
    C. october
    D. English language

18. All the items below are complete sentences *except* \_\_\_\_.
    A. Jimmy studies.
    B. Although Marie studied for the exam and hired a tutor.
    C. Jeffrey did not want to study but instead wanted to go surfing.
    D. Do not speak harshly to the patient.

19. What punctuation marks the end of a sentence?
    A. a period, comma, and dash
    B. a semicolon, a colon, and a question mark
    C. a period, a question mark, and an exclamation point
    D. a dash, a period, and a hyphen

20. Which of the following words is spelled correctly?
    A. beleive
    B. cemetary
    C. accomodate
    D. mathematics

## Grammar Review

*Correct the grammar, punctuation, or spelling in the following sentences if necessary.*

21. Its time for a coffee break.

22. Laura's supervisor asked her to separate the clean towels and washcloths from the dirty ones.

23. Your going to give an injection to the patient in Room 206B.

24. Do not loose your application.

25. They're coats are over their.

26. The pharmacist told me not to loose my reciept.

27. the luncheon is at noon first floor conference room.

28. I want to work in one of three cities, Atlanta, New York City, or Austin.

29. Dr. Evans said that I had three major problems in my essay spelling, punctuation, and passive verbs.

30. My sister in law is an occupational therapist.

## Critical Thinking Exercises

31. On a scale of one to ten, one being a poor communicator and ten being a successful communicator, how would you rate your communication skills? If you did not give yourself a 10 in communication skills, what can you do to improve your verbal, nonverbal, and written communication skills?

32. Public speaking is the number one fear reported by people in the United States. Do you fear getting up in front of people to deliver a speech or presentation? Think about the public speakers you have heard—for example, your instructor might speak in front of many people in a lecture hall. When were you excited about a lecture or presentation you observed? What was it about the speaker that interested you? When were you bored and restless during a presentation? Why?

33. If you are a poor speller, what can you do to ensure that your professional writing is free of spelling errors?

34. List at least five mistakes in grammar that you hear from your friends and the media on a regular basis.

35. Have you ever had the experience of calling a business or a healthcare facility and being treated rudely by the person who takes your call? Have you been put on hold for a long time? If you were answering the phone at that business or facility, how would your telephone etiquette differ from the person who took your call?

36. What were some of the things that caused you to be bored, inattentive, or annoyed in past meetings you have attended at work or for school activities? What can you do to counteract these feelings?

37. Are you bothered when someone approaches you and stands too close? Do you prefer to keep a large distance between yourself and others? How might these preferences affect your future healthcare career?

# Chapter

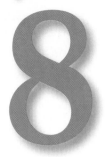

# 8

# Medical Terminology and Disease

## Terms to Know

acronyms
anatomical position
arteriosclerosis
atherosclerosis
body cavities
body mass index (BMI)
body planes
body system
cancer
carcinoma
combining form
combining vowel

dementia
inflammation
malignant
medical specialties
metastasis
myocardial infarction (MI)
neoplasm
prefix
suffix
word elements
word root

## Chapter Objectives

- Understand how medical words are constructed.
- Define *word roots*, *prefixes*, *suffixes*, *combining vowel*, and *combining form* and understand how each of these word elements can be used to form medical terms.
- Identify common abbreviations used in healthcare.
- Explain the importance of correct pronunciation and spelling of medical terminology.
- Identify medical specialties related to each body system.
- Describe classification of diseases by cause.
- Recognize terms used to describe diseases and the human body.
- Explain how cancers develop and metastasize.

Reinforce your learning with additional online resources
- **Practice** vocabulary with flashcards and interactive games
- **Assess** with posttests and image labeling
- **Expand** with activities and animations

Companion
*G-W Learning*

www.g-wlearning.com/healthsciences

**Study on the Go**

Use a mobile device to practice vocabulary terms and review with self-assessment quizzes.

Mobile
*G-W Learning*

www.m.g-wlearning.com

Has your doctor ever spoken to you using terms that were hard to understand or that you had never heard before? Sometimes it can seem like doctors and medical professionals speak a foreign language. Learning the language of medicine, called *medical terminology*, might feel overwhelming at first. However, if you wish to enter the medical field, you need to understand the basic rules for forming medical terms.

In ancient times, both the Greeks and Romans advanced the study and practice of medicine. Using the Greek and Latin languages, these early medical professionals named parts of the human anatomy, diseases, and treatments. First used centuries ago, these Greek and Latin terms remain a part of today's medical language (Figure 8.1).

| Term | Origin | Definition |
|---|---|---|
| artery | Latin, *arteria* | blood vessel that carries oxygen-rich blood away from the heart |
| phobia | Greek, *phobos* | irrational fear |
| vein | Latin, *vena* | blood vessel that carried oxygen-poor blood back to the heart |
| sperm | Greek, *sperma* | male sex cell that fertilizes the female's egg |

**Figure 8.1** Greek and Latin medical terms

**Did You Know?**

### Greek Contributions to Medical Terminology

The Greek father of medicine, Hippocrates, originated many medical terms. But the origin of medical terms varies. These terms may relate to history, mythology, poetry, geography, or physical objects. Psychology, the study of the mind, originates from the Greek term *psyche*, meaning "mind, soul, or love".

Estimates suggest that over 75% of modern medical terminology is of Greek origin. The Greek language also lends itself to easily building words from component parts. As a result, medical terminology can be built through classical roots that are easily understood.

## ‖Extend Your Knowledge‖

*Determining Term Origin*

Using a printed or online medical dictionary, find ten medical terms that have Latin origins and ten words that have Greek origins.

## *Building Medical Terms*

Medical words are like puzzles, with the **word elements** serving as the puzzle pieces. Each word element offers clues to the function, structure, or processes of the term as a whole. When the word elements are put together correctly, it is possible to determine the definition of the word by first defining each element.

Mastering medical terminology requires extensive review and practice. The time and effort you put into learning these words will pay off once you begin your healthcare career. You do not have to memorize every medical term right away. Instead, you can break down terms into their word elements

**word elements**
*the five parts used to form medical terms; includes the word root, prefix, suffix, combining vowel, and combining form*

to determine their overall definition. In a short time, you will do this automatically when introduced to a new term.

As you develop your medical vocabulary, you should keep in mind the five elements that may be used to form a word. Analyzing these word elements can help you understand the medical term as a whole. These five word elements include

1. word root;
2. prefix;
3. suffix;
4. combining vowel; and
5. combining form.

# Word Root

**word root**
*the body or the main element of a word*

The **word root** is the body, or the main part of the word. Examples of word roots include

- *cardi*, the word root for "heart";
- *nephr*, the word root for "kidney";
- *hepat*, the word root for "liver";
- *arthr*, the word root for "joint";
- *path*, the word root for "disease"; and
- *mast*, the word root for "breast."

## Word Root Characteristics

Every medical term contains a word root. The word root is the foundation of the medical term and gives the word its meaning. In some cases, a medical term may contain two or more word roots. When more than one word root is present in a term, the subsequent word roots follow immediately after the first. Refer to Table A in the reference section at the end of this chapter for a list of common word roots you will encounter when working in the healthcare field.

 *Check Your Understanding*

Table A provides numerous examples of medical terms formed by common root words. Review these examples and make a note of any terms you are familiar with. If you are not familiar with a word, look it up in your medical dictionary.

# Prefix

**prefix**
*the part of a word that comes before the word root; changes the meaning of the word root*

A **prefix** is the part of the word that comes before, or *precedes*, the word root. Prefixes change the meaning of the word root. Some common prefixes are

- *intra-* meaning "within";

- *trans-* meaning "across, through, or beyond";
- *sub-* meaning "under, below";
- *poly-* meaning "many"; and
- *electr-* meaning "electric."

## Prefix Characteristics

- A prefix attaches to the beginning of a word root and modifies the root's meaning (refer to Table B in the reference section at the end of this chapter). For example, in the term *autoimmune*, the prefix *auto-* means "self." Thus, adding the prefix signifies the immune response in the body is against itself.
- Not all medical terms include a prefix—it is an optional word element.
- A prefix can be a single letter (*a-*) or a group of letters (*hyper-*).
- A prefix is never the foundation of a medical term.
- When presented by itself, a prefix always ends with a hyphen to show it is just a word element, rather than a complete word. The hyphen disappears when the prefix joins another word element.

## Suffix

The **suffix** is the word element added after the word root to change its meaning. Examples:

- *-ectomy*, the suffix meaning "excision, surgical removal"
- *-itis*, the suffix meaning "**inflammation**"
- *-logy*, the suffix meaning "study of"
- *-gram*, the suffix meaning "record"

## Suffix Characteristics

- Every medical term includes a suffix (Table C).
- A suffix is always at the end of a medical term. A suffix attaches to the end of the word root and modifies its meaning.
- A suffix, like a prefix, can be a single letter (*-y*) or a group of letters (*-ectomy*).
- A suffix *cannot* be the foundation of a medical term.
- When presented by itself, a suffix always begins with a hyphen to show it is not a complete term. The hyphen is deleted when the suffix joins the word root.

Figure 8.2 includes common suffixes that mean "pertaining to." These suffixes might also be translated as "belonging to," "connected to," or "dependent on something." An example is the word *cutaneous*. When the word root *cutane/o* is joined with the suffix *-ous*, the newly formed term means "pertaining to the skin."

**suffix**
*the part of a word that is added after the word root to change its meaning*

**inflammation**
*term for redness, swelling, pain, tenderness, and heat affecting an area of the body; often a result of tissues reacting to injury*

| Suffix | Example |
|---|---|
| -ac,-al, -an, -ar | meningococcal (me-NIN-jah-KAHK-al) |
| -eal | peritoneal (PER-i-toh-NEE-al) |
| -iac, -ic, -ical | maniac (MAY-nee-ak) |
| -ine | intrauterine (IN-tra-YOO-ter-in) |
| -ose | sclerose (skle-ROHZ) |
| -ous | cutaneous (kyoo-TAY-nee-uhs) |
| -tic | septic (SEP-tik) |

**Figure 8.2**   Suffixes meaning, "pertaining to"

## Combining Vowel

**combining vowel**

*letter used to combine two word roots, or a word root and a suffix; usually an o*

A **combining vowel** is used to join two word roots, or is placed between a word root and a suffix. The most commonly used combining vowel is an *o*; however, there are some rare exceptions in which an *i* or *e* may be used as the combining vowel.

The combining vowel makes the word easier to pronounce. The combining vowel has no impact on the meaning of the word—it exists only to join word elements.

When a word root is combined with a suffix that begins with a vowel, the combining vowel is dropped from the new term. An example would be the word root and combining vowel *oste/o* (*oste* means bone). When the word root *oste/o* is combined with the suffix *-itis*, the combining vowel *o* is dropped. The word is spelled *osteitis*, meaning "inflammation of the bone."

## Combining Form

**combining form**

*term that describes a word root and a combining vowel used to form medical terms*

Lists of medical terms often present both the combining vowel and the word root, such as *oste/o*, *aden/o*, or *hyster/o*. When the word root and the combining vowel are joined, the result is called the **combining form**.

**Example**: arteri/o/scler/osis

Means "hardened artery walls." (Note: the *o* has been added because the suffix does not begin with a vowel.) *Arteri-* means "artery"; *scler* means "hardening"; and *osis* means "abnormal condition."

## *Combining Word Elements*

Once you are familiar with the five word elements, you can put them together to build a medical vocabulary (Figure 8.3).

**Example 1**: poly/arthr/itis

The term *polyarthritis* is composed of the prefix *poly-*, which means "many;" *arthr*, which means "joint;" and finally, the suffix *-itis*, meaning "inflammation of." Together these word elements create the term *polyarthritis*, which is defined as "inflammation of many joints."

It is important to note that not every medical term contains all five word elements. Some terms, for example, might have just a word root, combining vowel, and a suffix.

**Example 2**: cardi/o/logy

*Cardiology* is formed by combining the word root *cardi*, meaning "heart"; the combining vowel *o*; and *-logy*, the suffix, meaning "the study of." Together these word elements create the term *cardiology*, which means "the study of the heart."

Other medical terms have only a word root and a suffix with no combining vowel or prefix.

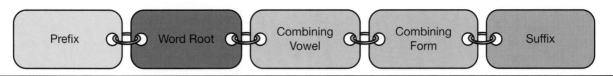

**Figure 8.3**   Combining word elements allows you to form a variety of medical terms.

**Example 3**: mast/ectomy

The term mastectomy is made up of the word root *mast,* meaning "breast," and the suffix *-ectomy,* which means "removal." Combing this word root and suffix gives us the term *mastectomy,* which can be defined as the "surgical removal of the breast."

It is important to learn and recognize the most common prefixes, suffixes, and word roots. Exceptions to general rules of medical terminology can be learned gradually as you become familiar with the basic structures of medical terminology.

## Singular and Plural Endings

Many medical terms originate from Latin and Greek words, a fact that affects their singular and plural forms. The rules for forming singular and plural forms of some medical terms follow rules of Greek and Latin rather than the English language.

For example, the heart has a right atrium and a left atrium. We do not call these two parts of the heart *atriums,* but rather the two *atria.* However, other words such as *biopsy* and *biopsies* change from singular to plural by following English language rules. Consider each medical term individually when changing from singular to the plural form (Figure 8.4).

| Terms ending in... | Singular Form | Plural Form |
|---|---|---|
| -a | bursa | bursae |
| -ax | thorax | thoraces |
| -ex or -ix | appendix | appendices |
| -is | metastasis | metastases |
| -ma | lipoma | lipomata |
| -nx | phalanx | phalanges |
| -on | ganglion | ganglia |
| -us | nucleus | nuclei |
| -um | ovum | ova |
| -y | artery | arteries |

**Figure 8.4**   Singular and plural endings

## *Pronunciation and Spelling of Medical Terms*

Medical terms can be difficult to pronounce, especially if you have never heard the word read aloud before. Even if you have heard a particular word, you might have heard different pronunciations. Another complication is that some words like *abduction* and *adduction* sound alike, but their meanings are completely different.

Clear pronunciation is important for effective communication in the medical environment. Remembering the following tips will help you properly pronounce difficult terms.

- *ch* often sounds like *k* as in "chronic" (KRO/nic)
- *g* sounds like *j* when the g comes before *e, i,* and *y* as in "genetics" (je/NE/tics)
- *i* is pronounced *eye* when it is added at the end of a word to make it plural as in "bacilli" (ba/SIL/eye)
- *pn* sounds like *n*, as though the p didn't exist as in "pneumonia" (nu/MO/ni/a)
- *ps* sounds like *s*, ignoring the *p* as in "psychiatry" (si/KI/a/tree)

Although the pronunciations of medical terms may vary, there is always only one accurate spelling. A medical dictionary is a valuable tool when determining the correct spelling of a term. Even experienced medical personnel occasionally use a dictionary.

If just one letter in a word is out of place, the meaning of the word can change. Small errors in spelling can result in serious mistakes. A misspelled word in a doctor's order could cause a patient to receive the wrong medication or treatment. A misspelling could also cause a misinterpretation by an insurance biller, possibly resulting in an unpaid insurance claim.

 *Check Your Understanding*

Write the correct spelling of these medical terms on a separate sheet of paper. Refer to Table A at the end of the chapter to check your answers.

1. neumonia
2. gynacology
3. artharitis
4. hepititis
5. hemitology
6. ileim
7. narkotic
8. leucemia
9. carcinigen
10. oncolagy

## Real Life Scenario

### Understanding Your Physician

Jeanette visits her family physician, Dr. Nolan, to discuss some health concerns. During her visit, the doctor is quite rushed, with a waiting room full of patients. Dr. Nolan answers Jeanette's questions using several medical terms she doesn't understand.

If you were in Jeanette's position, what would you do? Would you hesitate to burden the busy doctor with additional questions? Would you leave the office and look up the terms that confused you in a medical dictionary? Or would you ask Dr. Nolan to further explain the terms he has used or write them down? Would you consider switching to a new physician?

Remember the importance of clear, appropriate communication when you become a healthcare worker. When you speak to fellow healthcare workers, you will use medical terms. However, do not assume that your patients and their families understand medical vocabulary. Instead, use common terms so that you will be understood.

# Medical Abbreviations

The healthcare world is a fast-paced environment, and abbreviations may be used to speed up communication (Figure 8.5). Different medical facilities may have varying meanings for certain abbreviations. Hospitals often publish a list of acceptable abbreviations that may be used in the facility.

In some cases, abbreviations have caused confusion that leads to incorrect interpretations and results in serious errors. As a result, some healthcare facilities are moving toward restricting or eliminating the use of medical abbreviations.

Some abbreviations are called **acronyms**. An example of a common acronym is AIDS, which means *acquired immune deficiency syndrome*.

**acronyms**
*words formed from the first letters or parts of other words*

 **Check Your Understanding**

Match each abbreviation with its definition on a separate sheet of paper.

| | |
|---|---|
| 1. prescription | A. AIDS |
| 2. operating room | B. BS |
| 3. hepatitis B virus | C. UA |
| 4. acquired immune deficiency syndrome | D. ICU |
| 5. blood sugar | E. HBV |
| 6. urinalysis | F. CHF |
| 7. myocardial infarction | G. Rx |
| 8. congestive heart failure | H. ECG |
| 9. intensive care unit | I. OR |
| 10. electrocardiogram | J. MI |

| Abbreviation or Acronym | Meaning | Abbreviation or Acronym | Meaning |
|---|---|---|---|
| ABG | arterial blood gas | DOA | dead on arrival |
| ADL | activities of daily living | DOB | date of birth |
| AIDS | acquired immunodeficiency syndrome | Dx | diagnosis |
| AM | in the morning or before noon | ECG; EKG | electrocardiogram |
| Amb | ambulatory | ED; ER | emergency department; emergency room |
| ASAP | as soon as possible | EMG | electromyogram |
| ASHD | arteriosclerotic heart disease | ENT | ear, nose, and throat |
| BID, b.i.d. | twice a day | FBS | fasting blood sugar |
| BMR | basic metabolic rate | FDA | Food and Drug Administration |
| B/P, BP | blood pressure | Fe | iron |
| BS | blood sugar | FUO | fever of unknown origin |
| °C | centigrade, Celsius temperature | Fx | fracture |
| c̄ | with | GB | gallbladder |
| Ca | calcium | g | gram |
| CA | cancer | gtt | drop |
| Cath | catheter; catheterization | HBV | hepatitis B virus |
| cap | capsule | Hgb | hemoglobin |
| CBC | complete blood count | HIV | human immunodeficiency virus |
| cc | cubic centimeter | ICU | intensive care unit |
| CCU | coronary care unit | IV | intravenous |
| CHF | congestive heart failure | kg | kilogram |
| cm | centimeter | L&D | labor and delivery |
| CNS | central nervous system | L | left, liter |
| COPD | chronic obstructive pulmonary disease | lab | laboratory |
| CPR | cardiopulmonary resuscitation | LPN, LVN | licensed practical nurse, licensed vocational nurse |
| CSF | cerebrospinal fluid | lytes | electrolytes |
| CT scan | computerized axial tomography scan | mcg | microgram |
| CVA | cerebrovascular accident | MD | Doctor of Medicine |
| D&C | dilatation and curettage | mEq | milliequivalent |

**Figure 8.5**   Common medical abbreviations and acronyms

| Abbreviation or Acronym | Meaning | Abbreviation or Acronym | Meaning |
|---|---|---|---|
| mg | milligram | QID, q.i.d. | 4 times a day |
| MI | myocardial infarction | R | respiration, right |
| ml | milliliter | ROM | range of motion |
| mm | millimeter | R/O | rule out |
| MRI | magnetic resonance imaging | RT | right, radiation therapy |
| MRSA | Methicillin-resistant Staphylococcus aureus | Rx | prescription |
| N/A | not applicable, not available | $\bar{s}$ | without |
| NPO | nothing by mouth | Staph. | staphylococcus |
| OB/GYN | obstetrics/gynecology | STAT; stat. | immediately |
| OD | overdose, right eye | STI; STD | sexually transmitted infection, sexually transmitted disease |
| OR | operating room | T&A | tonsillectomy and adenoidectomy |
| ORTH | orthopedics | TIA | transient ischemic attack |
| oz | ounce | TID, t.i.d. | three times a day |
| PDR | *Physician's Desk Reference* | TPR | temperature, pulse, respirations |
| PID | pelvic inflammatory disease | UA | urinalysis |
| p.o. | by mouth | URI | upper respiratory infection |
| p/o | postoperative | UTI | urinary tract infection |
| preop | before surgery | VD | venereal disease |
| pt | patient | VS | vital signs |
| q | every | wt | weight |

**Figure 8.5**   (Continued)

## *Real Life Scenario*

### *Decoding a Medical Chart*

Peter is taking his father to see Dr. Wilson to discuss his father's upcoming surgery. With his father's permission, Peter asks to see his father's chart. Peter reads the following:

*Patient found to have a tumor in the colon following a colonoscopy. Biopsy done in pathology found to be a carcinoma, breaking through the colon wall. Surgery to follow in 10 days, with possible colostomy. Patient surgical history includes a T&A in 1970. Patient has chronic UTIs and had a mild MI in 2000.*

Using what you have learned in this chapter, translate this section from the father's chart. The tables at the end of this chapter, in particular, may be useful.

# Body Cavities, Positions, Directions, and Planes

Special terminology is used to describe the locations and movements of the human body's various parts. It is helpful to understand these terms and how to use them correctly before beginning your healthcare career. Medical professionals must write detailed reports after examining a patient, and their descriptions and diagnosis must be exact. For example, radiologists must be very specific when reporting what they see in X-rays, and insurance companies want precise details about diagnoses. It is very important that terms related to body cavities, specific locations on the body, and body planes become part of every healthcare worker's vocabulary.

**body cavities**
*spaces in the body that contain organs; the human body is divided into the dorsal and ventral cavities*

## Body Cavities

The human body is divided into several **body cavities**, or spaces that house internal organs (Figure 8.6). Of these body cavities, the dorsal cavity

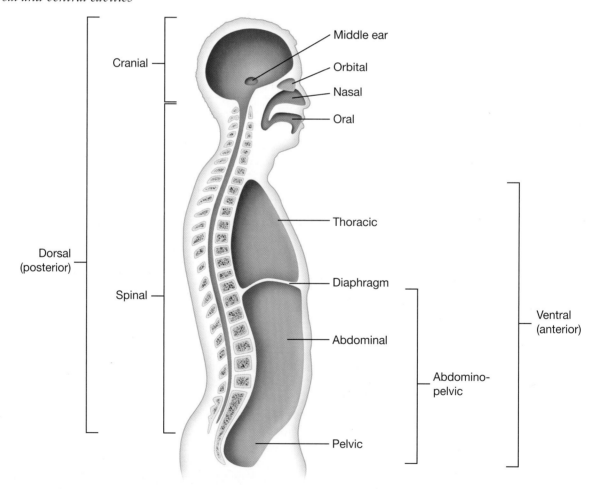

**Figure 8.6**    Body cavities hold organs and help define the anatomy of the human body.

(near the back) and the ventral cavity (near the front) are the two main divisions found in the body.

The dorsal cavity can be subdivided into the spinal and cranial cavities. The cranial cavity is located within the skull and holds the brain, large blood vessels, and nerves. The spinal cavity contains the spinal cord.

The ventral cavity is divided by the diaphragm into the thoracic (chest) cavity and the abdominopelvic cavity. Included in the thoracic cavity are the lungs, heart, major blood vessels, and part of the esophagus. Organs in the upper area of the abdominal cavity include the stomach, most of the intestines, the pancreas, liver, spleen, gallbladder, and kidneys. The lower part of the abdominopelvic cavity (often called the *pelvic cavity*) contains the bladder, urethra, reproductive organs, parts of the large intestine, and the rectum.

**anatomical position**
*a standing position in which the feet are parallel and the arms and hands are at the sides, palms facing out*

### Body Positions

Although the body can assume many positions, there are five common positions that may be mentioned in clinical assessments and treatments (Figures 8.7 and 8.8). These five positions include anatomical position, prone position, supine position, Fowler's position, and lateral position.

**Anatomical position** is an erect, standing position in which the person faces forward, with the feet parallel and arms hanging at the side, palms facing forward. This position is often considered the starting point when describing movement and directional terms of the human body. The prone position occurs when a person lies facedown, or on the stomach. The supine position calls for a person to lay faceup, or on the back. A person lying in a bed with the head of the bed elevated between 45° and 60° is in the Fowler's position. Finally, the lateral position features a body lying on its side.

## Directional Terms

When working in healthcare, you will often need to describe body directions. These directional terms are often used to describe movements, the relationship between body parts, or the location of a patient's symptom or problem. Directional terms are often used in physician orders, medical reports, insurance forms, and medical histories.

When studying the human body, you will often need to describe not only the location of a body part, but also the position of body parts in relation to other areas of the body (Figure 8.9). The front of the human body is called the anterior, or *ventral*, side. The back of the body is the posterior, or *dorsal*, side.

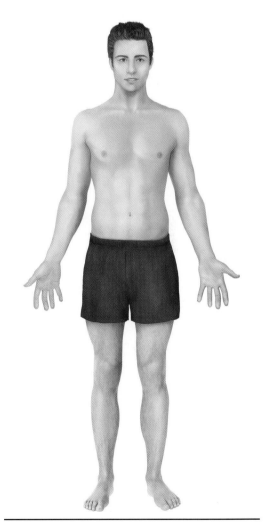

**Figure 8.7** Anatomical position is often used as the reference point when describing body movements.

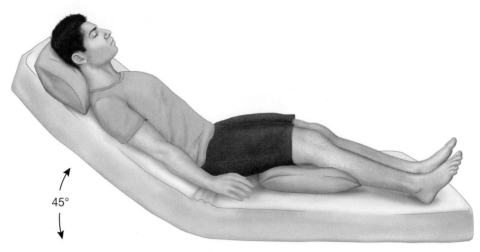

**A. Fowler position**

45°

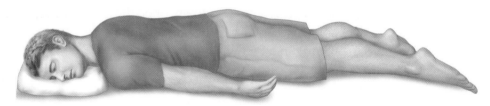

**B. Supine position**

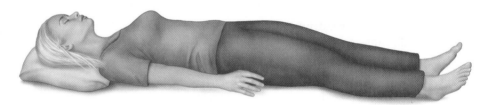

**C. Prone position**

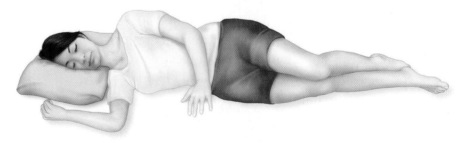

**D. Lateral position**

**Figure 8.8**   Patients are placed in various positions depending on the type of examination or treatment they are to receive.

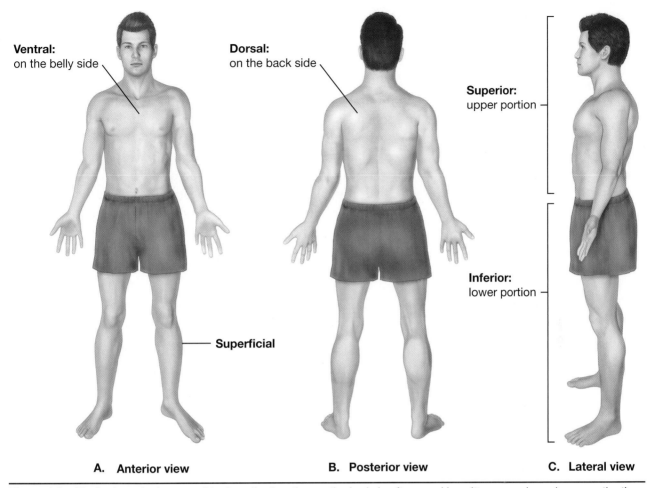

**Ventral:**
on the belly side

**Dorsal:**
on the back side

**Superior:**
upper portion

**Inferior:**
lower portion

**Superficial**

**A.   Anterior view**

**B.   Posterior view**

**C.   Lateral view**

**Figure 8.9**   Medical terminology used to describe location on the body is often used in written records such as a patient's medical history.

Other commonly used directional terms include superior, inferior, distal, and proximal. Areas closer to the head are described as *superior*. The *inferior* portion of the body is closer to the feet. The terms *distal* and *proximal* are used to describe the position of the appendages in relation to their point of attachment on the trunk. *Distal* indicates the farthest area from the point of attachment, and *proximal* means closer to the point of attachment. For example, the wrist is distal to the elbow, and the fingers are distal to the wrist. The knee is proximal to the ankle, but the ankle is proximal to the toes.

Directional terms are also used to describe the body's movement (Figure 8.10). For example, the term *abduction* means "movement of the limb away from the body." *Adduction* refers to "limb movement toward the body." *Flexion* (bending) increases the angle between joints, and *extension* (straightening) decreases the angle.

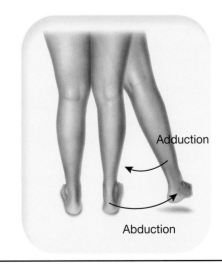

Adduction

Abduction

**Figure 8.10**   Directional terminology such as adduction and abduction describes the movement of the body.

**body planes**
*imaginary planes, or flat surfaces, that divide the body into sections; include sagittal, coronal, and transverse planes*

# Planes of the Body

To document information about their patients, medical professionals often refer to sections of the body in terms of anatomical planes. These **body planes** are imaginary lines drawn through the upright body (Figure 8.11).

Three commonly identified planes of the body include the sagittal, coronal, and transverse planes. The sagittal plane, a vertical plane, divides the body into *inexact* left and right sides. The midsagittal plane, or *median plane*, divides the body *evenly* into left and right sides. The coronal plane also divides the body vertically, but into front and back halves. Finally, the transverse plane separates the body into upper and lower parts. Planes of the body are often referred to in medical histories, physician's reports, and insurance forms as part of a detailed description of a patient's condition.

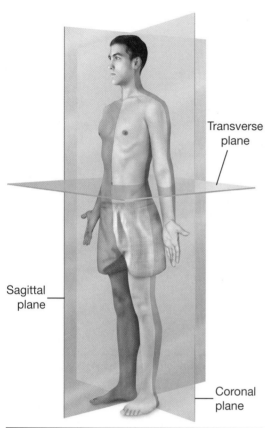

**Figure 8.11** The sagittal, transverse, and coronal planes can be used to divide the body and describe movements.

**body system**
*a group of organs working together to perform various functions and maintain homeostasis*

**medical specialties**
*specific areas of focus practiced by medical professionals, which are often named according to a body system*

# Systems of the Body

The body is divided into systems. A **body system** includes a group of organs working together to perform different functions. The body systems are discussed in detail in chapter 9.

# Medical Specialties

Because the medical field is so complicated, and there are so many diseases and disorders, physicians often develop a specialty to narrow their focus to a particular body system. This enables them to better treat their patients. **Medical specialties** are often defined by the body system to which they are connected (Figure 8.12).

Healthcare practices that are not directly related to a body system, but nevertheless have a specialty focus include:

- dentistry (dentist): the study and treatment of the teeth and gums
- geriatrics/gerontology (geriatrician): the study and treatment of the elderly
- dietetics (dietician): the study and use of nutrition, nutrients, and diet
- epidemiology (epidemiologist): the study of disease, disease-causing factors, and other public health problems, in an effort to prevent their occurrence or spread
- neonatology (neonatologist): the study and treatment of newborns
- oncology (oncologist): the study and treatment of cancer
- pediatrics (pediatrician): the study and treatment of infants and children
- pharmacology (pharmacologist): the study and use of drugs as medicines
- psychiatry (psychiatrist): the study and treatment of the mind

| Body System | Specialty |
|---|---|
| integumentary system | dermatologist |
| musculoskeletal system | orthopedist; orthopedic surgeon |
| nervous and sensory systems | neurologist; neurosurgeon; otolaryngologist (ENT physician); ophthalmologist |
| endocrine system | endocrinologist |
| respiratory system | pulmonologist |
| cardiovascular system | cardiologist; cardiac surgeon; hematologist |
| lymphatic and immune system | immunologist; internist; hematologist |
| gastrointestinal system | gastroenterologist |
| urinary system | urologist; nephrologist |
| reproductive system | obstetrician and gynecologist (OB/GYN); embryologist; urologist |

**Figure 8.12**   Medical specialties by body system

- radiology and nuclear medicine (radiologist): the use of X-rays, sound waves, and other forms of radiation and energy to diagnose disease

## Classification of Diseases by Cause

A disease is a disorder or abnormal condition of some part of the body's structure or function. The primary purpose of medicine is to treat disease. The study of disease and its treatment is one of the most interesting aspects of working in healthcare. Mastering medical terminology will allow you to easily identify terms related to disease and decipher their meaning (Figure 8.13). Breaking down terms related to disease often allows you to analyze them, but not all are easy to interpret.

The suffix *-osis*, meaning "abnormal condition," is often added to a word root to create a term pertaining to disease. So, an abnormal condition of a joint is *arthrosis*, and an abnormal condition of the kidney is called *nephrosis*.

Another suffix, *-pathy*, is used with a word root to construct a medical term that means "disease." *Cardiopathy* refers to a diseased condition of the heart, while *osteopathy* means a diseased condition of bone.

### Diagnosis

Diagnosis is both an art and a science. Even with the help of diagnostic software, doctors find that diagnosis is often a complex and difficult task. Although it is not always possible to determine what is making a person ill, diagnosis is one of the most interesting and important roles of the physician.

| Term | Breakdown | Definition |
|---|---|---|
| diagnosis | *dia-*, complete; *gnos*, knowledge; *-sis*, state of | act of determining the cause of a disease |
| prognosis | *pro-*, before; *gnos*, knowledge; *-sis*, state of | prediction of the probable outcome of a disease |
| idiopathic | *idio-*, unknown; *path*, disease; *-ic*, pertaining to | a disease of unknown cause |
| epidemic | *epi-*, upon; *dem*, people; *-ic*, pertaining to | a disease that spreads rapidly and affects a large number of people |
| endemic | *en-*, in; *dem-*, people; *-ic*, pertaining to | disease prevalent in a particular group of people or region |
| pandemic | *pan-*, all; *dem*, people; *-ic*, pertaining to | a disease that affects an unusually large number of the population |
| acute | *acu-*, sudden | a disease of sudden onset and short duration |
| chronic | *chron-*, time; *-ic*, pertaining to | a long-lasting disease |
| morbidity | *morbid*, disease; *-ity*, pertaining to | a diseased or unhealthy state |
| comorbidity | *co-*, together; *morbid*, disease; *-ity*, pertaining to | two or more coexisting diseases |
| mortality | *mortal*, death; *-ity*, pertaining to | number of deaths in a given population; the condition of being mortal |
| localized | *local-*, related to a particular area; *-ized*, to become | a disease, usually understood to be infectious or malignant that is confined to a certain area of the body |
| systemic | *system*, related to body system; *-ic*, pertaining to | a disease that affects a large part or most of the body |
| benign | *ben-*, good; *-ignis*, fire | noncancerous, not threatening |
| malignant | *mal-*, bad; *-ignis*, fire | cancerous, growing worse |
| congenital | *con-*, with; *-genic*, produced by or in; *-al*, pertaining to | a condition one is born with |

**Figure 8.13**   Common terms related to disease

| Term | Breakdown | Definition |
|------|-----------|------------|
| hereditary | *hered*, heir; <br> *-ary*, pertaining to | a disease inherited through the genes |
| sign | (no breakdown) | objective finding that can be seen by the examiner such as a rash, hair loss, or swelling |
| symptom | *sym-*, together; <br> *-ptom*, to fall or result | subjective findings that are experienced by the patient such as nausea, headache, or dizziness |
| syndrome | *syn-*, together; <br> *-drome*, to run | group of signs and symptoms appearing together that are typical of a certain disease |

**Figure 8.13**   Common terms related to disease (continued)

A diagnosis is made by studying a patient's medical history, listening to the patient's description of the illness, performing a physical examination, and analyzing the results of any diagnostic tests (Figure 8.14).

Diagnostic tests may include orders for diagnostic imaging such as those discussed in chapter 2. Laboratory testing of blood, urine, and other body fluids; and visual examinations using a scoped instrument (sometimes with a camera on the end) are diagnostic tests a medical professional may perform. For example, a bronchoscopy, or visual examination of the bronchial tubes, may be performed on a patient who has been coughing up blood. This diagnostic test is performed using a bronchoscope.

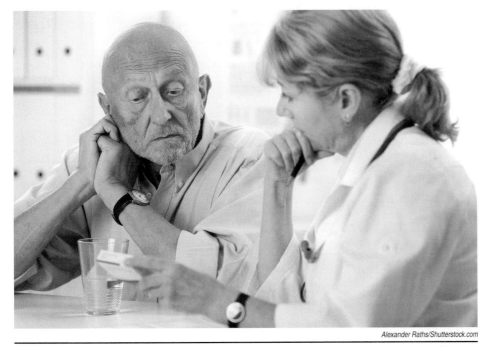

*Alexander Raths/Shutterstock.com*

**Figure 8.14**   Successful physicians understand the importance of possessing strong diagnostic skills.

Some examinations include a biopsy, or the removal of small pieces of tissue for microscopic examination. The term *biopsy* is composed of the word root *bi/o*, meaning "life" and *-opsy*, meaning "view of." Tissue and cells removed during a biopsy make it possible for medical professionals to perform laboratory examinations such as histology (*hist/o*, or "tissue"; *-logy*, meaning "study of") and cytology (*cyt/o* meaning "cells"; *-logy*).

A variety of treatment options exist, depending on a patient's diagnosis. Some diseases may require surgery. For example, if a biopsy reveals the presence of cancer, surgery is often ordered to remove the diseased tissue. Lung cancer may require a pneumonectomy (*pneumon/o*, or "lung"; *-ectomy*, meaning "removal"). A diagnosis of severe disease in the small intestine could require an ileostomy (*ile/o*, referring to the ileum; *-stomy*, meaning "new opening").

Other treatments for various diseases include medications, chemotherapy, radiation therapy, insertion of medical devices, dietary changes, physical therapy, lifestyle modifications, or psychotherapy. Physicians may also recommend incorporating yoga, meditation, or music therapy into a patient's treatment program.

## Disease Classifications

Diseases can be classified in different ways, but two of the more common methods include classifying by cause or by the affected body system. These classifications constantly overlap. For example, the disease tuberculosis is classified as an infectious disease, but when it attacks the lungs, tuberculosis is also a respiratory disease. Paraplegia, paralysis of the lower half of the body, is often a result of an accident that injured the spine. Therefore, it is a traumatic disease that affects the nervous system.

In this text, seven classifications of disease will be discussed:

- hereditary
- congenital
- environmental
- nutritional
- infectious
- degenerative
- traumatic

## Hereditary Disease

Hereditary disease results from abnormalities in the genes that carry a human's genetic information. There are thousands of hereditary diseases—many of which are caused by a flaw in a single gene, called a *monogenic disease*. According to the World Health Organization (WHO), about 10,000 monogenic diseases have been identified.

## Down Syndrome

One of the most common genetic diseases is Down syndrome, or *trisomy 21* (Figure 8.15). Down syndrome is a condition that occurs when three number 21 chromosomes are present, rather than the usual two. People born with this disease have varying degrees of mental disability. Physically, they may have a flat, broad face; folds of skin on the inner corners of the eyes; stunted growth; poor muscle tone; or atypical fingerprints. Babies born to parents past age 35 are more likely to be born with Down syndrome than babies born to younger parents.

## Sickle Cell Anemia

Sickle cell anemia is a common genetic disorder that primarily affects people of African and Mediterranean descent. This hereditary disease occurs when a child receives a sickle cell gene from each parent. Sickle cell anemia causes the red blood cells to take on a sickle, or crescent shape. The abnormally shaped red blood cells also have a sticky texture. Together, their shape and texture cause these red blood cells to clump together, block capillaries, and restrict blood flow to body tissue (Figure 8.16). Treatments vary based on an individual's symptoms, and often include blood transfusions to replace the sickle-shaped red blood cells with healthy ones.

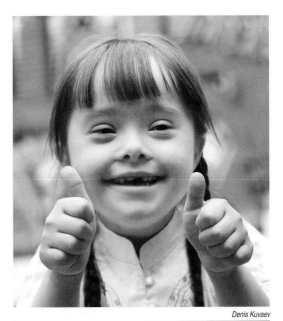

*Denis Kuvaev*

**Figure 8.15**   Down syndrome is the most common genetic disorder in the US.

# Congenital Disease

Congenital diseases, or *birth defects*, exist at birth but may not be evident until later. Congenital diseases are often the result of genetic disorders, so hereditary diseases may also be considered congenital. However, some congenital diseases are not considered hereditary. Such congenital diseases are the result of exposing the fetus to harmful substances such as drugs, chemicals, infectious disease, or radiation during development. The fetus is especially vulnerable during the first trimester (the initial three to four weeks of pregnancy). Exposure to rubella (German measles) in a non immunized mother during the first trimester results in a high incidence of congenital disease.

## Fetal Alcohol Syndrome

Consumption of alcohol during pregnancy has been linked to fetal alcohol syndrome, a condition that results in physical and mental deficiencies. Children suffering from fetal alcohol syndrome may have abnormalities in the head, face, heart, and extremities.

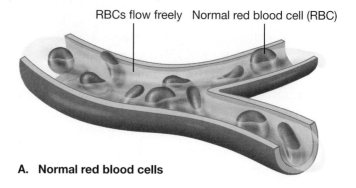

RBCs flow freely   Normal red blood cell (RBC)

**A.  Normal red blood cells**

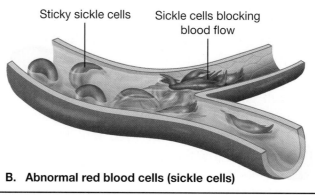

Sticky sickle cells    Sickle cells blocking blood flow

**B.  Abnormal red blood cells (sickle cells)**

**Figure 8.16**   Sickle-shaped red blood cells can block small blood vessels, halting blood flow.

## Cerebral Palsy

Cerebral palsy (CP) is a congenital disease characterized by permanent partial paralysis and lack of muscle coordination. Damage to the central nervous system, primarily during fetal development, can cause cerebral palsy. Infections in the pregnant mother such as maternal diabetes or anoxia (*an-*, or "lack of"; *-oxia*, meaning "oxygen") can cause cerebral palsy in the fetus. CP can also result from anoxia during birth as a consequence of the umbilical cord wrapping around the baby's neck during birth. Toddlers are also at risk of developing CP if they suffer a brain injury or infection.

 ### Check Your Understanding

Most physicians recommend that women who are planning to get pregnant should make an appointment with their obstetrician or primary care doctor to find out what vaccinations are needed. If the mother contracts chicken pox, mumps, measles (especially rubella), hepatitis B, or human papilloma virus (HPV) during her pregnancy, the consequences for the fetus are quite serious. Exposure to these diseases, particularly during the first trimester when the fetus is most vulnerable, can lead to congential diseases.

## Environmental Disease

Environmental diseases can result from exposure to air and water pollution; pesticides and other chemicals; the sun; asbestos; and radiation. Factors such as length, amount, and type of exposure as well as individual susceptibility contribute to the development of an environmental disease. Exposure to radiation, lead, pesticides, and other chemical hazards during pregnancy has been linked to birth defects.

**Did You Know?**

### Understanding Skin Cancer

There are three categories of skin cancer—basal cell **carcinomas**, squamous cell carcinomas, and malignant melanoma.

More than 90% of skin cancers appear on sun-exposed skin—especially the face, neck, ears, forearms, and hands. A change in color, size, shape, or texture of a mole can indicate skin cancer.

Basal cell and squamous cell carcinomas can cause serious illness and disfigurement, resulting from both the disease and the surgery performed to remove the diseased tissue. Melanomas cause more than 75% of all skin cancer deaths. This disease spreads to other organs if left untreated.

In order to avoid skin cancer, stay out of the sun. When spending time outdoors, you should wear sunscreen with a sun protection factor (SPF) of at least 50 (Figure 8.17).

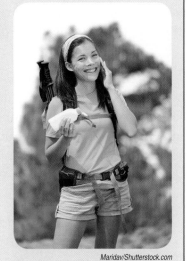

*Maridav/Shutterstock.com*

**Figure 8.17** Depending on a person's sensitivity to the sun, a sunscreen with a higher SPF might be necessary.

**carcinoma**
*cancerous tumor derived from epithelial cells*

Certain cancers are thought to be caused by toxins in the environment. Working with plastics in manufacturing and working around radiation puts people at a greater risk for cancer.

Because they filter the air we breathe, the lungs are particularly vulnerable to environmental diseases. Breathing asbestos has been linked to lung cancer. Secondhand smoke and environmental hazards in the workplace can also damage the lungs. For example, black lung disease is found in coal miners who regularly breathe coal dust. Pottery workers may develop silicosis, a lung disease caused by breathing the silica dust found in clay.

## Nutritional Disease

Nutritional diseases are the result of one or more of the following:

1. an inability to consume proper food and nutrients
2. an inability to absorb and utilize nutrients
3. overeating

**Think It Through**

How do you feel nutrition affects your health? Keep a food diary for a week to record your current eating patterns. Is your current diet meeting your nutritional needs? If not, what could you do to improve your eating habits?

**body mass index (BMI)**
*weight in kilograms divided by height in meters squared; a method of determining caloric nutritional status*

Malnutrition results from the inadequate intake of nutrients. This condition may result from a variety of causes, including inadequate food availability, fad diets, chronic alcoholism, or chronic illness such as cancer and AIDS. Disordered eating also causes malnutrition. Anorexia nervosa is an eating disorder in which a person fears weight gain, and therefore starves him or herself in order to control his or her weight. This voluntary starvation is sometimes accompanied by excessive exercise. Anorexia often leads to extreme weight loss and a weight well below normal for the affected individual's height and age. Bulimia nervosa, another dangerous chronic eating disorder, is characterized by binge eating followed by induced vomiting and the possible abuse of laxatives.

### Rickets

Rickets is a nutritional disease that occurs in children and adolescents. A prolonged deficiency of vitamin D causes osteomalacia (*oste/o*, meaning "bone"; -*malacia*, or "softening"). Osteomalacia is characterized by weakening of the bones, which can lead to bone fracture. Vitamin D is essential because it promotes the absorption of calcium and phosphorous from the gastrointestinal tract, which are necessary for bone growth and health.

### Obesity

Obesity is a medical condition in which a person has too much body fat. A **body mass index (BMI)** of 30 or higher indicates obesity. The causes of obesity include eating more calories than are burned; lack of exercise; unhealthy food choices and eating habits; a genetic predisposition; certain metabolic disorders, such as low thyroid function; and some medications. Being obese increases a person's chance of developing serious health issues such as heart disease, type 2 diabetes, osteoarthritis, and some cancers.

Losing even 5–10% of body weight can delay or prevent some of these diseases. To put this into perspective, an individual who weighs 200 pounds would benefit from losing even 10 or 20 pounds.

## Infectious Disease

In chapter 4, you learned about pathogenic microorganisms and the chain of infection. Infection occurs when pathogenic microorganisms enter the body, overcome the body's normal defenses, and multiply to the point that disease occurs. Bacteria, viruses, rickettsiae, protozoa, and fungi are pathogenic microorganisms that can cause disease.

Some infectious diseases can be transmitted from one person to another; these are called *communicable diseases*. The common cold is an example of a communicable, infectious disease. This disease is spread to others via virus-filled, airborne droplets produced by coughing or sneezing (Figure 8.18).

Serious infectious diseases are reported to county and state health departments, who will monitor the incidence—or number of cases—of the disease. By monitoring the prevalence of infectious disease, officials can quickly identify epidemics—or widespread growth of the disease. This enables officials to take steps to reduce the disease's impact on the population. Reporting disease cases also alerts officials to new infectious diseases. Organizations such as the National Institute of Allergy and Infectious Diseases (NIAD), the CDC, and WHO collect and share important information about infectious diseases.

### Hepatitis

Various forms of infectious hepatitis (*hepat-*, or "liver"; *-itis*, or "inflammation") are caused by a virus. Hepatitis A is spread through virus-infected feces that have contaminated food or water supplies. Hepatitis A is typically mild, although it can cause young children to become quite ill.

Hepatitis B is spread through contaminated blood by needlesticks and other sharps injuries, intravenous drug use, and sexual contact. Blood transfusions may also spread hepatitis B, but this is rare in the United States because donated blood is screened for diseases, including hepatitis B and C, syphilis, and HIV. This serious form of hepatitis can result in severe liver damage and even death.

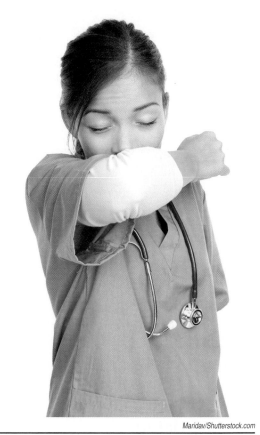

*Maridav/Shutterstock.com*

**Figure 8.18**  Sneezing or coughing into your arm can prevent the spread of infection.

Another form, hepatitis C, is often transmitted through contaminated needles, and is common among intravenous drug users. Hepatitis C can also cause liver damage and liver cancer.

Vaccines are available to protect against both hepatitis A and B viruses, but not for hepatitis C. Several less common types of infectious hepatitis exist beyond hepatitis A, B, and C.

### Tetanus

Not all infectious diseases are considered communicable. Tetanus, or *lockjaw*, is a potentially fatal disease that causes rigidity and severe contraction of muscles. This disease is caused by a bacterium found in the soil called *Clostridium tetani*. Rather than spreading from person to person, the tetanus bacterium enters the body through a cut or break in the skin.

## Degenerative Disease

Degenerative diseases, also known as *wear and tear diseases*, are those in which tissues or organs deteriorate over time. This may be due to normal body wear or to lifestyle choices.

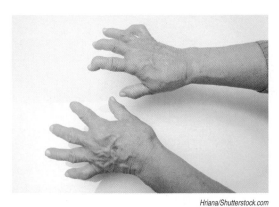

<small>Hriana/Shutterstock.com</small>

**Figure 8.19**   Arthritis is a painful condition that often affects the hands.

**atherosclerosis**
*buildup of plaque on the inner lining of an arterial wall over time*

**arteriosclerosis**
*hardening of arteries as a result of plaque buildup on an arterial wall*

**myocardial infarction (MI)**
*heart attack*

## Osteoarthritis

Osteoarthritis (*oste/o*, meaning "bone"; *arthr*, meaning "joint"; *-itis*, meaning "inflammation") is a chronic inflammation of the joints. This degenerative disease results in partial deterioration of the joint cartilage. In some cases, it may also cause abnormal formation of new bone at the joints. This is the most common type of arthritis, often occurring with age. Osteoarthritis typically affects the hands, feet, spine, and weight-bearing joints (Figure 8.19).

## Atherosclerosis and Arteriosclerosis

Another degenerative disease, **atherosclerosis** (*ather/o*, or "yellow plaque"; *scler/o*, or "hardening"; *-osis*, or "abnormal condition") is the buildup of plaque in the arteries. This plaque is composed of fats, cholesterol, triglycerides, calcium, and other substances found in the blood.

Over time, atherosclerosis develops into **arteriosclerosis**, or hardening of the arteries. Hardened plaque can block an artery, preventing the flow of blood to the heart, brain, kidneys, and other organs. Pieces of unstable plaque may also break loose from the wall of an artery, becoming circulating clots, or *thrombi*. A thrombus can plug another distant artery, potentially causing a sudden event such as a **myocardial infarction** (also known as a *heart attack*), or cerebral vascular accident (CVA), commonly called a *stroke*.

### Extend Your Knowledge

*Blood Pressure and Hypertension*

Blood pressure is the force of blood pushing against the walls of the arteries as the heart pumps blood.

Blood pressure is measured as either *systolic* or *diastolic*. Systolic blood pressure is the highest pressure in the arteries and results when the heart muscle contracts and pumps blood out of the body. Diastolic blood pressure is measured when the heart is at rest, filling with blood.

Blood pressure measurements are written with the systolic number above the line and the diastolic number below the line: $^{120}\!/_{80}$ millimeters of mercury (mmHg).

Prolonged periods of elevated blood pressure can damage the body, leading to a condition called *hypertension*. High blood pressure ($^{140}\!/_{90}$ is considered above normal) can lead to coronary artery disease, stroke, and kidney damage. People with high blood pressure can control it by living a healthy lifestyle and with medication.

**Did You Know?**

### What is Alzheimer's Disease?

Alzheimer's disease, a degenerative disease, is the most common form of **dementia**. Alzheimer's disease accounts for 50–80% of dementia cases.

Alzheimer's disease is characterized by confusion; mental deterioration; restlessness, especially near sundown; and the inability to speak and move well. Alzheimer's usually begins at age 65 or older. About five percent of cases are called *early onset*, meaning that the disease occurs at a younger age (usually in a person's 40s or 50s).

Alzheimer's disease prevents parts of brain cells from functioning correctly. Two abnormal structures called *plaques* and *tangles* build up inside cells, usually in a predictable pattern. Plaques and tangles can be seen on an MRI scan. The plaques and tangles first develop in areas related to memory before moving to other areas of the brain, destroying nerve cells in their path.

Researchers are working to uncover more details about the onset of Alzheimer's disease, how to slow its progression, and how to prevent it altogether. New treatments are rapidly being developed, but there is no cure for this disease.

**dementia**
*a disorder featuring a progressive loss of memory and other intellectual functions*

## Trauma

Trauma is any physical injury to the body caused by an accident or violence. Trauma may also be self-inflicted. Blunt force, sharp objects such as knives, gunshot wounds, poisons, animal bites or stings, blasts, suffocation, electrical shock, fire, or drowning may all lead to traumatic injury.

According to the National Center for Health Statistics (NCHS), traumatic injuries are the leading cause of death for people in the United States under 35 years of age. Motor vehicle accidents and falls are the most common accidents to cause trauma. Safety awareness is an extremely important part of reducing injury and death from trauma.

## *Cancer*

**Cancer** is a disease that occurs when an abnormal growth of cells multiply rapidly in the body. A **neoplasm** is a tumor that can be either malignant or benign. Cancer can occur in any part of the body and at any age, and there are a variety of causes.

While a normal human cell replicates itself exactly, stops reproducing when appropriate, and matures, a cancerous cell cannot do these things. Some unknown glitch in cancerous cells overrides the normal system of replication, maturation, and death. A cancer cell does not stop reproducing, nor is the body able to destroy these cells on its own. As a result, the high numbers of cancerous cells damage the part of the body where the cancer is growing.

**cancer**
*an abnormal growth of cells in the body that multiply rapidly and invade normal tissue*

**neoplasm**
*a tumor; can be either malignant or benign*

## Metastasis

Another unique quality of cancerous cells is their ability to move throughout the body. Normal cells stay together as they grow, keeping the cells in the correct location. Cancer cells, however, can lose the ability to stick together. As a result, cancerous cells may break off the primary tumor and spread throughout the body via the bloodstream. This process, called **metastasis**, allows new, or secondary, cancerous tumors to form in other areas of the body.

**metastasis**

*the spread of cancerous cells from their place of origin to other parts of the body via the bloodstream*

**malignant**

*term that describes a tumor that is threatening to life; cancerous*

## Common Cancers

Many types of cancer are diagnosed each year, with over 200 types identified. Cancer is a broad term that encompasses a number of **malignant** diseases. Each cancer has its own unique set of possible causes, symptoms, and treatment regimens. Early detection plays a key role in successful cancer treatment.

According to the American Cancer Society, the most common types of cancer are

1. non-melanoma skin cancers;
2. prostate cancer;
3. breast cancer;
4. lung cancer; and
5. colorectal cancer.

## Signs and Symptoms of Cancer

The American Cancer Society provides a list of the seven warning signs and symptoms of cancer. These signs and symptoms can be remembered by using the acronym **CAUTION**:

1. **Change** in bowel or bladder habits
2. **A sore** that does not heal
3. **Unusual** bleeding or discharge
4. **Thickening** or lump in the breast, testicles, or elsewhere
5. **Indigestion** or difficulty swallowing
6. **Obvious change** in the size, color, shape or thickness of wart, mole, or mouth sore
7. **Nagging cough** or hoarseness

Other signs and symptoms that should be investigated include

1. white patches in the mouth or white spots on the tongue;

2. unexplained weight loss;

3. fever;

4. fatigue;

5. pain; or

6. skin changes.

## Extend Your Knowledge

### Bone Marrow Transplants

Bone marrow transplants save thousands of lives each year. Because bone marrow produces blood cells, leukemia (a cancer of the blood) and some lymphomas (cancer of the lymphatic system) can be treated with a bone marrow transplant. Healthy bone marrow is also used to treat several types of bone marrow diseases. Without treatment, both of these diseases can result in death.

The transplantation process begins with large doses of chemotherapy or radiation to destroy the abnormal stem cells in the bone marrow. Healthy marrow is then infused into the patient's bloodstream. If successful, the new bone marrow migrates to the cavities of the large bones, and begins producing normal blood cells.

The donated bone marrow must match the genetic makeup of the patient's own marrow as perfectly as possible. Today, many people are waiting for a bone marrow transplant because a suitable donor cannot be found. Bone marrow registries exist to test potential donors' bone marrow for compatibility with a patient awaiting transplant.

 *Check Your Understanding*

Approximately 85% of lung cancer is caused by smoking. People who smoke are 15 to 30 times more likely to get lung cancer than nonsmokers.

Make a list of as many reasons as you can think of not to smoke. The health risks associated with smoking are no secret, so why do you think people continue to smoke? What diseases might specifically be caused by smoking? Why is it so difficult for most people to quit smoking?

# *Medical Terminology Reference Tables*

| Common Word Roots | | |
|---|---|---|
| **Word Root** | **Meaning** | **Example** |
| acr/o | extremities | acromegaly (AK-roh-MEG-a-lee) |
| aden/o | gland | adenopathy (AD-ee-NAHP-a-thee) |
| albin/o, alb/o | white | albinism (AL-bigh-nizm) |
| angi/o | vessel | angioma (an-jee-OH-ma) |
| arteri/o | artery | arteriogram (ar-TER-ee-oh-gram) |
| arthr/o | joint | arthritis (ar-THRIGH-tis) |
| audi/o | hearing | audiology (AW-dee-AHL-oh-jee) |
| aur/o | ear | auriform (AW-ri-form) |
| bi/o | life | biology (bigh-AHL-oh-jee) |
| blephar/o | eyelid | blepharitis (BLEF-a-RIGH-tis) |
| brachi/o | arm | antibrachial (AN-tee-BRAY-kee-al) |
| bronchi/o | bronchial | bronchial pneumonia (BRAHNG-kee-al noo-MOH-nee-a) |
| bucc/o | cheek | buccal cavity (BOOK-al) |
| carcin/o | cancer | carcinogen (kar-SIN-oh-jen) |
| cardi/o | heart | cardiologist (KAR-dee-AHL-oh-jist) |
| cephal/o | head | cephalogram (SEF-a-loh-gram) |
| cerebr/o | brain | cerebrospinal fluid (SER-ee-broh-SPIGH-nal) |
| cervic/o | neck | cervical collar (SER-vi-kal) |
| chol/e | bile | cholecystic (KOH-leh-SIS-tik) |
| cholecyst/o | gallbladder | cholecystectomy (KOH-leh-sis-TEK-toh-mee) |
| chondr/o | cartilage | chondrotomy (kahn-DRAHT-oh-mee) |
| chrom/o | color | chromatosis (KROH-ma-TOH-sis) |
| col/o, colon/o | colon | colonoscopy (KOH-lahn-AHS-koh-pee) |
| cost/o | ribs | costectomy (kahs-TEK-toh-mee) |
| crani/o | skull | craniotomy (KRAY-nee-AHT-oh-mee) |
| cutane/o | skin | cutaneous (kyoo-TAY-nee-uhs) |
| cyan/o | blue | cyanotic (SIGH-a-NAHT-ik) |

**Table A**   Common word roots used in the medical field

| Common Word Roots | | |
|---|---|---|
| *Word Root* | *Meaning* | *Example* |
| cyst/o | bladder | cystogram (SIS-toh-gram) |
| cyt/o | cell | cytoplasm (SIGH-toh-plazm) |
| dacry/o | tear | dacryocyst (DAK-ree-oh-SIST) |
| dactyl/o | fingers; toes | dactylitis (DAK-ti-LIGH-tis) |
| dent/i | tooth | dentistry (DEN-tis-tree) |
| derm/o, dermat/o; derma | skin | dermatology (DER-ma-TAHL-oh-jee) |
| enter/o | intestine | enteritis (EN-ter-IGH-tis) |
| erythr/o | red | erythrocyte (e-RITH-roh-sight) |
| esophag/o | esophagus | esophagectomy (eh-SAHF-a-JEK-toh-mee) |
| fasci/o | band; fibrous | fasciitis (fa-SIGH-tis) |
| gastr/o | stomach | gastrocele (GAS-troh-sel) |
| gingiv/o | gum | gingivitis (JIN-ji-VIGH-tis) |
| gloss/o | tongue | glossospasm (GLAHS-oh-spazm) |
| gluc/o, glyc/o | sugar; sweet | glycogen (GLIGH-koh-jehn) |
| gynec/o, gyn/o | woman | gynecology (GIGH-neh-KAHL-oh-jee) |
| hem/o, hemat/o, hema | blood | hematology (HEE-ma-TAHL-oh-jee) |
| hepat/o | liver | hepatitis (HEP-a-TIGH-tis) |
| hist/o | tissue | histology (his-TAHL-oh-jee) |
| home/o | same; similar | homeostasis (HOH-mee-oh-STAY-sis) |
| hydr/o | water | hydrophobia (HIGH-droh-FOH-bee-a) |
| hyster/o | uterus | hysterectomy (HIS-ter-EK-toh-mee) |
| icter/o | jaundice | icteric (ik-TER-ik) |
| idi/o | unknown; individual; distinct | idiopathic (ID-ee-oh-PATH-ik) |
| ile/o | ileum (part of the small intestine) | ileitis (IL-ee-IGH-tis) |
| kerat/o | cornea; scaly | keratotomy (KER-a-TAHT-oh-mee) |
| lact/o | milk | lactation (lak-TAY-shuhn) |
| lapar/o | abdomen | laparotomy (LAP-a-RAHT-oh-mee) |
| leuk/o | white | leukemia (loo-KEE-mee-a) |
| lingu/o | tongue | lingual (LING-gwal) |

**Table A**   Common word roots used in the medical field (continued)

| Common Word Roots | | |
|---|---|---|
| **Word Root** | **Meaning** | **Example** |
| lip/o | fat | liposuction (LIP-oh-SUHK-shuhn) |
| lith/o | stone | lithology (li-THAHL-oh-jee) |
| mast, mast/o | breast | mastitis (mas-TIGH-tis) |
| melan/o | black | melanoma (MEL-a-NOH-ma) |
| mening/o, meningi/o | membrane that surrounds the brain and spinal cord | meningitis (MEN-in-JIGH-tis) |
| mon/o | one; single | monocyte (MAHN-oh-sight) |
| myc/o | fungus | mycology (migh-KAHL-oh-jee) |
| myel/o | spinal cord; bone marrow | myelogram (MIGH-eh-loh-gram) |
| my/o | muscle | myopathy (migh-AHP-a-thee) |
| narc/o | stupor; sleep | narcotic (nar-KAHT-ik) |
| nas/o | nose | nasopharynx (NAY-zoh-FAIR-ingks) |
| necr/o | death | necropsy (NEK-rahp-see) |
| nephr/o | kidney | nephritis (ne-FRIGH-tis) |
| neur/o | nerve | neuritis (noo-RIGH-tis) |
| ocul/o | eye | oculist (AHK-yoo-list) |
| onc/o | tumor | oncology (ahng-KAHL-oh-jee) |
| oophor/o | ovary | oophorectomy (OH-ahf-oh-REK-toh-mee) |
| ophthalm/o | eye | ophthalmologist (AHF-thal-MAHL-ah-jist) |
| orch/o, orchi/o | testicle | orchiopexy (OR-kee-oh-PEK-see) |
| orth/o | straight | orthopedics (OR-thoh-PEE-diks) |
| oste/o | bone | osteoma (AHS-tee-OH-ma) |
| ot/o | ear | otology (oh-TAHL-ah-jee) |
| path/o | disease | pathologist (pa-THAHL-ah-jist) |
| ped/o (Latin) | foot | pedograph (PED-oh-graf) |

**Table A**    Common word roots used in the medical field (continued)

| Common Word Roots | | |
|---|---|---|
| *Word Root* | *Meaning* | *Example* |
| ped/o (Greek) | child | pediatrician (PEE-dee-a-TRISH-an) |
| pharyng/o | throat | pharyngoplasty (fa-RING-goh-PLAS-tee) |
| phleb/o | vein | phlebotomist (fle-BAHT-oh-mist) |
| phot/o | light | photolysis (foh-TAHL-i-sis) |
| pleur/o | relating to the pleura, a membrane that encompasses the lungs | pleurisy (PLOOR-i-see) |
| pneum/o, pneumon/o | air; lungs | pneumonia (noo-MOH-nee-a) |
| proct/o | rectum | proctoscope (PRAHK-toh-scohp) |
| psych/o | mind | psychologist (sigh-KAHL-ah-jist) |
| pulmon/o | lung | pulmonitis (POOL-moh-NIGH-tis) |
| pyel/o | renal pelvis | pyelonephritis (PIGH-eh-loh-neh-FRIGH-tis) |
| py/o | pus | pyogenic (PIGH-oh-JEN-ik) |
| rhin/o | nose | rhinopathy (righ-NAHP-a-thee) |
| salping/o | tube | salpingolysis (sal-ping-GAHL-i-sis) |
| scler/o- | hardening | scleroderma (SKLEH-roh-DER-ma) |
| semin/i | seed | seminal (SEM-i-nal) |
| seps/o | poison; infection | sepsis (SEP-sis) |
| somat/o | body | somatogenic (SOH-mat-oh-JEN-ik) |
| splen/o | spleen | splenomegaly (SPLEE-noh-MEG-a-lee) |
| thorac/o | chest | thoracotomy (THOH-ra-KAHT-ah-mee) |
| thromb/o | clot | thrombosis (thrahm-BOH-sis) |
| trache/o | trachea | tracheostomy (TRAY-kee-AHS-tah-mee) |
| ur/o, ur/i | urine | urology (yoo-RAHL-ah-jee) |
| vas/o, vascul/o | blood vessel | vasoconstriction (VA-soh-kahn-STRIK-shuhn) |

**Table A**   Common word roots used in the medical field (continued)

## Prefixes for Medical Terms

| Prefixes | Meaning | Example |
|----------|---------|---------|
| a-, an- | without; lack of; absent | asepsis (a-SEP-sis) |
| ab-, abs- | from; away | abscess (AB-ses) |
| ad- | near; toward | adrenal (a-DREE-nal) |
| ante- | before; forward | antenatal (AN-tee-NAY-tal) |
| anti- | against | antiseptic (AN-ti-SEP-tik) |
| auto- | self | autoimmune (AW-toh-i-MYOON) |
| bi- | two; twice | bicellular (bigh-SEL-yoo-lar) |
| brady- | slow | bradycardia (BRAD-ee-KAR-dee-a) |
| contra- | against; opposite | contraception (KAHN-tra-SEP-shuhn) |
| de- | lack of; down; away from | dehydration (DEE-high-DRAY-shuhn) |
| di- | two | dimorphic (digh-MOR-fik) |
| dia- | through; between | diarrhea (DIGH-a-REE-a) |
| dys- | painful; difficult | dysmenorrhea (DIS-men-oh-REE-a) |
| ecto- | outside | ectomorph (EK-toh-morf) |
| endo- | within; inner | endometrium (EN-doh-MEE-tree-uhm) |
| en- | in; inside | encapsulated (en-KAP-syoo-lay-ted) |
| epi- | upper; above | epiglottis (EP-i-GLAHT-is) |
| eu- | good; normal | euphoric (yoo-FOR-ik) |
| ex-, extra | out; away from | extrahepatic (EKS-tra-heh-PAT-ik) |
| hemi- | half | hemiplegia (HEM-ee-PLEE-jee-a) |
| hyper- | over; above; increased | hyperactive (high-peh-RAK-tiv) |
| hypo- | under; beneath; decreased | hypotension (HIGH-poh-TEN-shuhn) |
| inter- | between | intercostal (IN-ter-KAHS-tal) |

**Table B**   Prefixes used to form medical terms

| Prefixes for Medical Terms | | |
|---|---|---|
| *Prefixes* | *Meaning* | *Example* |
| intra- | within; into | intramuscular (IN-tra-MUHS-kyoo-lar) |
| macro- | large | macrocyte (MAK-roh-sight) |
| mal- | bad; poor | malabsorption (MAL-ab-SORP-shuhn) |
| mega- | large | megacephaly (MEG-a-SEF-a-lee) |
| meta- | change; beyond | metachromatic (MET-a-kroh-MAT-ik) |
| micro- | small | microscope (MIGH-kroh-skohp) |
| multi- | many | multi-infarct (in-FARKT) |
| neo- | new | neoplasm (NEE-oh-plazm) |
| pan- | all | pangenesis (pan-JEN-e-sis) |
| para- | alongside; abnormal | paraplegia (PAIR-a-PLEE-jee-a) |
| peri- | surrounding | pericarditis (PER-i-kar-DIGH-tis) |
| poly- | much; many | polycystic (PAHL-ee-SIS-tik) |
| post- | behind; after | postpartum (pohst-PAR-tuhm) |
| pre- | before; in front of | premenstrual (pree-MEN-stroo-al) |
| pseudo- | false | pseudotumor (SOO-doh-TOO-mer) |
| retro- | behind; backward | retrosternal (RET-roh-STER-nal) |
| semi- | half | semicircular (SEM-ee-SIR-kyoo-lar) |
| sub- | under; below | subacute (SUB-a-KYOOT) |
| supra- | upper; above | supraventricular (SOO-pra-ven-TRIK-yoo-lar) |
| tachy- | rapid | tachycardia (TAK-i-KAR-dee-a) |
| trans- | across; through | transfusion (trans-FYOO-zhuhn) |
| ultra- | beyond; excess | ultramicroscopic (UL-tra-migh-kroh-SKAHP-ik) |
| uni- | one | unicellular (YOO-ni-SEL-yoo-lar) |

**Table B**   Prefixes used to form medical terms (continued)

| Suffixes for Medical Terms | | |
|---|---|---|
| **Suffixes** | **Meaning** | **Example** |
| -algia | pain | neuralgia (noo-RAL-jee-a) |
| -cele | hernia | cystocele (SIS-toh-sel) |
| -cide | kill | germicide (JER-mi-sighd) |
| -crine | to secrete; separate | endocrine (EN-doh-krin) |
| -ectomy | removal; excision | hysterectomy (HIS-ter-EK-toh-mee) |
| -emia | blood condition | leukemia (loo-KEE-mee-a) |
| -esthesia | nervous sensation | anesthesia (AN-es-THEE-zee-a) |
| -form | resembling; in the shape of | auriform (AW-ri-form) |
| -gene, -genic | production, origin | neurogenic (NOO-roh-JEN-ik) |
| -gram | record | myelogram (MIGH-eh-loh-gram) |
| -graph | instrument for recording | cardiograph (KAR-dee-oh-graf) |
| -iasis | abnormal condition | cholelithiasis (KOH-lee-li-THIGH-a-sis) |
| -ism | process; condition | hyperthyroidism (high-per-THIGH-royd-izm) |
| -itis | inflammation of | appendicitis (a-PEN-di-SIGH-tis) |
| -lepsy | seizure | epilepsy (EP-i-LEP-see) |
| -logy | study (process of) | biology (bigh-AHL-oh-jee) |
| -lysis | breakdown; destruction | hemolysis (hee-MAHL-i-sis) |
| -mania | obsessive preoccupation | monomania (MAHN-oh-MAY-nee-a) |
| -megaly | enlargement | splenomegaly (SPLEE-noh-MEG-a-lee) |
| -meter | measure | thermometer (ther-MAHM-eh-ter) |
| -oma | tumor | lipoma (li-POH-ma) |
| -opia | vision | amblyopia (AM-blee-OH-pee-a) |

**Table C**   Suffixes used to form medical terms

| Suffixes for Medical Terms | | |
|---|---|---|
| *Suffixes* | *Meaning* | *Example* |
| -opsy | view | autopsy (AW-tahp-see) |
| -orexia | appetite | anorexia (AN-oh-REK-see-a) |
| -osis | condition; usually abnormal | neurosis (noo-ROH-sis) |
| -pathy | disease | arthropathy (ar-THRAHP-a-thee) |
| -penia | too few | leukopenia (LOO-koh-PEE-nee-a) |
| -phobia | fear | photophobia (FOH-toh-FOH-bee-a) |
| -plasm | formation | ectoplasm (EK-toh-plazm) |
| -plasty | operative revision | rhinoplasty (RIGH-noh-PLAS-tee) |
| -plegia | paralysis | hemiplegia (HEM-ee-PLEE-jee-a) |
| -renal | kidney | suprarenal (SOO-pra-REE-nal) |
| -rrhea | hemorrhage; flow | diarrhea (DIGH-a-REE-a) |
| -sclerosis | hardening | arteriosclerosis (ar-TER-ee-oh-skler-OH-sis) |
| -scope | instrument to examine | microscope (MIGH-kroh-skohp) |
| -scopy | visual examination | microscopy (migh-KRAHS-koh-pee) |
| -some | body | chromosome (KROH-moh-sohm) |
| -spasm | contraction | cardiospasm (KAR-dee-oh-spazm) |
| -stasis | stoppage | hemostasis (HEE-moh-STAY-sis) |
| -stomy | new opening | colostomy (koh-LAHS-toh-mee) |
| -tomy | process of cutting | lobotomy (loh-BAHT-oh-mee) |
| -type | picture; classification | genotype (JEN-oh-tighp) |
| -uria | urination; presence in the urine | hematuria (HEE-ma-TYOO-ree-a) |
| -y | process; condition | gastroenterology (GAS-troh-EN-ter-AHL-ah-jee) |

**Table C**   Suffixes used to form medical terms (continued)

# Chapter Review and Assessment

## Summary

The healthcare world uses its own language. Familiarizing yourself with medical prefixes, suffixes, word roots, the combining vowels, and the combining forms will help you succeed as a healthcare worker. Using common medical abbreviations is vital to understanding medical terminology.

Mastering medical terminology will also help students better understand the parts of the body, which are commonly divided into body systems. Body systems and their components can often be paired with medical specialties. Working in a particular medical specialty requires a healthcare worker to possess extra knowledge of that body system and its related terminology, diseases, and disorders.

It is also important to familiarize yourself with common diseases and disorders. Understanding the classifications of disease by cause, which include hereditary, congenital, environmental, nutritional, infectious, degenerative, or trauma-related, is helpful. Cancer is a prevalent disease that can affect all parts of the body. Early detection through recognition of the signs and symptoms of cancer is a key factor in successful treatment.

In addition to learning the basic word elements, healthcare professionals are often expected to learn terms related to body cavities, positions, directions, and planes. Such terms must be used properly to explain the exact location of a symptom or describe a patient's anatomy. Insurance forms require precise language about the patient's medical status.

Mastery of medical terminology takes study, repetition, and drills. Although proper medical terminology must be used when working with other medical professionals and filling out paperwork, remember that patients are probably not familiar with this language. Do not use medical language when explaining something to a patient. Instead, explain things using terms they can understand.

## Review Questions

*Answer the following questions using what you have learned in this chapter.*

### Short Answer

1. Identify the five word elements used in medical terminology.
2. Explain the purpose and use of prefixes and suffixes in medical terminology.
3. Why might a combining vowel be dropped when forming a medical term?
4. Why is it critical that all medical terms are spelled correctly in a patient's medical history?
5. Describe anatomical position.
6. What is an acronym?
7. Describe the sagittal, transverse, and coronal planes of the body.
8. Identify four diagnostic tests.
9. What is congenital disease?
10. Identify the differences between hepatitis A, B, and C.

### True or False

11. *True or False?* An epidemic is a disease that spreads rapidly and affects a large number of people.
12. *True or False?* A common way to classify disease is by cause.
13. *True or False?* Sickle cell anemia is an enviornmental disease.
14. *True or False?* All infectious diseases are transmitted from person to person.
15. *True or False?* A fetus is most vulnerable to disease during the first trimester.
16. *True or False?* Black lung disease is an example of an environmental disease.
17. *True or False?* The transverse plane divides the body into right and left sides.
18. *True or False?* Oncologists study and treat cancer.

## Multiple Choice

19. The red blood cells of patients with sickle cell anemia take on a(n) _____ shape.
    A. oblong
    B. crescent
    C. rectangular
    D. heart

20. The American Cancer Society lists the seven warning signs of cancer. Which of the following is not included in that list?
    A. acne
    B. nagging cough or hoarseness
    C. a sore that does not heal
    D. unusual bleeding or discharge

21. The five word elements used in medical terminology include prefixes, suffixes, _____.
    A. combining vowels, combining forms, and vocabulary terms
    B. word roots, combining vowels, and combining consonants
    C. word roots, combining vowels, and combining forms
    D. combining vowels, word roots, and plural forms

22. A(n) _____ is a specialist in nervous system diseases.
    A. nephrologist
    B. endocrinologist
    C. orthopedist
    D. neurologist

23. The suffix _____ means "inflammation of."
    A. -osis
    B. -cide
    C. -rrhea
    D. -itis

24. When in Fowler's position, the patient is _____.
    A. lying on his or her back, with the head of the bed raised about 45°, and knees elevated
    B. standing erect and facing forward with arms at the sides and palms facing forward
    C. lying face up
    D. lying on his or her side

25. Which of the following terms means "toward the front"?
    A. posterior
    B. superior
    C. dorsal
    D. anterior

26. The prefix _____ means "bad" or "poor."
    A. *tachy-*
    B. *pseudo-*
    C. *ecto-*
    D. *mal-*

27. Inferior means _____.
    A. "closer to the feet"
    B. "on the belly side"
    C. "close to the head"
    D. "limb movement toward the body"

28. The suffix *-osis* means _____.
    A. "origin"
    B. "formation"
    C. "view of"
    D. "abnormal condition"

## Critical Thinking Exercises

29. After studying medical terminology, what do you feel is the most difficult part of learning this new language? What can you do to overcome any obstacles to learning?

30. How might the use of abbreviations lead to errors in a healthcare facility?

31. Research a specific type of cancer online. How does the incidence of cancer differ between men and women? What are the signs and symptoms of this particular disease?

32. Research the incidence of sexually transmitted infection in your area. Make a bar graph showing the different STIs and the number of reported cases. Why do you think one disease might be more prevalent than another?

33. Research the seven different causes of disease listed in this chapter. Describe a disease in each category that was not discussed in this chapter. Discuss not only the cause of the disease, but also the symptoms and prognosis (likely outcome). Can anything be done to prevent these diseases?

# *Additional Practice*

## Defining Medical Terms

*Identify the meaning of the following prefixes, suffixes, and word roots.*

1. acr/o
2. chrom/o
3. -pathy
4. ot/o
5. path/o
6. -stomy
7. -scopy
8. -tomy
9. onc/o-
10. -penia
11. tachy-
12. ultra-
13. uni-
14. py/o
15. hyper-
16. hypo-
17. myc/o
18. -opsy
19. -osis
20. idi/o

## Singular or Plural Endings

*Identify the plural form of the following medical terms.*

21. thorax
22. appendix
23. metastasis
24. cardiologist
25. bursa
26. phalanx
27. ovum
28. artery
29. ganglion
30. vein

*Identify the singular form of the following medical terms.*

31. nuclei
32. lipomata
33. ganglia
34. biopsies
35. atria

## Medical Terms and Abbreviations

*Provide the equivalent medical term or abbreviation for each English term or phrase provided.*

36. removal of a breast
37. removal of an ovary
38. inflammation of the liver
39. red blood cell
40. white blood cell
41. abbreviation for heart attack
42. abbreviation for cancer
43. a doctor who treats women
44. removal of a gallbladder
45. acquired immune deficiency

*Provide the meaning of the following abbreviations.*

46. CPR
47. D&C
48. CA
49. Ca
50. CCU
51. QID
52. T&A
53. FBS
54. g
55. OB/GYN

## Medical Specialties

*Match the medical specialty with its description.*

56. a doctor who treats infants and children

57. a physician who treats diseases of the eye

58. a doctor who specializes in the nervous system

59. a doctor who treats newborns

60. one who treats the skin

61. a doctor who specializes in the gastrointestinal system

62. a doctor who specializes in disorders of the ears, nose, and throat

63. a physician who specializes in the cardiovascular system

64. a physician who treats the elderly

65. a physician who specializes in the skeletal system

A. gerontologist
B. gastroenterologist
C. otolaryngologist
D. orthopedist
E. pediatrician
F. neurologist
G. cardiologist
H. dermatologist
I. ophthalmologist
J. neonatologist

## Spelling Challenge

*Correct the spelling of these medical terms.*

66. carsinoma

67. melignent

68. kneeoplasm

69. meocardial infraction

70. cutetaneous

71. elektrokardiogram

72. Fouler's position

73. hepatytus

74. jerryatrics

75. peteiatrics

## Terms Related to Disease

*Match each medical term with its meaning.*

76. non-cancerous

77. long-lasting disease

78. a disease confined to a certain area of the body

79. cancerous

80. disease affecting an unusually large number of the population

81. a disease of sudden onset and short duration

82. prediction of the probable outcome of a disease

83. act of determining the cause of a disease

A. chronic
B. acute
C. pandemic
D. prognosis
E. diagnosis
F. localized
G. benign
H. malignant

# Chapter

# Science

## Terms to Know

lymph

anatomy
antibody
antigen
bone marrow
cell membrane
central nervous system
   (CNS)
chromosome
cytoplasm
deoxyribonucleic acid
   (DNA)
differentiation
endocrine glands
homeostasis
hormones
human reproduction
hypothesis
immunity
joints
ligaments

lymphocyte
metabolism
nucleus
organs
peripheral nervous
   system (PNS)
pH scale
phagocytosis
physiology
puberty
respiration
science
scientific method
sexually transmitted
   infection (STI)
stem cells
tendons
tissues

## Chapter Objectives

- Define *science.*
- Identify the six steps of the scientific method and understand how the process can be used to solve a problem.
- Identify categories of science that are relevant to healthcare.
- Define *anatomy* and *physiology.*
- Describe basic parts of the human cell.
- Identify how cancer cells differ from normal cells.
- Discuss the importance of the discovery of DNA.
- Explain the difference between cells, tissues, organs, and body systems.
- Identify the body systems discussed in this chapter, including their main organs and representative diseases.
- Explain the significance of Maslow's hierarchy of needs.
- Identify the four types of growth and development that occur in every life stage.
- Discuss the various life stages of the human being.
- Describe some specialties related to life stages.

Reinforce your learning with additional online resources
- **Practice** vocabulary with flashcards and interactive games
- **Assess** with posttests and image labeling
- **Expand** with activities and animations

www.g-wlearning.com/healthsciences

Companion
G-W Learning

**Study on the Go**
Use a mobile device to practice vocabulary terms and review with self-assessment quizzes.

www.m.g-wlearning.com

Mobile
G-W Learning

# Studying Science

What is **science**? How does it apply to healthcare careers? Science is a system of acquiring knowledge through observation and experimentation to describe the natural world.

Modern medicine is based on well-established laws, principles, and practical findings in many scientific areas of study, including chemistry, physics, biology, anatomy, and physiology. Pursuing a career in the healthcare field means that, in most cases, you have been exposed to many science courses throughout your education.

Depending on the career that you choose, you may study disciplines that fall into the category of the natural sciences. The natural sciences comprise disciplines that study the physical world, including biology, physics, chemistry, and geology, but excluding social sciences and the abstract sciences such as mathematics.

## Science Disciplines Related to Healthcare

There are numerous disciplines, or specialized areas, that fall under the broad category of science. Many science courses are relevant when studying for a career in healthcare. Whether you are hoping to go into the research field in an effort to discover new medical uses for lasers, or you want to work in the financial office of a hospital, you will encounter science disciplines. Depending on the type of degree you wish to pursue, you will be required to take at least two or three science courses (Figure 9.1). These courses may include anatomy and physiology, biology, chemistry, botany, bioengineering, health sciences, physics, or computer science.

Education for most healthcare careers focuses on how the human body works (or animal bodies, in the case of veterinary medicine). Studying the inner workings of the human body will help you provide patients with the proper care—analyzing medical records, treating wounds, or administering medication. Knowing how your body works will improve your ability to maintain good health. This knowledge will also help you be an educated partner to your physician when solving potential health problems in the future.

# The Scientific Method

In order to derive conclusions about the world around them, scientists use the **scientific method** to logically formulate, test, and evaluate a problem or hypothesis. A **hypothesis** is an idea or a suggestion often intended to explain something, the cause of which is unknown.

The application of the scientific method has resulted in many medical discoveries. These discoveries relate to the functions of the human body; diagnosis and treatment of disease; as well as the development of new drugs and machines used in patient care. Physicians use the scientific method to arrive at diagnoses and to determine the appropriate treatment to use.

**science**
*system of acquiring knowledge through observation and experimentation to describe the natural world*

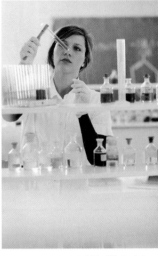

*dotshock/Shutterstock.com*

**Figure 9.1** Developing a strong science background will be beneficial in your future healthcare career.

**scientific method**
*a method designed to logically formulate, test, and evaluate a problem or hypothesis*

**hypothesis**
*an idea or a suggestion often developed to explain something, the cause of which is unknown*

Medical advances such as new surgical procedures and vaccines have been made by applying the scientific method. The scientific method can be used for problem solving in school or at work. The scientific method may also be helpful when evaluating information found on the Internet, in newspapers, or given to you by friends or coworkers.

## The History of the Scientific Method

No one person can be said to have invented the scientific method. Elements of this method can be traced back to ancient people who found it to be a natural way of obtaining reliable knowledge. The accomplishments of the individuals listed below contributed to the development of the scientific method:

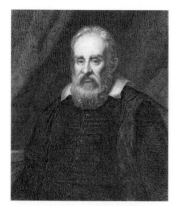

*Georgios Kollidas/Shutterstock.com*

**Figure 9.2**   Galileo Galilei

- Aristotle (384–322 BCE), a Greek philosopher who is one of history's great thinkers, worked to find reliable knowledge by studying phenomena, or observable facts and events.
- Roger Bacon (1214–1294) was an English philosopher and Franciscan friar. Bacon was influenced by writings of Muslim scientists. He described a cycle of observation, hypothesis, experimentation, and verification that led to many important discoveries.
- Galileo Galilei (1564–1642) was an Italian physicist, mathematician, astronomer, and philosopher (Figure 9.2). He is often described as the father of the scientific method because he put together pieces of the method that were developed by others. Galileo developed a system that combined observation, hypothesis, mathematical deduction (starting from a broad idea and narrowing the idea down to a hypothesis), and confirmation.
- Francis Bacon (1561–1626), an English philosopher, statesman, scientist, and author, played a very important role in the advancement of scientific thought (Figure 9.3). Bacon proposed a research method called *induction*—reasoning that moves from specific observations to broader generalizations. Bacon also urged scientists to keep records of experiments and exchange data to share newly discovered knowledge.

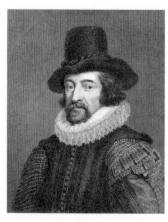

*Georgios Kollidas/Shutterstock.com*

**Figure 9.3**   Frances Bacon

- René Descartes (1596–1650) was a French philosopher, mathematician, and physicist (Figure 9.4). Descartes developed the use of mathematical methods in scientific inquiry. His goal was to add elements of precision and certainty to many fields of study.

Thanks to these great thinkers, and many who followed, the world has a framework for developing and executing scientific investigation that produces accurate and reliable findings. The medical field, in particular, has benefitted greatly from the development of the scientific method.

Other intellectuals who helped to refine the scientific method include Sir Isaac Newton, Charles Darwin, Albert Einstein, and Benjamin Franklin.

# Using the Scientific Method

The six steps of the scientific method are initiated by asking a question. Each step is listed below, along with an example that highlights how the scientific method can be applied in an everyday situation.

1. **The question**: The goal of research using the scientific method is to find an answer to an important question. The question should be worthwhile and able to be answered through the collection and analysis of data.

   > During a fishing trip, Brandon slips while climbing down to the river and twists his ankle. The experience is painful, causing Brandon to ask, "What have I done to my ankle?"

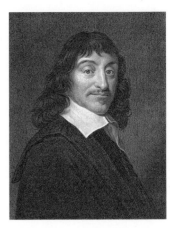

*Georgios Kollidas/Shutterstock.com*

**Figure 9.4** René Descartes

2. **Hypothesis**: A hypothesis is an educated guess as to what your research will reveal about the question you have asked. By the end of the process, a hypothesis will either be confirmed or rejected.

   > Brandon suspects that he has sprained his ankle.

3. **Research and collecting data**: Research involves recording observations and collecting data to determine whether your hypothesis is accurate.

   > Because Brandon is out of town and cannot consult his family physician, he decides to treat the sprain by icing his ankle. The ice seems to help, and Brandon wraps his ankle securely with a bandage to prevent the ankle from moving. At this point, Brandon's assumption that his ankle is sprained seems to be reasonable.

4. **Interpreting the data**: Examine the collected data and establish whether it is sufficient to begin determining the result of your study. If not, further research may be required to come to an accurate result and conclusion.

   > Two weeks have passed since the accident and Brandon continues to have ankle pain. The swelling in his ankle has increased, and Brandon finds it difficult to walk. Brandon decides to visit a local clinic to have the ankle evaluated.

5. **Results**: After collecting and interpreting the data, it is possible to determine the results of a study. Was the hypothesis confirmed? Did the interpretation of the data collected reveal that it was incorrect?

   > An X-ray shows that Brandon has a cracked bone in his ankle. His original ankle sprain hypothesis was proven false and rejected.

6. **Conclusion:** The conclusion of a study consists of a concise statement expressing the key findings of the study.

   > Surgery is immediately performed on Brandon's ankle to repair the broken bone. A plate is attached to the bone to prevent it from shifting its position.

Scientists working to solve healthcare problems often use the scientific method. These scientists are asking questions related to the diagnosis and treatment of disease, as well as developing safe drug therapies and diagnostic machines for their patients. After drawing conclusions and either rejecting or confirming their hypothesis based on their use of the scientific method, scientists often share their results with others. Such communication can inspire additional experiments and often results in exciting discoveries in healthcare.

 *Check Your Understanding*

Think of a problem that could be solved by using the scientific method. Divide a piece of paper into two columns. In the left column, list the six steps of the scientific method. In the right column, follow the example of Brandon's sprained ankle and use the steps to solve your problem.

# *Human Anatomy and Physiology*

Figure 9.5 illustrates components that make up the human body. Each component is critical to understanding how the body functions. **Anatomy** is the study of the structure of the body. **Physiology** involves the study of the function of the body. The first body component discussed will be the smallest—the human cell.

## Cells

The human body is built on a foundation composed of approximately five trillion microscopic cells. Cells vary according to their specific function. Bone, muscle, skin, and blood are made up of different types of cells, a phenomenon called **differentiation**. Cells can be flat, round, irregularly shaped, or threadlike. All cells can reproduce, use oxygen, utilize nutrients, produce energy, eliminate wastes, and maintain their shape.

As Figure 9.6 shows, the human cell has several components. With the exception of mature red blood cells, all human cells have a **nucleus**. The nucleus is the "brain" of the cell that directs all of its activities. Inside of the nucleus are 23 paired (46 total) **chromosomes** that contain genetic information, or *deoxyribonucleic acid* (DNA).

Every cell is held together by an outer layer called the **cell membrane**. The cell membrane is selectively permeable, meaning it controls what enters and exits the cell. Inside of every cell is the **cytoplasm**, a transparent, gel-like substance that is usually composed of 70–90% water and houses all of the organelles, the microscopic functional units of the cell. Structures such as the mitochondria and ribosomes are organelles; each performs a specific function in the cell.

**anatomy**
*the study of the structure of the body*

**physiology**
*the study of the function of the body*

**differentiation**
*process through which cells of the body vary according to their specific function*

**nucleus**
*the "brain" of a cell; directs all activities and contains genetic information*

**chromosome**
*threadlike structure found in the nucleus of most living cells; carries genetic information*

**cell membrane**
*the outer layer of a cell that holds the cell together*

**cytoplasm**
*transparent, gel-like substance inside of every cell; cellular activities occur here*

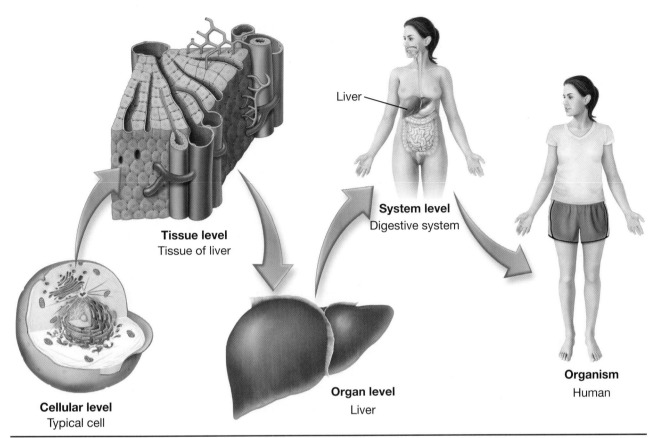

**Tissue level**
Tissue of liver

**System level**
Digestive system

**Organism**
Human

Liver

**Cellular level**
Typical cell

**Organ level**
Liver

**Figure 9.5** From the smallest cell to the most complex organ system, each component of the human body plays an important role in making the body function.

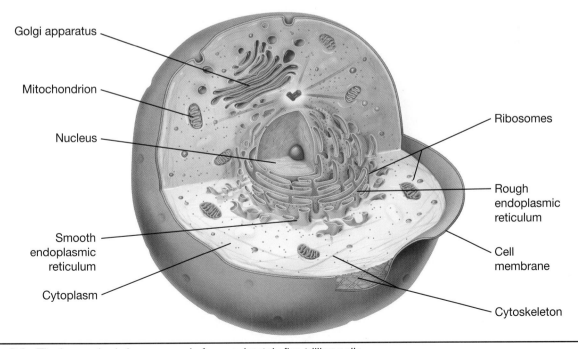

Golgi apparatus

Mitochondrion

Nucleus

Ribosomes

Rough endoplasmic reticulum

Smooth endoplasmic reticulum

Cell membrane

Cytoplasm

Cytoskeleton

**Figure 9.6** The human body is composed of approximately five trillion cells.

---
**Extend Your Knowledge**

*What's in a Cell?*

Organelles are all of the structures within the cell's cytoplasm. Organelles help to carry out the life processes in the cell. Research the organelles shown in Figure 9.6 and create a table that describes the function of each.

---

**deoxyribonucleic acid (DNA)**
*genetic material shaped like a double helix; part of all living cells*

**stem cells**
*cells in the body that evolve into specific cells in a particular organ system*

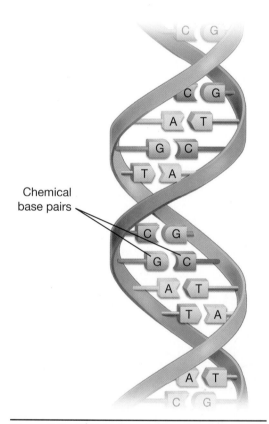

Chemical base pairs

**Figure 9.7**   DNA is described as the *molecule of life.*

## Deoxyribonucleic Acid (DNA)

**Deoxyribonucleic acid**, or *DNA*, is found in every cell of the human body. DNA is shaped like a twisting ladder composed of chemical base pairs, called a *double helix* (Figure 9.7).

DNA resides on chromosomes in the nucleus of a cell, sections of which are called *genes*. The structure of DNA was not known until James Watson, an American scientist, and Francis Crick, a British researcher, discovered the famous double helix. This was a major scientific breakthrough.

In 2003, the Human Genome Project, an international research initiative, successfully mapped the DNA sequence of a human, known as the *human genome*. Mapping the human genome allows researchers to better understand the genetic factor of human disease. Researchers identified and mapped approximately 20,000 to 25,000 genes located on the DNA helix. This development may enable researchers to discover damaged genes causing genetic disorders and, hopefully, eliminate those disorders.

## Stem Cells

All cells in the body begin as undifferentiated **stem cells**. Stem cells mature into differentiated cells, meaning that they evolve to function in a particular organ system. For example, white blood cells develop to fight infection, while mature red blood cells carry oxygen and carbon dioxide through the body.

After an embryo develops, adult stem cells can be found throughout the human body. Stem cells have been found in tissues such as the brain, bone marrow, blood, blood vessels, and the skin.

## Tissue

**tissues**
*groups of cells that work together to accomplish the same task*

Just as there are many different kinds of cells in the human body, there is also an assortment of **tissues** of various shapes and sizes. Body tissues are groups of cells that work together to accomplish the same task. There are four types of tissues:

- connective tissue
- epithelial tissue
- muscle tissue
- nervous tissue

## Connective Tissue

Connective tissue helps hold body parts together. The most common of all body tissues, connective tissue is found in bones, organs, muscles, nerves, and skin. Connective tissue holds body parts together by forming fine webs of tissue that provide support and structure.

Connective tissue is composed of collagen fibers and elastic fibers. Collagen fibers are densely packed, and are arranged in a parallel construction to provide the tissue strength. Elastic fibers enable connective tissue to stretch.

**Cartilage.** An example of connective tissue is cartilage. Cartilage is a flexible connective tissue found in the rib cage, the ear, the nose, the bronchial tubes, and the joints between bones. Cartilage is not as hard and rigid as bone, but is stiffer and less flexible than muscle.

## Epithelial Tissue

Epithelial tissue covers the external and internal body surfaces. The skin consists of epithelial tissue. The linings of internal organs are made of this tissue as well.

## Muscle Tissue

Muscle tissue allows the body to move. The three kinds of muscle tissue are skeletal, cardiac, and smooth muscle. Skeletal muscle is attached to bones and facilitates movement by contracting and relaxing. The walls of the heart are composed of cardiac muscle, while the walls of other organs are composed of smooth muscle.

## Nervous Tissue

Nervous tissue reaches all parts of the body but is concentrated in the spinal cord and brain. Nervous tissue can be likened to a messenger sending messages throughout the body. Neurons—cells found in nervous tissue—are responsible for generating, sending, and receiving electrical signals (or messages) to all parts of the body.

# Organs

As tissues are groups of similar cells, **organs** are two or more groups of tissues working together. Every organ in the human body performs one or more specific functions. For example, the stomach is made up of connective, epithelial, muscle, and nervous tissue. Although there is typically only one of each organ, some organs occur in pairs, such as the kidneys or the lungs.

**organs**
*two or more groups of tissues working together to perform specific functions*

### *Real Life Scenario*

#### *Finding an Organ Donor*

Kim's kidneys have failed and her doctor has put her on hemodialysis, a treatment that simulates the work of the kidneys by mechanically filtering waste from the blood.

Kim needs a kidney transplant, and both her sister and brother are willing to donate one of their kidneys to Kim. To do so, they must go through a procedure known as *tissue typing* to determine if their tissues are compatible with Kim's, a quality called *histocompatibility*.

Tissue typing examines the antigens found on the surface of cells found in kidney tissue. Antigens are molecules found on cells that react to foreign molecules, triggering a response that can lead to organ rejection. A donor's antigens must match the recipient's antigens for an organ transplant to be successful.

To test for histocompatibility, blood is drawn and tests are performed on the blood cells to determine compatibility. In Kim's case, her sister was a compatible donor, and Kim received a healthy kidney.

The only transplant that does not require tissue typing is a corneal transplant. A cornea (the transparent, dome-shaped tissue that covers the iris and pupil of the eye) does not have its own blood supply, and therefore lacks antigens that may cause a negative response or rejection.

Some organs are called *vital organs*. Vital organs are those without which the human body cannot survive. These organs include the brain, heart, liver, and lungs (you must have at least one functioning lung to survive). Organs that you *can* live without are called *non-vital organs*. These include the appendix, gallbladder, and spleen.

**Did You Know?**

#### *Living with One Kidney or Lung*

Did you know that you can live successfully with only one lung or one kidney? For example, some people are only born with a single kidney (in this case, the left kidney is often missing). When one organ of the pair is missing, the remaining kidney or lung increases in size and compensates for the loss of the other organ.

## *The Body Systems*

Human body functions are controlled by groups of organs known as the *body systems*. A body system consists of organs that work together to accomplish a more complex task than a single organ can perform. For example, the urinary system removes wastes, controls the body's fluid balance, and ensures electrolyte balance in the blood. (Electrolytes are a mixture of sodium, potassium, chloride, and biocarbonate ions that affect metabolic processes of the body.) To accomplish these tasks, the kidneys eliminate wastes and substances that may upset fluid and electrolyte balance. Waste and other substances cannot be removed without the cooperation of the kidneys, bladder, urethra, and ureters.

If one organ is not functioning properly, the entire system, or even the body as a whole, will be affected. An example of this is a poorly functioning heart. When the heart is not functioning properly, insufficient amounts of blood is pumped to the lungs to gather oxygen. This means that the rest of the body does not get proper amounts of oxygen. In this case, the failure of one organ may cause oxygen deprivation throughout the entire body.

Each of the body systems plays an important role in maintaining **homeostasis**. Homeostasis is a state of internal balance achieved by adjusting the physiological systems of the body. Individudal systems work to achieve homeostasis, but sometimes homeostasis cannot be maintained without two body systems working together. All body systems are related and some body systems overlap, such as the endocrine and reproductive systems, which share organs like the ovaries and testes.

**homeostasis**
*state of internal balance achieved by adjusting the physiological systems of the body*

## The Integumentary System

The integumentary system covers and protects the body. Functions of the integumentary system include

- regulation of body temperature;
- production of vitamin D from sunlight;
- excretion of minor amounts of waste materials in sweat; and
- transmission of sensory information for pain, touch, pressure, and temperature.

The integumentary system includes the skin, sebaceous glands, sweat glands, fingernails, and hair.

### *The Skin*

The skin is the largest organ in the body. The average adult body has almost 21 square feet of skin. The skin has three layers of tissue (Figure 9.8):

1. **Epidermis.** The visible layer of skin, the epidermis, lacks blood vessels and nerve cells. Everyday activities such as bathing and moving around cause the body to shed about 500 million cells of the epidermis each day. These cells must continuously replace themselves.

2. **Dermis.** Located below the epidermis, the dermis is a layer of dense, irregular, connective tissue. Capillaries, muscles, nerve endings, hair follicles, sweat glands, and sebaceous (oil) glands can all be found in the dermis. This layer helps your skin move with you. Age and frequent suntanning decrease the dermis' firmness.

3. **Subcutaneous.** This layer of skin (the epidermis and dermis are the cutaneous layers) is primarily composed of lipocytes (or *fat cells*), which manufacture and store large amounts of fat. This skin layer is important because it protects deeper tissues of the body, acts as a heat insulator, and stores energy.

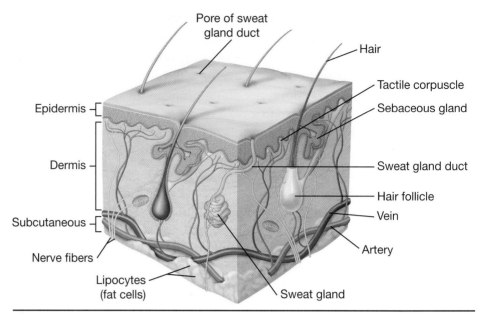

**Figure 9.8** The skin covers and protects the entire body.

**Sebaceous Glands.** Visible only by microscope, these small glands are responsible for depositing an oily secretion on the hairs that cover the skin. They are found in all parts of the skin covered by hair, with the exception of the soles of the feet and palms of the hands. The acidic nature of these glands helps destroy some pathogens on the skin's surface. The oily secretion of sebaceous glands also keeps the skin from drying out.

**Sweat Glands.** Sweat glands, also referred to as *sudoriferous glands*, play an important role in regulating body temperature. There are two types of sweat glands: *apocrine* and *eccrine*. Apocrine sweat glands secrete sweat at the hair follicles in the groin, anal regions, and armpits. Eccrine sweat glands are located all over the skin, being more prominent on the palms, feet, forehead, and upper lip.

### Hair and Fingernails

Body hair doesn't just contribute to our physical appearance, it also serves several important purposes. Body hair helps regulate body temperature, functioning as a sensor to detect skin changes. Hair in the nose helps to filter out dust and other small particles, while the eyelashes protect our eyes from foreign objects.

Both hair and fingernails are composed of the protein *keratin*. As specialized epithelial cells grow out and over the nail bed, they become keratin. The *cuticle* of the nail is a fold of tissue at the nail root. The nails' pinkish color comes from blood vessels beneath them, while the half-moon shaped area is a result of a thicker layer of cells at the nails' base.

There are many diseases and disorders associated with the integumentary system. Some of these include eczema, dermatitis, psoriasis, and skin cancer. There are also various diseases associated with a virus that affect the integumentary system. These diseases are commonly known as *chicken pox*, *shingles*, *cold sores*, *genital herpes*, and *human papilloma virus (HPV)*.

## The Musculoskeletal System

Together, the skeletal and muscular systems form the framework that holds the human body together. While these systems are sometimes considered separately, they are known collectively as the musculoskeletal system. The musculoskeletal system consists of bones, joints, and muscles.

### Bones

The skeleton is composed mainly of bones, as well as cartilage and joints (Figure 9.9). There are four types of bones:

- **Long bones.** These bones are longer than they are wide. Long bones are found in arms and legs.
- **Short bones.** About the same size in length and width, short bones are mostly found in ankles and wrists.
- **Flat bones.** These bones are thinner than both short and long bones. These bones can be flat or curved and are plate-like in appearance. Examples of flat bones include the skull, sternum (or *breastbone*), and ribs.
- **Irregular bones.** These are odd-shaped bones that do not fit into the other bone categories. These bones are needed to connect other bones. Examples of irregular bones are vertebrae (found in the spinal column) and coxal (hip) bones.

Long bones are covered with a tough, fibrous connective tissue called *periosteum*. Periosteum contains blood vessels to provide nutrients to the bone cells. Each bone has bulbous ends called *epiphyses*. The region between two bone ends, or *shaft* of the bone, is called the *diaphysis*. The diaphysis is hollow and acts as a storage area for **bone marrow**. Bone marrow is soft, blood-forming tissue that comes in two types—yellow and red. Yellow marrow stores fat, while red bone marrow is needed for the production of blood cells.

**bone marrow**
*soft, spongy, blood-forming tissue found inside bones*

**Did You Know?** *How Many Bones are in the Human Body?*

The average adult human has 206 bones in her body. An infant can have between 300 and 350 bones at birth. Some of these bones fuse together as the infant grows. When some bones fuse and become one bone (such as the bones that comprise the skull), the total number of bones drops to 206.

The human body continues to build new bone tissue throughout a person's life, but also constantly tears down old bone. *Osteoblasts* are specialized cells that form bones. *Osteoclasts* tear down bone material and help move calcium and phosphate into the blood.

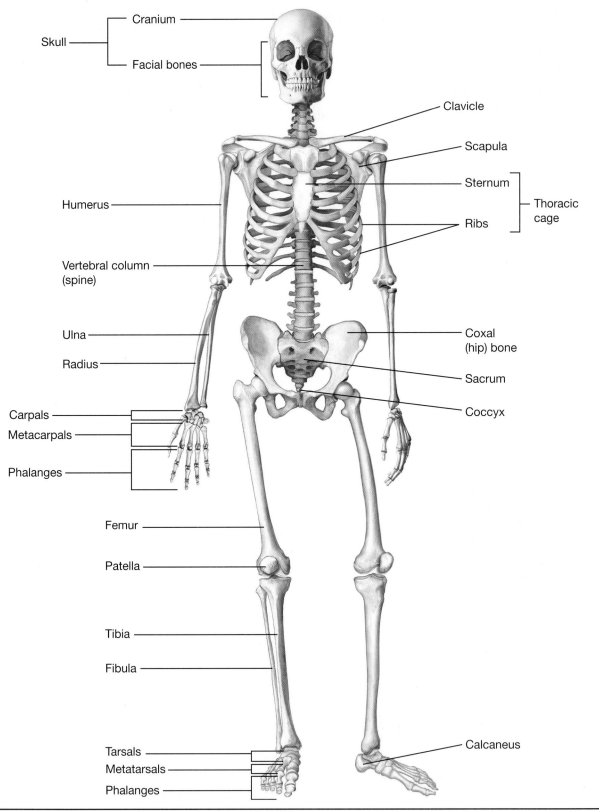

**Figure 9.9** The human skeleton is composed of two parts—the appendicular and axial skeleton (shown here in red). Bones of the axial skeleton provide support, while the appendicular bones provide movement of the appendages.

About 10% of the body's bone tissue is torn down and rebuilt each year. This process of breaking down and rebuilding bone (called *bone remodeling*) continues into a person's 40s with no net gain or loss of bone mass. In later life, bone loss can outweigh bone growth.

Exercise is one of the best ways to slow bone loss and prevent muscle, bone, or joint problems. A moderate exercise program can help the body maintain strength and flexibility and the bones stay strong. A well-balanced diet with adequate amounts of calcium is especially important. Women in particular must be careful to get enough calcium and vitamin D as they age to avoid osteoporosis, a disease characterized by softening of the bones.

Breaks in a bone are called *fractures*. Fractures are common injuries associated with the skeletal system. Four of the common classifications of fractures are greenstick, stress, comminuted, and spiral. Scoliosis, an abnormal lateral curvature of the spine, is another disorder associated with the bones.

**Think It Through**
Research the various fractures mentioned in the text. What factors influence the type and severity of a fracture? Are some bones more susceptible to certain types of fractures? If so, why?

## Joints

Without **joints**, or *articulations*, the human body could not move. When two or more bones come together, a joint is formed. Joints are held together by connective tissue called **ligaments**. Ligaments are tough, white bands that connect bone to bone. **Tendons** attach muscles to bones.

There are several types of joints:
- **Amphiarthroses.** These joints move only slightly; for example, the joints between vertebrae in your spine are amphiarthroses joints.
- **Synarthroses.** Joints that do not move are synarthroses joints. The fibrous joints between the skull bones are an example of synarthroses.
- **Synovial joints.** These joints are covered with a membrane that contains a fluid lubricant, making movement easy. Hip and knee joints are synovial joints.

Joint pain or injury can be attributed to several diseases or disorders. Joint dislocation, arthritis, and bursitis are some conditions related to the joints.

**joints**
*physical point of connection between two bones; articulation*

**ligaments**
*tough bands of fibrous tissue that connect bone to bone*

**tendons**
*fibrous tissues that connect muscles to bone*

## Muscles

There are more than 600 individual muscles in the human body. Figure 9.10 shows a selection of these muscles. Muscles account for about 40% of the total body weight of an adult human. Muscles usually act in groups to help the body move. There are three types of muscles in the human body:
1. Cardiac muscles control the contractions of the heart.
2. Smooth muscles facilitate movements that we do not control. These muscles are *involuntary muscles* that move the organs and systems of the body, such as the digestive system.
3. Skeletal muscles can move at our will and are also called *voluntary muscles*. These muscles are responsible for the movement of the skeletal system.

Common muscle-related diseases include fibromyalgia and muscular dystrophy. The muscles can also suffer from strain, contusion, cramps, delayed-onset muscle soreness (DOMS), tendinitis, and shin splints.

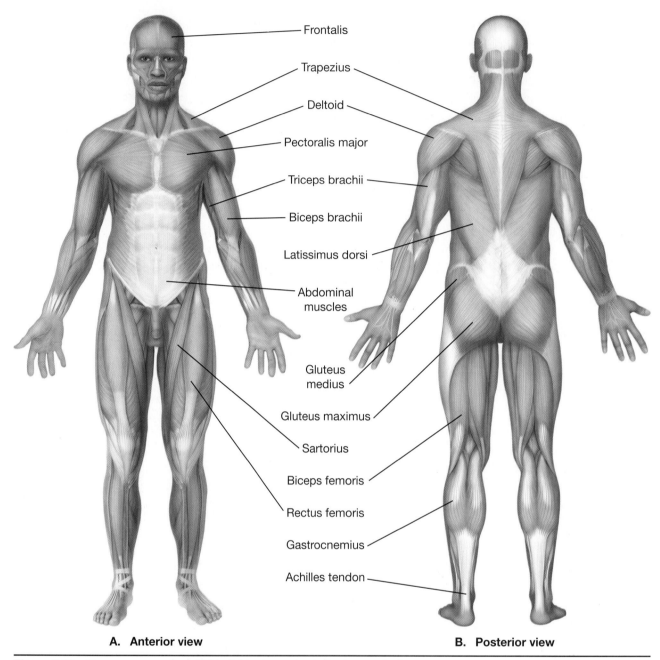

**A. Anterior view**    **B. Posterior view**

Frontalis
Trapezius
Deltoid
Pectoralis major
Triceps brachii
Biceps brachii
Latissimus dorsi
Abdominal muscles
Gluteus medius
Gluteus maximus
Sartorius
Biceps femoris
Rectus femoris
Gastrocnemius
Achilles tendon

**Figure 9.10**    There are more than 600 individual muscles in the human body.

## The Nervous System

The nervous system directs the functions of all other body systems through nerve impulses generated by neurons, or *nerve cells*, located throughout the body. The nervous system contains two parts—the **central nervous system (CNS)** and the **peripheral nervous system (PNS)** (Figure 9.11).

Dementia, Alzheimer's disease, epilepsy, multiple sclerosis, Parkinson's disease, cerebral palsy, cardiovascular accident (stroke), and meningitis are all diseases or disorders of the nervous system.

**central nervous system (CNS)**

*part of the nervous system that includes the brain and the spinal cord*

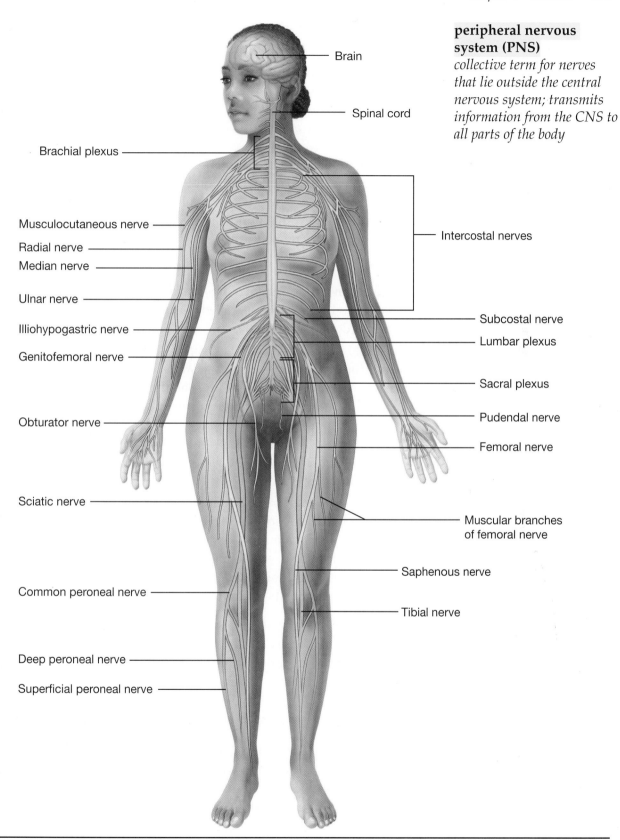

Brain

Spinal cord

Brachial plexus

Musculocutaneous nerve

Radial nerve

Median nerve

Ulnar nerve

Illiohypogastric nerve

Genitofemoral nerve

Obturator nerve

Sciatic nerve

Common peroneal nerve

Deep peroneal nerve

Superficial peroneal nerve

**peripheral nervous system (PNS)**
*collective term for nerves that lie outside the central nervous system; transmits information from the CNS to all parts of the body*

Intercostal nerves

Subcostal nerve

Lumbar plexus

Sacral plexus

Pudendal nerve

Femoral nerve

Muscular branches of femoral nerve

Saphenous nerve

Tibial nerve

**Figure 9.11** Together, the CNS and PNS direct the functions of all other body systems.

### Neurons

The CNS and PNS work together to send messages that direct all of our body movements and functions to the brain. These messages are carried to the correct areas of the brain by neurons. All activity in the body is controlled by more than 100 billion neurons throughout the body.

Neurons produce an electrical impulse that moves down the extension of the nerve cell, or the *axon*. Dendrites extend out from the neuron's cell body and stimulate the neuron by collecting and responding to different types of stimuli. The axon is surrounded by a protective myelin sheath, which affects the rate at which electrical transmissions travel through the neuron. There is a terminal bundle at the end of the axon that sends nerve impulses to neighboring neurons.

### The Central Nervous System (CNS)

The central nervous system (CNS) is made up of the brain and the spinal cord. Three thin layers of tissue, called *meninges*, cover and protect the brain and spinal cord. The bones of the spinal column also protect the spinal cord.

The spinal cord is considered a "super-highway" for information coming to and from the central nervous system. Nerves of the spinal cord convey messages to and from the brain. The thalamus, an important part of the brain, relays sensory messages between the brain and spinal cord. The spinal cord extends from the brain stem and passes through the spinal column. Injury to the spinal cord can result in paralysis and the loss of voluntary muscle function.

Many important structures of the brain contribute to the function of the CNS (Figure 9.12). For example, the hypothalamus—a small gland that works as part of both the CNS and endocrine system—exercises control over the pituitary gland and body functions such as emotions, appetite, body temperature, and sleep.

**Cerebrum.** The cerebrum is involved in the processing of memory and learning. The cerebrum also controls voluntary movements and interpretation of the senses. Spaces within the cerebrum called *ventricles* contain cerebrospinal fluid (CSF), a watery fluid that bathes the brain and spinal cord and serves as a cushion to help protect them from injury.

**Brain Stem.** The brain stem plays an important role in the CNS. It is a stalk-like structure that connects the cerebrum with the spinal cord.

The brain stem is divided into three sections: the cerebellum, the pons, and the medulla oblongata. The cerebellum coordinates muscle activity and balance. The pons serves as a bridge, connecting the cerebrum and cerebellum with the rest of the brain. The medulla oblongata contains

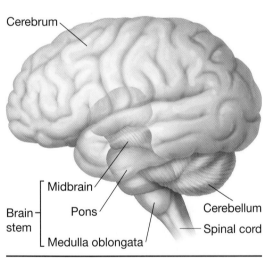

Cerebrum

Midbrain

Brain stem

Pons

Medulla oblongata

Cerebellum

Spinal cord

**Figure 9.12** As the director of the nervous system, the brain is both structurally and functionally complex.

important centers that regulate vital activities of the body. The medulla oblongata's respiratory center controls breathing, its cardiac center slows the heart when it beats too fast, and the vasomotor center controls blood pressure by narrowing or enlarging blood vessels.

## The Peripheral Nervous System (PNS)

While the CNS controls the activity of the brain and spinal cord, the PNS transmits information to all other parts of the body. The PNS contains all of the nerves and ganglia (the junction where two nerves meet) outside of the brain and spinal cord.

Twelve pairs of cranial nerves relay impulses to and from the left and right sides of the brain. These nerves enable the sense of smell, sight, hearing, taste, and facial sensations. They also control eye movements, balance, and communication between the brain and various organs. Thirty-one pairs of spinal nerves carry signals throughout the body.

**Did You Know?**

### Brain Surgery

The brain has no pain receptors. Neurosurgeons can operate on the brain while the patient is awake, and the patient will not feel any pain. Having the patient awake can ensure that the complicated surgery doesn't affect any vision or motor control functions.

# The Sensory System

The sensory system is a part of the nervous system that consists of sensory receptors such as the eyes, ears, and the senses of taste, smell, and touch. These receptors transmit information from internal and external environments to the brain, where it is processed.

## The Eyes

The eyes enable one of the most useful senses—vision (Figure 9.13). Each eye (commonly called the *eyeball*) is set into an orbital socket (or *eye socket*) in the skull. Eyelids and eyelashes cover the eye and aid in eye protection. Tears produced in the lacrimal gland help rid the eye of foreign matter that might cause irritation. The white of the eye, called the *sclera*, is the outer lining. The front part of the sclera is called the *cornea*.

The colored portion of the eye is called the *iris*. In the center of the iris is an opening called the *pupil*. Muscles of the iris control the amount of light allowed into the eye through dilation (enlarging) and contraction (shrinking) of the pupil.

Located behind the pupil is the lens, which focuses light rays on the retina. The retina is the innermost coating of the eye, which is filled with specialized nerve endings that sense vision. The nerve endings of the retina send impulses to the optic nerve located at the back of the eye. Once

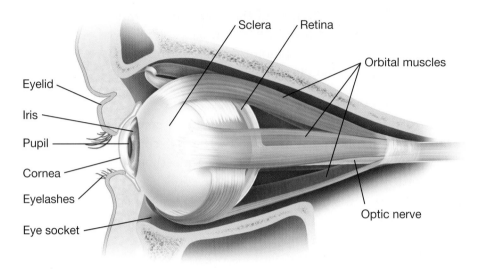

Sclera    Retina

Orbital muscles

Eyelid

Iris

Pupil

Cornea

Eyelashes

Eye socket

Optic nerve

**Figure 9.13**    Specialized internal structures of the eye send messages to the brain, creating the sense of sight.

the optic nerve receives a picture, it communicates this information to the brain so that the brain can interpret what the eye is seeing.

Cataracts, conjunctivitis (also known as *pink eye*), glaucoma, and macular degeneration are all diseases and disorders of the eye.

### The Ear

The ear has two important functions: hearing and maintaining the body's sense of balance, or *equilibrium*. The ear is divided into three main parts—the outer (external) ear, the middle ear (sometimes called the *tympanic cavity*), and the inner (internal) ear (Figure 9.14).

The outer ear is made up of the lobe and the auricle, which is also called the *pinna*. The auricle is the outer portion of the ear that leads to the ear canal, or *external auditory canal*. At the end of the ear canal is the eardrum, or *tympanic membrane*. The tympanic membrane is a very thin membrane, measuring approximately 0.1 millimeters thick. It separates and transmits sound between the outer ear and the middle ear.

The middle ear is a space containing three small bones (collectively referred to as *ossicles*). The ossicles include the malleus (*hammer*), incus (*anvil*), and stapes (*stirrup*). These bones transmit and amplify sound waves the eardrum receives from the outside world.

The Eustachian tube is also a part of the middle ear. These tubes work to equalize pressure on both sides of the eardrum. The Eustachian tubes also connect the middle ear and the pharynx, which helps match the pressure in the ear and pharynx with the outside world. This connection causes your ears to pop when the pressure in an airplane cabin changes as the plane starts to land. This connection also allows disease-causing bacteria, especially in children, to travel from the throat to the middle ear via the Eustachian tubes, resulting in a middle ear infection.

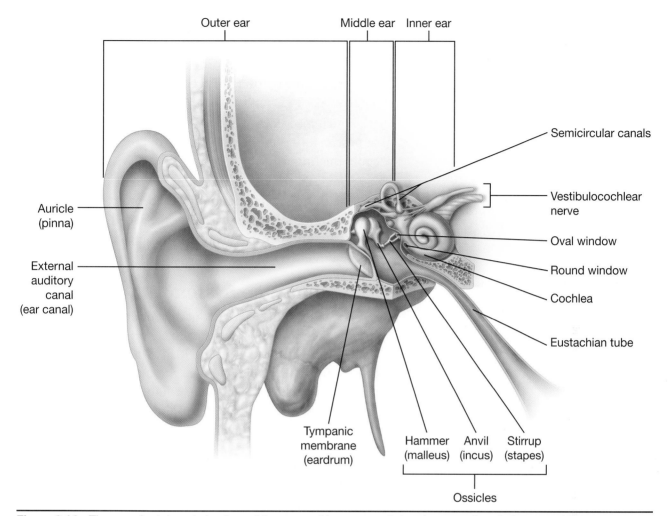

**Figure 9.14** The complex internal structure of the ear enables a person's hearing as well as their sense of balance.

The inner ear has two membrane-covered outlets into the middle ear—the oval window and the round window. The inner ear houses a snail-shaped organ called the *cochlea*, which contains thousands of hair-like nerve endings that carry sound vibrations through the auditory nerve to the brain. This is the actual process of hearing. Semicircular canals in the inner ear transmit signals to the cerebellum. The cerebellum interprets impulses from these canals to maintain balance with signals coming to the brain from the vestibulocochlear nerve.

Deafness, presbycusis (age-related deafness), and tinnitus are disorders of the ear. Various ear infections are also possible, and include external otitis (*swimmer's ear*), otitis media (*middle ear infection*), and labyrinthitis (*inner ear infection*).

## Taste, Smell, and Touch

Receptors found in various locations throughout the body contribute to our sense of taste, smell, and touch. These receptors absorb environmental

**endocrine glands**
*glands that secrete chemical substances called hormones, which regulate body functions; part of the endocrine system*

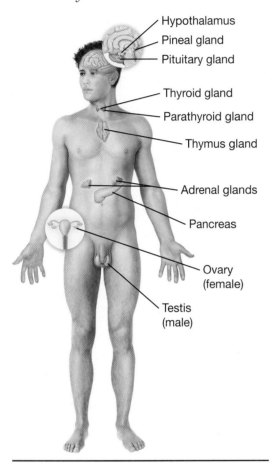

**Figure 9.15** Endocrine glands are found in various locations throughout the body.

Hypothalamus
Pineal gland
Pituitary gland
Thyroid gland
Parathyroid gland
Thymus gland
Adrenal glands
Pancreas
Ovary (female)
Testis (male)

**hormones**
*chemicals secreted by endocrine glands to regulate body functions*

**metabolism**
*term for the chemical processes occurring within a living organism that maintains life*

changes and send that information to the brain through nerve impulses. The brain then processes and interprets the messages.

Taste receptors are located in the tongue and are called *taste buds*. The sense of smell is made possible by olfactory receptors located in the upper part of the nasal cavity.

Touch receptors are small, rounded bodies called *tactile corpuscles* found in the skin, the tip of the tongue, and especially the fingertips.

Some diseases that affect our sense of taste and smell include rhinitis, burning mouth syndrome, and oral candidiasis (commonly known as *thrush*). Also, the nasal septum (the structure that divides the right and left air passages) can be deviated or perforated.

## The Endocrine System

The endocrine system contains **endocrine glands** that secrete chemical substances called **hormones** to help regulate body functions (Figure 9.15). The endocrine system affects growth and developement; energy balance; reproduction; water and electrolyte balance; and **metabolism**. Your metabolism includes all of the complicated chemical processes by which cells produce energy needed to support and sustain life.

The glands in the endocrine system secrete hormones into the bloodstream. Hormones influence the activities of tissues and cells throughout the body. Every endocrine gland produces or secretes specialized hormones that create a unique response in the body (Figure 9.16).

Some common diseases and disorders of the endocrine system include Addison's disease, Cushing syndrome, hyperthyroidism, hypoglycemia, hypothyroidism, and diabetes mellitus (commonly known as *diabetes*).

### Extend Your Knowledge

#### Diabetes Mellitus

There are two forms of diabetes mellitus—type I and type II. Type I diabetes mellitus is also known as *juvenile-onset* because symptoms appear when the patient is a child. Type II diabetes is also known as *adult-onset*, as symptoms do not appear until the patient reaches adulthood. Using resources in your school's library or on the Internet, list the symptoms of type I and II diabetes mellitus. Compare the two types and identify ways to prevent or manage these endocrine disorders. Then describe the difference between a diabetic coma and insulin shock.

| Endocrine Gland | Function |
|---|---|
| **Adrenal gland** | affects metabolism and growth; monitors electrolyte and fluid balance |
| **Hypothalamus** | stimulates or inhibits pituitary secretions; integrates responses from nervous system |
| **Ovaries** | contributes to development of female sex characteristics, including the menstrual cycle and reproductive functions |
| **Pancreas** | maintains blood glucose levels ; islets of Langerhans secrete the hormones glucagon and insulin |
| **Parathyroid glands** | maintains blood calcium levels |
| **Pineal gland** | releases the hormone melatonin to control sleep |
| **Pituitary gland** | regulates and aids in the secretion of essential hormones |
| **Testes** | produces testosterone in males |
| **Thymus gland** | stimulates the production of T and B cells to aid in the immune response |
| **Thyroid gland** | produces thyroxine ($T_4$) and triiodothyronine ($T_3$) to regulate the metabolism of proteins, carbohydrates, and fats |

**Figure 9.16**   Functions of endocrine glands

## The Respiratory System

Every cell in the human body needs oxygen to survive. The role of the respiratory system is to supply that oxygen to the cells and remove carbon dioxide, a gaseous waste product of the body. This process is referred to as **respiration**, or *breathing*.

Oxygen enters the body through the mouth and nose. This process is called *inhalation* (inspiration). The process of forcing air out of the lungs, is called *exhalation* (expiration).

The respiratory system is divided into the upper respiratory tract and the lower respiratory tract (Figure 9.17). Components of the upper respiratory tract include the nose, nasal cavity, paranasal sinuses, pharynx, and larynx. The lower respiratory tract includes the trachea and lungs, which house the bronchi, bronchioles, and alveoli. Figure 9.18 lists the various parts of the respiratory system and the function of each.

After oxygen enters the body through either the nose or mouth, it travels through each structure of the respiratory system before arriving at the alveoli. The alveoli are clusters of microscopic air sacs. Oxygen diffuses, or travels through the thin walls of the alveolar sacs to the capillaries that surround the sacs. Red blood cells in the single cell wall of the capillary absorb the oxygen while sending carbon dioxide out of the capillary. Carbon dioxide is sent to the alveoli through the capillary's single-celled walls, to be exhaled by the respiratory system. This process is called *gas exchange*.

The respiratory system is susceptible to several serious conditions and diseases in addition to the common cold and flu. These include asthma,

**respiration**
*the act of supplying oxygen to the cells and removing carbon dioxide; also called breathing*

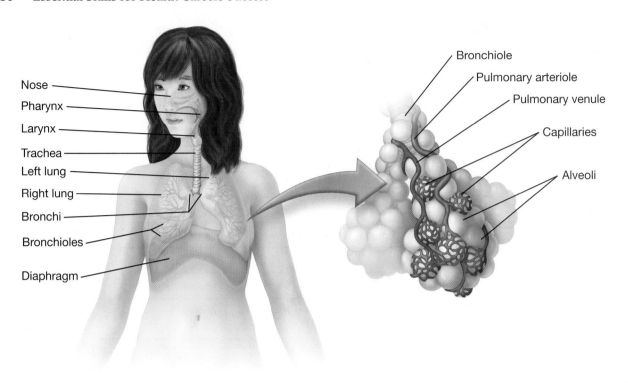

**Figure 9.17**    The respiratory system supplies oxygen to the body's cells and removes carbon dioxide.

| Structure | Function |
|---|---|
| **Alveoli** | transport oxygen and carbon dioxide to and from red blood cells in capillaries; main site of gas exchange |
| **Bronchi** | air passages located between the trachea and bronchioles |
| **Bronchioles** | conduct airflow between the bronchi and alveoli |
| **Diaphragm** | moves down (contracts) to promote inspiration; moves up (relaxes) to force air from the lungs during expiration |
| **Epiglottis** | a flap that closes and covers the trachea when food or water is ingested to prevent them from entering the lungs |
| **Larynx (voice box)** | routes air through vocal cords to produce speech |
| **Lungs** | houses the structures and tissues that conduct gas exchange |
| **Nasal cavity** | filter inspired air; provide sense of smell |
| **Oral cavity (mouth)** | inspired and expired air travels through the mouth when the nose is blocked or in the case of mouth-breathers |
| **Paranasal sinuses** | warms and moistens inhaled air |
| **Pharynx (throat)** | passageway that transports air from the nose and mouth to the trachea |
| **Trachea (windpipe)** | passageway for air between the pharynx and the bronchi |

**Figure 9.18**    Structure and function of the respiratory system

chronic obstructive pulmonary diseases (COPD), lung cancer, pulmonary embolism, pneumonia, and tuberculosis.

# The Cardiovascular System

The cardiovascular system's main responsibility is to circulate, or move blood throughout the body so that the blood can deliver oxygen and nutrients to the body's cells and remove waste materials like carbon dioxide. The blood also transports hormones secreted by the endocrine system. The heart, arteries, and veins are the main organs of this system.

Because of the cardiovascular system's important, life-sustaining role, cardiovascular disease or disorder is often serious, and even life-threatening. Heart disease is the leading cause of death in the United States. Some common diseases and disorders of the cardiovascular system include myocardial infarction (heart attack), aneurysm, atherosclerosis, heart murmurs, hypertension (high blood pressure), and endocarditis.

## The Heart

The normal adult heart beats 72 to 82 beats per minute. This organ is about the size of a clenched fist, weighing 8 to 10 ounces in women and 10 to 12 ounces in men. The heart is located in the thoracic cavity, under the breastbone (or *sternum*).

The heart has four chambers: the upper chambers, or *atria* (plural for *atrium*); and the lower chambers, or *ventricles*. The upper chambers receive blood coming into the heart, while the lower chambers pump blood out of the heart.

The *septum* divides the heart vertically into right and left halves. The interatrial septum separates the right and left atria, and the thick interventricular septum divides the two ventricles. The walls of the septum prevent oxygen-rich blood from mixing with oxygen-poor blood.

> **Did You Know?**
>
> **Heart Statistics**
>
> Every day, the heart beats about 100,000 times, sending approximately 2,000 gallons of blood pumping through the body. The heart performs an incredible job—keeping blood flowing through 60,000 miles of blood vessels to feed the organs and tissues of the body. Any damage to the heart can reduce its efficiency, forcing the heart to work harder to continue supplying the body's much-needed blood.

The heart consists of three layers. The outer layer is called the *pericardium* and is a double-layered sac. The middle layer, the myocardium, is the muscle of the heart. The endocardium, which lines the heart chambers and valves, is the innermost layer of the heart.

**Valves of the Heart.** The heart has four valves, which ensure that blood flows in only one direction (Figure 9.19). The two atrioventricular valves (*AV valves*)

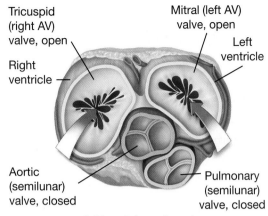

Tricuspid (right AV) valve, open

Right ventricle

Mitral (left AV) valve, open

Left ventricle

Aortic (semilunar) valve, closed

Pulmonary (semilunar) valve, closed

**A. Ventricles relaxed**

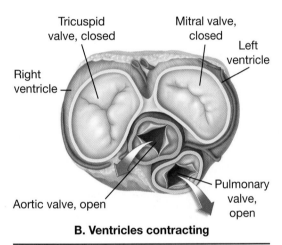

Tricuspid valve, closed

Right ventricle

Mitral valve, closed

Left ventricle

Aortic valve, open

Pulmonary valve, open

**B. Ventricles contracting**

**Figure 9.19** The four valves of the heart allow blood to flow in only one direction.

are located between the atria and the ventricles. When these valves open, they allow blood to travel from the atria into the ventricles. If closed, the AV valves prevent blood from flowing backward into the atria as the ventricles contract.

The AV valve on the right side of the heart is called the *tricuspid valve*. On the left side of the heart, the AV valve is called the *mitral valve*, or *bicuspid valve*.

The two valves that separate the ventricles from the lungs and rest of the body are called the *semilunar valves*. One of the semilunar valves is the pulmonary valve, which is located at the opening of the pulmonary artery on the right side of the heart. The aortic valve, the second semilunar valve, is located at the opening of the aorta on the left side of the heart.

**Blood Flow through the Heart.** To fully understand how the heart performs its critical function, you should understand the step-by-step flow of blood through the heart (Figure 9.20). Remember that this process is happening on both sides of the heart at the same time.

1. Deoxygenated blood enters the right atrium from the inferior and superior vena cava.
2. Deoxygenated blood flows through the tricuspid valve into the right ventricle.
3. The right ventricle contracts, forcing the pulmonary valve to open and deoxygenated blood to flow into the pulmonary artery.
4. The right and left pulmonary arteries carry the deoxygenated blood to the lungs.
5. Oxygen-rich blood travels through the pulmonary veins and into the left atrium.
6. The left atrium fills with blood, forcing the mitral valve to open.
7. Oxygenated blood flows through the mitral valve into the left ventricle.
8. The left ventricle contracts, forcing the mitral valve to close and the aortic valve to open.
9. Oxygen-rich blood travels through the aorta to the rest of the body.

**Blood Vessels.** The heart pumps blood through the blood vessels to all parts of the body. There are three types of blood vessels that transport blood throughout the cardiovascular system. These three types include arteries, capillaries, and veins:

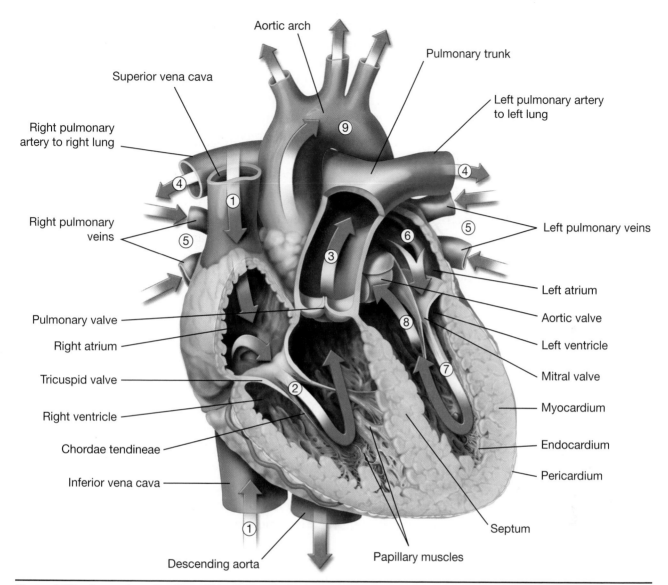

**Figure 9.20** As you trace the flow of blood through the heart, note that the blue arrows represent deoxygenated blood, while the red arrows represent oxygenated blood.

- **Arteries.** With the exception of the pulmonary arteries (which carry oxygen-poor blood to the lungs), all arteries in the body carry oxygen-rich blood away from the heart. Arterial blood is bright red in color because of the oxygen it carries. Arterial walls are thick because they have to withstand the pumping force of the heart. Arteries branch into arterioles, which connect arteries to capillaries. The aorta is the largest artery in the body. Coronary arteries branch off the aorta to supply blood to the walls of the heart. Blockage of a coronary artery may result in coronary artery disease and a heart attack.
- **Capillaries.** Capillaries are microscopic, thin-walled blood vessels. Nutrients pass from the bloodstream to the cells of the body via the

capillaries. The body's cells take in oxygen and nutrients from the blood through the thin capillary walls, and transfer waste and carbon dioxide to the blood cells in the capillaries.

- **Veins.** Veins are vessels that carry oxygen-poor blood from the capillaries back to the heart. Smaller veins, called *venules*, carry blood from the capillaries to the veins. At that stage, the blood is called *venous blood*. Venous blood is a darker red color than arterial blood. Veins have thinner walls than arteries, and valves that help to prevent the backward flow of blood. These valves keep venous blood moving forward to the heart.

**Electrical Activity of the Heart.** The conduction system of the heart is responsible for controlling the rate, rhythm, and strength of heart beats, or *contractions*. This system conveys electrical impulses that facilitate proper heart function. Included in the conduction system are two areas of nodal tissue and a network of fibers.

The sinoatrial node, or *SA node*, is located at the top of the right atrium of the heart. The SA node sends out an electrical impulse telling the heart to contract between 60 and 100 beats per minute (bpm).

The SA node fires an electrical impulse that causes the atria to contract. The impulse is also carried to the atrioventricular node (*AV node*). The AV node is a very dense network of fibers that delays the electrical impulse briefly (up to a tenth of a second). When the electrical impulse leaves the AV node, it is carried through a collection of conducting fibers called the *bundle of His* and into the ventricular septum. The bundle of His then divides into the right and left bundle branches and forms conduction fibers called the *Purkinje fibers*. The Purkinje fibers transmit the impulse to the ventricles, stimulating their contraction.

## Extend Your Knowledge

### The Electrocardiogram

When adults have a checkup, they are often given an electrocardiogram (also known as an *ECG* or *EKG*). An electrocardiogram records the electrical activity of the heart (Figure 9.21).

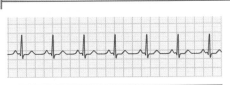

**Figure 9.21**   An ECG illustrates the electrical activity of the heart. This example shows a normal ECG.

## The Lymphatic and Immune Systems

The lymphatic system and immune system share some of the same structures and functions. Both systems work to prevent and fight disease and destroy any pathogens that find their way into the body.

The lymphatic system helps the body remove and destroy waste products, dead blood cells, pathogens, poisons, cancer cells, and other debris.

This system also absorbs fats and fat-soluble vitamins from the gastrointestinal system to deliver nutrients to the body's cells. The immune system facilitates all types of **immunity**, or the ability to resist pathogens.

The lymphatic system is connected to the cardiovascular system by a network of capillaries. As Figure 9.22 shows, the key parts of the lymphatic system include lymphatic capillaries, lymphatic vessels, lymph nodes, lymphatic ducts, tonsils, the thymus gland, and the spleen.

**immunity**
*ability to resist pathogens*

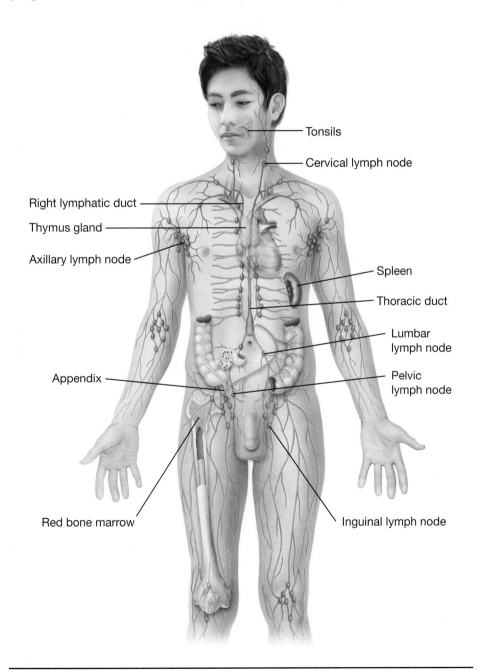

**Figure 9.22** The lymphatic system fights foreign invaders that may cause infection and disease.

### Lymphatic Capillaries

These vessels extend into spaces between body tissues and blood vessels. Lymphatic fluid, called **lymph**, begins as blood plasma that has leaked into tissues from blood vessel capillaries. Lymph contains two types of white blood cells, waste products, and foreign matter from the cells. The lymph travels through the capillaries to lymphatic vessels.

### Lymphatic Vessels

These vessels, which resemble veins, move the lymph from body tissues to the lymphatic trunks. These trunks deposit lymph into the veins, where it once again becomes plasma—the liquid component of the blood.

### Lymph Nodes

Small, bean-shaped lymph nodes lie along the lymphatic vessels. Concentrated in the abdomen, armpit, chest, elbows, groin, and knees, lymph nodes filter bacteria, viruses, and other waste out of the lymph. They also house white blood cells called **lymphocytes**. These cells are crucial in helping the body defend itself from pathogenic microorganisms.

### Lymphatic Ducts

There are two main lymphatic ducts—the right lymphatic duct and the thoracic duct. The right lymphatic duct is a vessel that carries lymph from the right side of the body, draining the right arm and the right side of the neck and chest. The thoracic duct drains the rest of the body.

### The Spleen

Located behind the stomach, the spleen filters waste products and microorganisms from the blood. The spleen also manufactures two types of white blood cells—lymphocytes and monocytes—to help defend the body against pathogens. The spleen also destroys non-functioning red blood cells and stores red blood cells. Certain infections or traumatic blows to the abdomen may damage the spleen. A person can live without a spleen, but they will be more susceptible to infection than they were before it was removed.

### The Thymus Gland

Also part of the endocrine system, the thymus gland is soft and has two lobes. The thymus gland is located beneath the breastbone, at the level of the heart. This gland is large during early childhood and gradually shrinks until it becomes very small in adulthood. The thymus houses T lymphocytes (*T cells*) while they mature. T cells provide immunity and are essential for destroying foreign invaders.

### Tonsils

Composed of lymphatic tissue rich with lymphocytes, the tonsils are located at the back of the nasal cavity, above the roof of the mouth. The tonsils are typically large in childhood and shrink during early adulthood.

---

**lymph**
*colorless fluid from the body's tissues that carries white blood cells; collects and transports bacteria to the lymph nodes for destruction; carries fats from the digestive system*

**lymphocyte**
*white blood cell that destroys pathogenic microorganisms*

The tonsils filter tissue and bacteria. On occasion, the tonsils can become overwhelmed by the bacteria they filter, which results in an infection. Infected tonsils become enlarged, make swallowing difficult, and lead to a sore throat and swollen lymph nodes, a condition known as *tonsillitis*. Frequent tonsillitis may be treated by surgically removing the tonsils to prevent further infection. The pharyngeal tonsil (also called the *adenoid*) lies at the back of the throat and opens into the nasal cavity. The adenoid can also become enlarged and infected.

### The Immune System

The immune system is closely linked to the lymphatic system, and the two systems share several organs. The immune system's main job is to defend against intruders, most commonly bacteria and viruses.

The human body has many types of defenses against disease. The skin serves as a physical barrier for pathogens attempting to enter the body. Cilia, tiny hair-like tissues in the nose, also stop infectious invaders. Substances such as gastric juices in the stomach serve as chemical barriers. Specialized white blood cells attack and ingest pathogens in the bloodstream.

Human beings are born with some natural immunity. For instance, people with a healthy immune system are not as susceptible to various bacteria found in the soil. However, these bacteria can harm people with a compromised immune system. Immunity can also be acquired. Once we have had a certain disease, our bodies are sensitized to that disease. The body may know how to destroy that disease if it attacks again. Vaccinations also produce acquired immunity.

White blood cells (leukocytes) found in the plasma play an important role in the immune system. There are five types of white blood cells (Figure 9.23). These types are classified by the presence of spots, or *granules*, in their cytoplasm. Those with granules are known as *granulocytes* and those without are known as *agranulocytes*.

**Antigens and Antibodies.** When a potentially harmful foreign molecule enters the body, that molecule is called a foreign **antigen**. Some examples of foreign antigens include microorganisms, splinters, or poison. Our bodies have their own antigens—other antigens are marked as foreign when they do not match the body's antigens.

A healthy immune system responds quickly to foreign antigens. This response begins when white blood cells produce **antibodies**, which are active in the immune response once foreign antigens are discovered in the body. White blood cells surround, ingest, and destroy the invader as part of a process called **phagocytosis**. Chemicals are released to stimulate inflammation, fever, and the production of pus. Pus is a thick, yellow-white substance composed of white blood cells, dead tissue, and cellular debris. Inflammation, fever, and the presence of pus are all signs that the immune system is working.

**antigen**
*any foreign substance, either outside or inside the body, that causes the immune system to produce antibodies*

**antibody**
*a protein produced by the immune system; circulates in the plasma in response to the presence of foreign antigens*

**phagocytosis**
*process in which white blood cells surround, ingest, and destroy a foreign invader*

| Type | Percentage of WBCs | Function |
|------|--------------------|----------|
| **neutrophil** 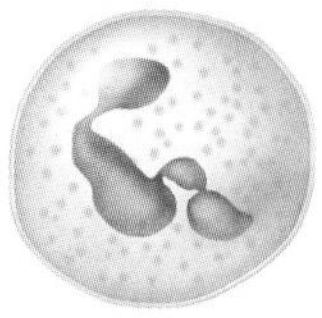 | 55%–77% | kills bacteria and fungi using phagocytosis |
| **eosinophil** 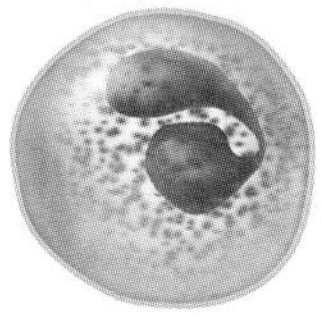 | 1%–3% | active in the allergic response; destroys parasites |
| **basophil** 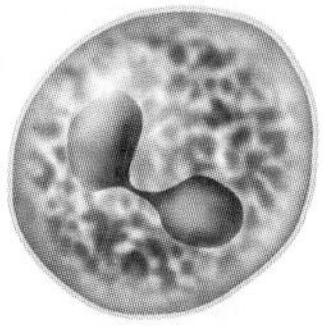 | <1% | releases histamine as part of an allergic response |
| **lymphocyte** 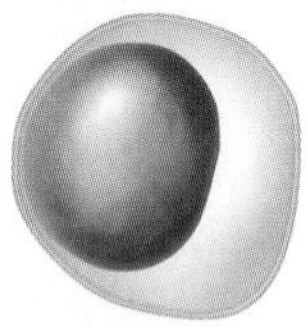 | 25%–33% | B cells produce antibodies; T cells and natural killer cells fight cancerous tumors and viruses |
| **monocyte** 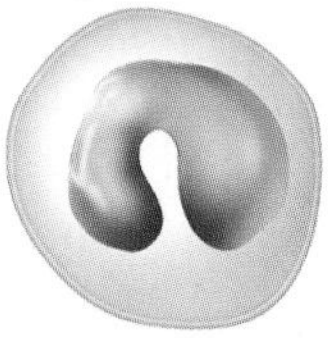 | 2%–10% | performs phagocytosis; morphs into macrophage that removes dead cell debris and attacks microorganisms |

**Figure 9.23**   White blood cells play a major role in the immune response.

There are many diseases and disorders related to the lymphatic and immune systems. Because the immune system is responsible for fighting pathogens, diseases that affect this system can be particularly dangerous. If the immune system is not functioning as it should, the rest of the body systems are at risk for other infections. Allergies, tonsillitis, infected adenoids, and infectious mononucleosis (also called *mono*) are some common diseases related to the lymphatic and immune systems. Untreated tonsillitis can have serious consequences, such as chronic infection and hearing loss. More serious ailments include AIDS, rheumatoid arthritis, leukemias, and lymphomas.

# The Gastrointestinal System

The gastrointestinal system, also called the *digestive system*, includes many organs working together to ingest and break down food. The gastrointestinal system is responsible for absorbing the nutrients your body needs, and disposing of the waste (Figure 9.24).

The process of digestion includes many steps. First, food enters the body via the mouth (*oral canal*), and is broken down by both mechanical and chemical means. The food travels down the gastrointestinal tract (commonly called the *GI tract*) via the esophagus.

Mechanical breakdown of food is completed by chewing and also through churning in the stomach. Chemical breakdown occurs in the stomach and small intestine, where acids and enzymes (proteins that speed up chemical reactions) break apart food molecules. Nutrients from the food molecules are absorbed primarily in the small intestine. The major function of the large intestine is to absorb water. The feces, or remaining materials not absorbed in the digestive process, are expelled from the body via the rectum.

## The Liver and Gallbladder

The liver and gallbladder are accessory, or *supporting*, organs of digestion. The liver has many functions, mostly relating to the body's metabolism—the production and processing of various chemicals. The liver helps maintain a stable, healthy internal environment in the body. The functions of the liver include

- secretion of bile, a brownish-green fluid that helps digest fats;
- monitoring and filtering the blood to remove toxins, destroy old red blood cells, and maintain normal blood concentrations of glucose, fats, and amino acids;
- nutrient breakdown, such as converting carbohydrates to fats; and
- storage of proteins, glycogen (a form of glucose), iron, and vitamins, as well as blood proteins (clotting factors) that are critical in helping the blood to clot.

The liver also has an extensive blood supply, enabling it to accomplish its many tasks.

The gallbladder stores bile secreted by the liver. The gallbladder also delivers bile to the small intestine when it is needed to help break down fats. Humans can live without a gallbladder, but cannot survive without a liver.

## The Pancreas

The pancreas is another accessory organ of digestion. Like the liver, the pancreas has both digestive and metabolic functions. The pancreas also makes two important hormones—insulin and glucagon. Insulin lowers blood glucose (sugar) levels, while glucagon raises blood glucose levels.

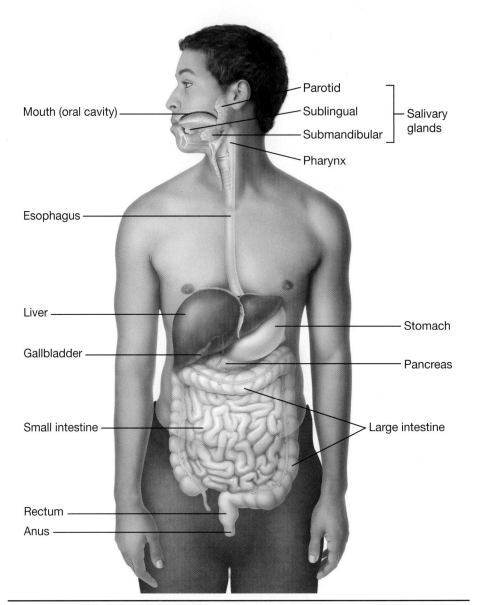

**Figure 9.24**    Structure and organs of the gastrointestinal system

Cirrhosis of the liver, gastroenteritis, hepatitis, ulcerative colitis, hiatal hernias, and ulcers are all common diseases and disorders of the gastrointestinal system.

## The Urinary System

The urinary system filters blood, excretes wastes, and regulates blood pH and volume. The urinary system includes two kidneys, two ureters, a single urethra, and the urinary bladder. Disorders such as kidney stones, chronic kidney disease, and urinary tract infections (UTIs) can cause inflammation or obstruction of the organs in this system. Consequences of these disorders may result in temporary organ malfunction or permanent organ damage.

## Urine Production

The urinary system must complete three important processes in order to produce urine:

1. **Filtration.** The blood is filtered in order to separate important, beneficial substances—glucose and amino acids—from waste substances— ammonia and certain drugs. This filtering helps identify substances that need to be eliminated as urine.

2. **Reabsorption.** As filtration takes place, beneficial substances are moved back into the blood so they can be reabsorbed by the body.

3. **Secretion.** The final step in this process is achieved when the urinary system secretes waste from the body in the form of urine.

## Structures of the Urinary System

The chief organs in the urinary system are the pair of bean-shaped kidneys (Figure 9.25). Each about the size of a fist, the kidneys are located dorsally to the upper abdomen. The kidneys are a very complex filtration system. As you may recall from chapter 8, the word *renal* refers to the kidneys.

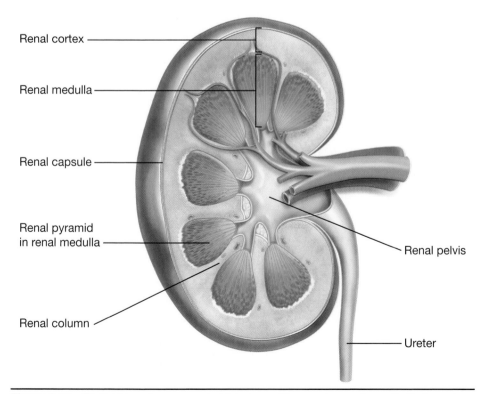

Renal cortex

Renal medulla

Renal capsule

Renal pyramid in renal medulla

Renal column

Renal pelvis

Ureter

**Figure 9.25** Each kidney has approximately one million nephrons, the units that create urine.

Covered by the renal capsule, the interior of the kidney is divided into three parts:

- the cortex (outer layer)
- the medulla (middle layer)
- the pelvis (innermost layer)

Blood is filtered in the cortex of the kidney. Erythropoietin, a hormone necessary for red blood cell production, is produced in the renal cortex. The renal medulla contains a number of triangle-shaped areas called *pyramids*. Urine is collected in the pyramids, separated by renal columns. The renal pelvis serves as a funnel for the urine. The pelvis is divided into two or three large collecting cups, called *major calyces*, which then branch into several *minor calyces*. Urine continually drains through the pyramids into the calyces.

The major filtering mechanisms in the kidney are called nephrons. Blood enters each kidney through the renal artery and leaves through the renal vein. Inside the kidney, the renal artery branches into smaller arteries, which lead to the microscopic nephrons. Each kidney contains about one million nephrons, some in the cortex and some in the medulla.

The renal pelvis empties into the ureters—two tubes approximately six or seven inches in length, that carry urine to the urinary bladder, or *bladder*. The urinary bladder is a hollow, muscular organ that stores urine to be eliminated. The bladder can hold approximately 500 milliliters of urine when moderately full before it empties. The walls of the bladder can stretch and allow the bladder to hold twice as much as it holds when considered full. When the bladder is stretched, nerve endings are stimulated and signal the brain that the bladder is full.

Urine is eliminated from the body by way of the urethra, a tube of smooth muscle with a mucous lining. The female urethra is about 1.5 inches long, whereas the male urethra is 8 inches long. The process of excreting urine is often called *voiding*.

### Acid-Base Balance

The kidneys maintain a balance between acids (*acidity*) and bases (*alkalinity*) in the body. All chemicals in the body fall into one of three categories—acid, base, or neutral. *Acidic* and *basic* are terms for the extreme ends of the spectrum. A substance that is neither an acid nor a base is called *neutral*.

**pH scale**
*system for measuring a substance's acidity or alkalinity; ranges from 0 to 14*

The level of a substance's acidity or alkalinity is measured on the **pH scale**. The scale ranges from 0 to 14, with acids falling on the lower end of the scale and bases on the upper end. The normal pH of human blood falls within a tight range of 7.35 to 7.45.

If the kidneys sense that the blood's pH level is above or below the normal range, buffering agents will be excreted to maintain the acid-base balance. A buffering agent might make the blood more acidic or basic, depending on the pH. The regulation of blood pH is another example of how the body achieves homeostasis.

Common disorders and diseases of the urinary system include acute and chronic kidney failure, cystitis (inflammation of the bladder), kidney stones, various infections of parts of the kidney, incontinence, and urethritis.

 *Check Your Understanding*

1. Which body system is connected to the cardiovascular system by a network of capillaries?
2. Name the five types of white blood cells found in the body.
3. Describe the difference between antigens and antibodies.
4. Describe the difference between chemical and mechanical breakdown in the gastrointestinal system.
5. Which organ produces urine?

## The Reproductive System

The reproductive system allows humans to reproduce, or create offspring. The reproductive system is controlled by hormones and, as a result, shares some organs with the endocrine system.

Unlike other body systems, the reproductive system does not begin to function at birth. Rather, reproductive functions only begin once the system has matured. This maturation takes place during a process called **puberty**. Puberty usually lasts several years, and begins between the ages of 8 and 14 (typically beginning earlier in females than in males). Puberty is an indication that sexual reproduction is possible.

**Human reproduction** occurs when the male sex cell (sperm) and female sex cell (ova, or *egg*) unite to create a new human being. This process is known as *fertilization*. After fertilization, a fetus takes approximately 40 weeks to develop, at which point the mother will give birth.

The reproductive system is also unique because different structures compose this system depending on your gender (Figures 9.26 and 9.27). Because females may become pregnant and give birth, the female reproductive system has more functions than the male reproductive system. Refer to Figures 9.28 and 9.29 for a description of the various reproductive organs and structures.

Common disorders and diseases of the reproductive system include **sexually transmitted infections (STIs)** and reproductive tract infections (RTIs) in both females and males. Various cancers affect the reproductive systems, including ovarian cancer and uterine cancer in women, and testicular cancer in men. Functional problems may also exist, such as male impotence.

**puberty**
*a stage of life beginning between the ages of 8 and 14; indicates sexual reproduction is possible*

**human reproduction**
*process that occurs when the male sex cell and female sex cell unite to create a new human being*

**sexually transmitted infection (STI)**
*an infection transferred from one person to another through sexual contact*

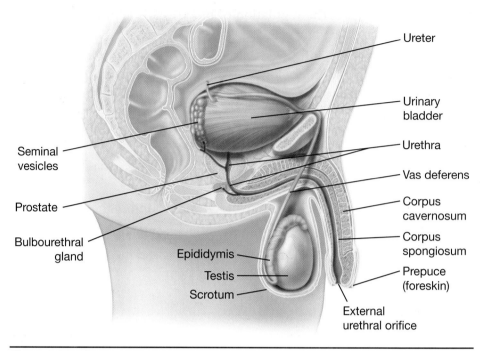

**Figure 9.26**   The male reproductive system

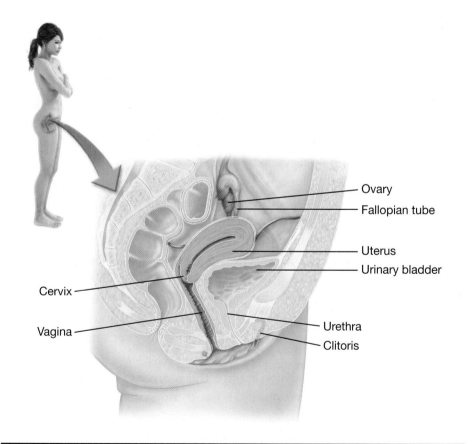

**Figure 9.27**   The female reproductive system

| Male | Function |
|---|---|
| **Bulbourethral glands** | lubricate penis for insertion by secreting small amounts of fluid just before emission of the semen |
| **Corpus cavernosum and corpus spongiosum** | sponge-like expandable erectile tissue (capable of being raised to an upright position) |
| **Epididymis** | site of sperm maturation and storage; holds the testes in place |
| **Penis** | delivers sperm to the female reproductive tract |
| **Prepuce (foreskin)** | protects the sensitive glans (head) of the penis |
| **Prostate gland** | secretes fluid into the urethra to buffer the acid in urine and the vagina |
| **Scrotum** | houses the testes and associated ducts |
| **Seminal vesicles** | produces secretions that amount for about 60% of the total volume of semen; supply energy for the sperm |
| **Testes** | produce sperm and the male sex hormone, testosterone |
| **Urethra** | transports sperm and urine out of the body |
| **Vas deferens** | carries sperm to the urethra |

**Figure 9.28** Structures and functions of the male reproductive systems

| Female | Function |
|---|---|
| **Cervix** | lower, narrower part of the uterus;  allows flow of menstrual blood from the uterus into the vagina, directs sperm into the uterus during intercourse; supports the uterus |
| **Endometrium** | receives and nourishes the fertilized ova; thickens and sheds as part of the menstrual cycle |
| **External genitalia** | lubricates the entrance to the vagina; produce pleasurable sensations during sex; protect the reproductive tract from infectious agents |
| **Fallopian tubes** | bring the ova to the uterus; common site for fertilization |
| **Mammary glands** | produce milk in nursing mothers |
| **Ovaries** | produce female sex hormones and ova (or *eggs*) |
| **Uterus** | receive and nourish a fertilized egg; house the fetus during gestational development; expel the fetus using muscular contractions during childbirth |
| **Vagina** | passageway for menstrual flow, semen, and the fetus during childbirth; acidic nature of the vagina helps prevent bacterial infections |

**Figure 9.29** Structures and functions of the female reproductive systems

**Reproductive System Facts**

- The largest cell in the female body is the ovum (or *egg*), found in the ovaries.
- A mature ovum has a life span of 12 to 24 hours.
- In her lifetime, a woman can give birth up to 35 times.
- A female infant is typically born with about 600,000 immature ova in her ovaries.
- The fallopian tubes are only as wide as the head of a pin.
- A healthy male can produce about 500 million sperm each day.
- Sperm lives for approximately 36 hours.

# Human Growth and Development

Human growth and development begins at conception and ends at death. During an individual's lifetime, certain needs must be met for growth and development to progress successfully. In addition to knowing how the physical body functions, healthcare workers must be aware of the various stages of human growth and development. This knowledge will help healthcare workers meet their patients' needs and provide quality healthcare. Each stage of life brings unique challenges and changes.

## Maslow's Hierarchy of Needs

In 1943, American psychologist Abraham Maslow proposed that healthy humans have a certain number of needs. These needs are arranged in a hierarchy, or an organized system of ranking people or things. Maslow's system is often represented as a five-level pyramid. The base of the pyramid represents the most basic human needs. If these basic needs are not met, the higher-level needs toward the top of the pyramid may not be realized (Figure 9.30).

## Four Types of Growth and Development

Throughout the stages of life, every person encounters four types of growth and development:

- physical (body growth)
- mental (development of the mind)
- emotional (feelings)
- social (interacting and relating to others)

Each type of change occurs during every life stage. Growth and development varies greatly among all individuals. Physical bodies, mental development, and social

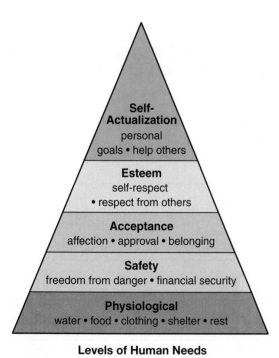

**Levels of Human Needs**

**Figure 9.30**  Maslow believed that basic needs must be mastered before an individual can progress up the pyramid to the higher-level needs.

interaction may grow at different rates. For instance, emotional maturity differs from person to person, and social interaction can range from extreme shyness to dramatic extroversion.

## Life Stages

There are many different ways to classify the stages of human life. Each stage presents its own challenges. For our purposes, the following stages are discussed: prenatal, infancy, childhood (early and late), adolescence, adulthood (early, middle, and late), and death.

### Prenatal: Fertilization until Birth

The prenatal stage spans the period from fertilization until birth. During the first nine weeks of development, the fertilized egg is in the embryo stage. After the embryo stage is the fetus stage, which lasts until birth.

Prenatal development occurs during approximately forty weeks of pregnancy. Pregnancy is divided into trimesters, or three-month periods. During the first trimester, a large liver and bones begin to form, kidneys produce urine, and the lower trunk muscles develop. In the second trimester, the ribs and major body systems develop. Before the third trimester, survival outside the mother is difficult. Growth and organ development are rapid during the third trimester.

> **Did You Know?**
>
> ### Prematurity and Development
> Babies born at 23 weeks of gestation have a 17% rate of survival. A large percentage of surviving children born before 26 weeks show a high level of disability.

### Infancy: Birth until One Year

Infancy is the time between birth and the first birthday. During the first month of life, the baby is considered a *neonate*. After these first 30 days, the baby is called an *infant* until reaching the first birthday (Figure 9.31).

The infancy stage brings dramatic and rapid changes to the human. The baby begins to roll over, crawl, walk, and grasp objects. Mental development brings responses to cold, hunger, and pain through crying. The baby also begins to recognize surroundings and people. Emotionally, the baby is able to show anger, distrust, happiness, and excitement. During infancy, the baby is dependent on others for all of its needs.

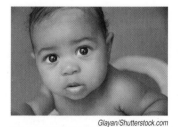

*Glayan/Shutterstock.com*

**Figure 9.31** Infancy lasts from birth until the first birthday.

### Early Childhood: One to Six Years

Early childhood is defined as the time between one year and six years (Figure 9.32). Children in this stage who are between one and three years of age are called *toddlers*. A toddler needs constant attention. Most toddlers

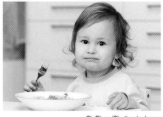

*Sk Elena/Shutterstock.com*

**Figure 9.32** Early childhood is marked by many physical and mental developments including walking, talking, and using utensils when eating.

walk by fifteen months, and can run easily, throw a ball, and scribble with a crayon by the age of two.

During early childhood, physical development is slower than in infancy. Mental development includes verbal growth, short attention span, asking questions, recognizing letters, and, in some cases, beginning to read. Children develop self-awareness and can recognize the effect they have on others. Children can become impatient and frustrated when trying to do something beyond their capabilities. Younger children may be self-centered, but typically transform into sociable six-year-olds. The child also develops strong attachments to parents during this stage.

### Late Childhood: Six to Twelve Years

The period of time from six to twelve years of age is the late childhood stage (Figure 9.33). Preadolescence, or *prepubescence*, is often defined as the years from age ten to age twelve. Children in this age group are sometimes referred to as *preteens*.

Physical development at this stage is slow and steady. Muscle coordination becomes well developed, and some children master physical activity requiring complex motor-sensory coordination. Mentally, the child is developing quickly, as much of their life revolves around school. Reading and writing skills advance, and abstract concepts like loyalty, values, honesty, and morals become understood.

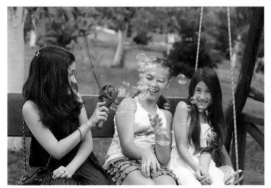

*Olesia Bilkei/Shutterstock.com*

**Figure 9.33** Activities become more group-oriented as an individual enters late childhood. Preteens tend to seek the approval of their family and friends.

Emotional development brings greater independence and a more defined personality during this stage. Many preteens replace fear with the ability to cope. Socially, activities become more group-oriented and the opinions of others become more important. Preteens need reassurance, parental approval, and acceptance by their peers.

### Adolescence: Twelve to Twenty Years

The adolescent stage of development can be full of excitement and exploration. It is also a time for tremendous physical and psychological changes that can cause anxiety and conflict.

Physical development during this stage is accelerated. Puberty leads to the development of secondary sexual characteristics. Both boys and girls experience the growth of underarm and pubic hair. Girls' breasts begin to develop and their hips widen, while boys experience muscle growth and facial hair development. Girls also begin to menstruate and boys produce sperm and semen (the fluid that contains sperm). Hormones surge, weight control may become an issue, and acne may influence the teenager's physical appearance and social interactions.

Mental development may include reasoning, abstract thinking, and critical thinking. Adolescents often do not see the connection between behavior and consequences, leading them to make potentially bad decisions. In this stage of life, teenagers must learn to make decisions and accept responsibility for negative actions.

A teenager's emotions can be stormy and conflict with those around them. During this stage, teenagers may also develop concern for the welfare of others, and may become involved in community service projects.

Social development revolves around a teenager's peers, who hold a great influence. Adolescents often feel tremendous pressure to look good. Body image is often influenced by flawless, unrealistic examples presented in the media. As a result, eating disorders can be a problem among adolescents. Bullying, a common problem among adolescents, can lead to hurt feelings and dangerous behaviors including suicide.

## Real Life Scenario

### Teenage Rebellion

Judith and her husband Ken wonder why their sweet, loving daughter Sophie is changing. At fourteen, Sophie is not interested in spending time with her parents, announcing that she doesn't want to go on the family vacation this year. Sophie spends more and more time in her room, texting her friends and playing loud music. Recently, Ken sent Sophie back to her room to change out of an outfit he felt was inappropriate for school.

Should these parents be worried about Sophie's recent attitude changes? When should parents become concerned about teen behavior?

### Early Adulthood: Twenty to Forty Years

With the advent of early adulthood, the individual has completed physical development. Muscles are fully developed and coordination is at its peak. Young adults often seek additional education, choose their careers, and achieve financial and physical independence as part of their mental development. All of these challenges can make this stage a stressful time in a person's life.

Socially, this age group may move away from peers and spend more time with others who have similar life paths. Many individuals find a partner and start a family during this stage.

Today, this stage in life is very different than in the past, when people got married in their late teens or early twenties. Economic strains may find young adults living at home until their late twenties. This may cause young adults to delay the start of their own family, and parenting may not begin until a person's thirties or even early forties. Health issues are less common during this period.

### Middle Adulthood: Forty to Sixty-Five Years

People in middle adulthood, or *middle-age*, are active and productive, but may begin to notices signs of aging (Figure 9.34). Hair begins to thin or go gray; skin isn't as smooth as it once was; muscle tone may be lacking; hearing loss may be noticeable; eyesight may weaken; and weight gain may

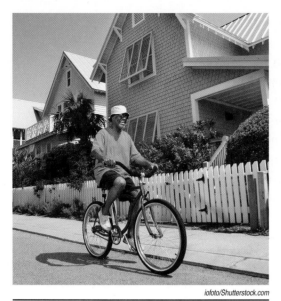

iofoto/Shutterstock.com

**Figure 9.34** Many people find middle adulthood to be a rewarding, active period of their lives.

occur. Middle-aged adults continue to develop mentally, becoming confident decision makers and troubleshooters.

This stage can become a time of contentment and satisfaction with life. Children may become independent, leaving their parents with more personal time. The health of many middle-aged people is still fairly good, but signs of future problems can come to light. These signs may include high cholesterol, arthritis, diabetes, and other problems resulting from obesity and lack of exercise.

### Late Adulthood: Sixty-Five Years and Up

During these years, all body systems begin to show signs of aging. Advances in geriatrics, a branch of medicine concerned with problems associated with old age, have successfully extended this stage of life for many people.

In late adulthood, wrinkles and age spots begin to appear, and the skin begins to dry. Muscles lose tone and strength, and the bone disease osteoporosis can lead to an increased incidence of bone fracture, especially of the hip. Memory loss can occur during this stage, but many people remain mentally active. Travel, volunteerism, and social activities can enhance this stage of life.

Emotional development during this stage can vary greatly among individuals. Some people slip into depression because of loss of identity after retirement or the death of a spouse and friends. The reality of one's own death is also something one must face. Physical infirmities can lead to increased dependence on others, which is very difficult for most people. These infirmities may mean a person must move to a retirement community or seek assisted-living arrangements. Today, many retirement communities offer a broad range of life-affirming activities.

### Death and Dying

Death is the final stage of growth. Death is often accompanied by grief—either the person's own grief at the loss of their life, or the grief of their family and friends. Dr. Elisabeth Kübler-Ross (1926–2004), a Swiss-American psychiatrist, observed that there are five stages of grief. The stages may not occur in a strict order, and some people may not progress through them all. These stages include:

1. **Denial.** The refusal to believe death is coming.
2. **Anger.** Feelings of negativity develop and may be directed at a person's own illness or body. Individuals may also experience feelings of resentment toward others.
3. **Bargaining.** A person wants more time, and proposes deals or exchanges (usually with a higher power, family members, or their doctor) in order to extend life.

4. **Depression.** Struggling with the loss of life can cause people to become sad, withdrawn, and disinterested in activities.

5. **Acceptance.** The reality of death is understood and accepted. If a person reaches this stage, death can be a peaceful experience.

In the decades after Dr. Elisabeth Kübler-Ross first shared these findings, her concepts have been largely accepted by the public. Research continues to examine and build upon the findings of Kübler-Ross.

Research in this field has brought about many changes in the way the dying are treated. For instance, hospice services are now widely available. Hospices operate with a philosophy that focuses on bringing comfort, self-respect, and tranquility to the dying. The dying are often given palliative care, which relieves and prevents the suffering of patients in the last stages. This service is available to the terminally ill in their homes as well as in hospice facilities.

 *Check Your Understanding*

1. What is the difference between the embryo stage and the fetus stage?
2. At what point is a baby called an infant rather than a neonate?
3. What is preadolescence?
4. Name the five stages of grief.

## Specialties Related to Life Stages

Each stage of human life brings with it very specific needs. In the past, a family doctor treated all stages. Today, specialties have developed to concentrate on the needs that arise during each stage of life. Figure 9.35 illustrates many specific occupations related to life stages.

| Life Stage | Specialties |
| --- | --- |
| **Prenatal** | obstretrician; perinatologist; medical geneticist |
| **Infancy** | pediatrician; neonatologist; neonatal nurse |
| **Early childhood** | pediatrician; pediatric nurse |
| **Late childhood** | pediatrician; pediatric nurse |
| **Adolescence** | sports medicine; endocrinologists; dermatologists; psychologists |
| **Early and middle adulthood** | internists; specialists such as neurologists, cardiologists, or gynecologists |
| **Late adulthood** | internist; geriatric medicine; hospice physician; hospice nurse |

**Figure 9.35** Specialties related to life stages

# Chapter Review and Assessment

## Summary

Science is a system of acquiring knowledge through observation and experimentation to describe the natural world. Modern medicine is based on many scientific disciplines, and the student who wants a career in healthcare must take science courses.

The scientific method is used to obtain reliable knowledge. The method can be used throughout the medical field to diagnose illness, invent new therapies, design and develop new technologies, and discover new drug treatments.

In order to understand the human body, it is helpful to study anatomy and physiology. This subject matter focuses on the form and function of the human body. The body is divided into various organ systems that complete specific tasks and processes. These systems include the integumentary, musculoskeletal, nervous, sensory, endocrine, respiratory, cardiovascular, lymphatic and immune, gastrointestinal, urinary, and reproductive systems.

Understanding how the human body works, the various stages of growth and development, and the concepts described in Maslow's hierarchy of needs will help healthcare workers effectively meet the needs of their patients. The stages of growth and development include prenatal, infancy, early childhood, late childhood, adolescence, early adulthood, middle adulthood, and late adulthood. In each stage there will be physical, mental, emotional, and social challenges and changes. Death and dying is studied as the final life stage. There are many professional specialties that focus on specific life stages.

## Review Questions

*Answer the following questions using what you have learned in this chapter.*

### Short Answer

1. Name four categories of science that are relevant to healthcare.

2. Name three men whose accomplishments and discoveries contributed to the development of the scientific method.

3. List the six steps of the scientific method.

4. Describe the pathway of blood through the heart.

5. What is the difference between anatomy and physiology?

6. What is the function of the pancreas?

7. Name four organs of the lymphatic system.

8. What are the differences between arteries, veins, and capillaries?

9. Name three endocrine glands.

10. What is the difference between inspiration and expiration?

### True or False

11. *True or False?* DNA is found inside the nucleus of the cell.

12. *True or False?* The term *neonate* refers to a baby up to one year old.

13. *True or False?* Geriatrics is a branch of medicine specializing in problems associated with old age.

14. *True or False?* Multiple sclerosis is a disease of the gastrointestinal system.

15. *True or False?* Physiology is the study of the structure of the body.

16. *True or False?* Capillaries are larger than veins.

17. *True or False?* Eustachian tubes are found in the eye.

18. *True or False?* The skin is the largest organ of the body.

19. *True or False?* The urinary system is the body system most heavily involved in removing carbon dioxide from the body.

20. *True or False?* The aorta divides the heart into two parts.

## Multiple Choice

21. Which of the following statements is incorrect?
    A. Human beings have 23 pairs of chromosomes.
    B. DNA stands for *deoxyribonucleic acid*.
    C. DNA has been called the *molecule of life*.
    D. DNA was discovered in the early 1900's.

22. Which of the following statements is correct?
    A. A hospice facility serves the terminally ill.
    B. People can receive hospice care in their own homes.
    C. Hospice care includes relief from pain.
    D. All of the above.

23. Which of the following structures is part of the eye?
    A. iris
    B. pupil
    C. retina
    D. All of the above.

24. The _____ is *not* a part of the lymphatic system.
    A. thoracic duct
    B. spleen
    C. heart
    D. thymus gland

25. Basophils, lymphocytes, and _____ are all types of white blood cells.
    A. neutrophils
    B. stem cells
    C. antibodies
    D. cytoplasms

26. Bone marrow can be either red or _____.
    A. blue
    B. yellow
    C. green
    D. orange

27. _____ muscles control voluntary movements.
    A. Coarse
    B. Skeletal
    C. Cardiac
    D. Smooth

28. Which of the following is *not* a stage of death or dying?
    A. acceptance
    B. denial
    C. anger
    D. questioning

29. Functions of the integumentary system include all of the following *except* _____.
    A. vitamin B production from sunlight
    B. regulation of body temperature
    C. excretion of minor amounts of waste material in sweat
    D. transmission of sensory information such as pain, touch, and pressure

30. _____ is a disease of the integumentary system associated with a virus.
    A. A cold sore
    B. Chicken pox
    C. Human papilloma virus (HPV)
    D. All of the above.

31. Which of the following is *not* a part of the respiratory system?
    A. alveoli
    B. lungs
    C. trachea
    D. pons

32. Which of the following is *not* a part of the female reproductive system?
    A. vagina
    B. cervix
    C. ureters
    D. fallopian tubes

## Critical Thinking Exercises

33. Give an example of how you might use the scientific method to solve a problem.

34. What science courses have you taken? Which science courses interest you the most? Which courses do you plan to take and why?

35. Identify two body systems whose organs work together. What is their common task? How do they integrate their processes?

36. Research the layers of the meninges that cover the brain and spinal cord. Describe the characteristics and function of each.

37. As you consider the path of your future healthcare career, is there a particular life stage you would like to focus on? Does working with the elderly interest you most, or would you prefer to work with teens? Explain your choice.

# Chapter

# 10

# Math

## Terms to Know

12-hour clock
24-hour clock
addition
algebra
base ten system
Celsius temperature
  scale (°C)
common denominator
database
decimal numbers
division
English system of
  measurement
equations
Fahrenheit temperature
  scale (°F)
fractions

mean
median
metric system of
  measurement
mixed numbers
mode
multiplication
nominal numbers
ordinal numbers
percentage
prime number
proportion
ratio
spreadsheet
subtraction
whole numbers

## Chapter Objectives

- Explain the different forms of numbers, including whole, mixed, decimals, and fractions.
- Perform basic mathematical computations such as addition, subtraction, multiplication, and division.
- Understand the uses of fractions, decimal fractions, percentages, and ratios in the healthcare environment.
- Perform computations using fractions, decimal fractions, percentages, and ratios.
- Explain how algebra can be applied to problem solving in healthcare.
- Demonstrate how to use a calculator to perform functions of addition, subtraction, multiplication, and division.
- Explain the possible functions of graphs and charts when displaying healthcare information.
- Identify the importance of the metric system in healthcare, and recognize key terms and prefixes used in the metric system.
- Demonstrate how to convert Fahrenheit temperatures to Celsius temperatures.
- Explain how the 24-hour clock works and why it is used in healthcare facilities.

Reinforce your learning with additional online resources
- **Practice** vocabulary with flashcards and interactive games
- **Assess** with posttests and image labeling
- **Expand** with activities and animations

Companion
*G-W Learning*

www.g-wlearning.com/healthsciences

**Study on the Go**
Use a mobile device to practice vocabulary terms and review with self-assessment quizzes.

Mobile
*G-W Learning*

www.m.g-wlearning.com

No matter which healthcare field you choose for your career, you will be required to perform some math calculations when doing your job. Of course, there are professions in the medical field such as pharmacists, physicians, or registered nurses that will require more math skills than others. But at the minimum, you will be required to know how to add, subtract, multiply, divide, and use the metric system. You will also be expected to understand and use decimals, fractions, and ratios. It is important that you are comfortable performing these basic math calculations.

This chapter begins with a review of important math skills. If you find this review too easy, answer the *Basic Math Review* questions in the *Additional Practice* section at the end of the chapter. If you are able to correctly answer these questions, and you feel confident using a calculator, skip to the section of the chapter entitled *Data Analysis*. The student workbook and a companion website associated with this textbook program contain additional math problems to help you review various math skills important in most health professions.

## Numbers and the Base Ten System

The number system used for counting based on groups of ten is called the **base ten system**. Numbers that have more than one digit are defined by their place value. For example, the number 9,234,567 is read as: nine million, two hundred thirty-four thousand, five hundred, sixty-seven. If you understand the base ten system, you know that you can break that number down to 9 millions, 2 hundred thousands, 3 ten thousands, 4 thousands, 5 hundreds, 6 tens, and 7 ones. You could illustrate the number 9,234,567 as:

$$9,000,000 + 200,000 + 30,000 + 4,000 + 500 + 60 + 7$$

- the ones digit shows the number of ones (1)
- the tens digit shows the number of tens (10)
- the hundreds digit shows the number of hundreds (100)
- the thousands digit shows the number of thousands (1,000)
- the ten thousands digit shows the number of tens of thousands (10,000)
- the hundred thousands digit shows the number of hundreds of thousands (100,000)
- the millions digit shows the number of millions (1,000,000)

**base ten system**
*numbering system used for counting that is based on multiples of ten*

✓ *Check Your Understanding*

Read the following numbers out loud and identify the place value of each number. For example, how many ones, tens, hundreds, and thousands are in each number?

1. 540
2. 4,321
3. 98
4. 200,000
5. 4,444,444

6. 106
7. 2,435
8. 111,222
9. 12,432,000
10. 4

## Types of Numbers

There are different types of numbers and each type is used for its own special purpose. The following descriptions of numbers will help you to understand the differences between types.

### Whole Numbers

**whole numbers**
*numbers used for counting; do not contain decimal points or fractions; integers*

**Whole numbers** (also called *integers*) are the numbers you use to count, including zero. Whole numbers do not have decimal points and are not fractions or negative numbers. Examples of whole numbers include 1, 5, 10, 13, 20, and 0. Another name for whole numbers is *cardinal numbers*. A cardinal number (1, 2, 3, for example), is different from an ordinal number.

### Ordinal Numbers

**ordinal numbers**
*numbers that place objects in a series in order*

When objects are placed in order, you use **ordinal numbers** to tell their position. If ten students were ranked according to their grade on their health occupations final, you would say that the student who got the top grade was in first place, the next student was in second place, and so on.

The first ten ordinal numbers are first, second, third, fourth, fifth, sixth, seventh, eighth, ninth, and tenth. They can also be written as $1^{st}$, $2^{nd}$, $3^{rd}$, $4^{th}$, $5^{th}$, $6^{th}$, $7^{th}$, $8^{th}$, $9^{th}$, and $10^{th}$.

### Decimal Numbers

**decimal numbers**
*numbers expressed with a decimal point; values left of the decimal are whole numbers and values to the right are fractions*

**Decimal numbers** are expressed with a decimal point separating whole numbers and decimal fractions. Whole numbers appear to the left of the decimal point. Decimal fractions, or numbers with a value that is less than 1, appear to the right of the decimal point.

Examples: 10.5, 5.54, 3.1416, 152.71

### Fractions

**fractions**
*numbers composed of a numerator on top and a denominator on the bottom; indicates part of a whole*

**Fractions** are numbers defined as one or more parts of a whole number. Using fractions is an easy way to show portions less than one. Fractions are used to express parts of a whole, like the numbers that appear to the right of the decimal point in decimal numbers. Fractions are used in cooking, building, sewing, the stock market, and many other places.

Examples: 1/2, 3/4, 5/8

## Mixed Numbers

**Mixed numbers** are whole numbers with a fraction included.

Examples: 32¾, 1½, 416½

**mixed numbers**
*whole numbers followed by a remaining fraction*

## Negative Numbers

Negative numbers are less than zero, but are not a fraction or a decimal. Negative numbers are also called *negative integers*.

Examples: –5, –100, –235

## Percentages

The term *percent* means *per hundred*. When you use a **percentage**, you are working with a number by dividing it into 100 parts. For example, a dollar can be divided into 100 pennies. One penny is 1/100th of a dollar. Sometimes, it is easier to express a percentage using the percent sign (%). For example, seven pennies can be expressed as 7% of a dollar.

**percentage**
*a number divided into 100 parts; expressed with the percent sign (%)*

## Prime Numbers

A **prime number** is a number that is only divisible by itself and 1. If you try to divide a prime number by any other number, you will have a number and a fraction left over. A prime number must be a whole number greater than 1 (Figure 10.1).

**prime number**
*a number that is only divisible by itself and 1*

## Nominal Numbers

**Nominal numbers** name something—a telephone number, a house number, or a zip code. Nominal numbers do not show quantity or rank. They are used only to identify something.

**nominal numbers**
*numbers that name or identify something*

Examples: 417 Fern Avenue
The zip code for my hometown is 01796.
My office phone number is 708-967-5732.

| 2 | 3 | 5 | 7 | 11 | 13 | 17 | 19 | 23 | 29 | 31 | 37 | 41 | 43 | 47 | 53 | 59 | 61 | 67 |
|---|---|---|---|---|---|---|---|---|---|---|---|---|---|---|---|---|---|---|
| 71 | 73 | 79 | 83 | 89 | 97 | 101 | 103 | 107 | 109 | 113 | 127 | 131 | 137 | 139 | 149 | 151 | 157 | 163 |
| 167 | 173 | 179 | 181 | 191 | 193 | 197 | 199 | 211 | 223 | 227 | 229 | 233 | 239 | 241 | 251 | 257 | 263 | 269 |
| 271 | 277 | 281 | 283 | 293 | 307 | 311 | 313 | 317 | 331 | 337 | 347 | 349 | 353 | 359 | 367 | 373 | 379 | 383 |
| 389 | 397 | 401 | 409 | 419 | 421 | 431 | 433 | 439 | 443 | 449 | 457 | 461 | 463 | 467 | 479 | 487 | 491 | 499 |

**Figure 10.1** Prime numbers

# *Adding Whole Numbers*

**addition**

*the process of combining two or more numbers to obtain their total value*

**Addition** is the process of combining two or more numbers. The numbers being added together are called *addends*. The addends of a written addition problem are separated by an addition sign (+). The answer to an addition problem is called the *sum* and comes after an equal sign (=) in addition problems.

Examples: 5 + 4 = 9
4 + 6 = 10

When adding numbers that contain two or more digits, it is best to write numbers in a column, aligning the place value of the digits such as the ones, tens, or hundreds. Make sure the numbers in each column line up beneath one another. This alignment helps you add the correct numbers together. Always add the numbers in the right column first, before moving to the columns to the left.

Example:

```
   21
+  37
─────
   58
```

This problem can be rewritten as:

```
    2 tens and  1 ones
+   3 tens and  7 ones
────────────────────────
    5 tens and  8 ones   = 58
```

Sometimes, addition problems require you to carry over digits to the left.

Example:

```
   36
+  45
```

First add the ones column (6 + 5 = 11) and carry the remaining 1 to the tens column. Then, add the tens column.

```
   1
   36
+  45
─────
   81
```

Example:

```
   788
+   57
──────
   845
```

Add the ones column and carry over the *1* to the tens column. Then, add the tens column, and carry the *1* to the hundreds column.

```
  11
  788
+  57
─────
  845
```

## *Real Life Scenario*

*Supply Inventory*

1. Carlos works in a doctor's office. One day, he is asked to take inventory of disposable office surgery trays in the office. He finds 10 trays in exam room A's closet, 8 in exam room B's closet, and 24 in the supply cupboard. How many trays are in the doctor's office?

2. Carlos is then asked to take inventory of boxes of alcohol swabs in the office. He counts 20 boxes in exam room A's closet, 18 in exam room B's closet, 12 in the reception room drawers, and 9 in the supply cupboard. How many boxes of alcohol swabs are in the office?

3. Finally, Carlos must total the number of patients that were seen by the doctor over the course of the week (5 days). There were 20 patients seen on day 1, 35 on day 2, 40 on day 3, 34 on day 4, and 21 on day 5. How many patients did the doctor see over the course of five days?

# *Subtracting Whole Numbers*

**Subtraction** is the opposite of addition. When numbers are subtracted, one number is taken away from another. Simple subtraction is written as $6 - 2 = 4$, with the minus sign (–) indicating subtraction. The answer obtained in a subtraction problem is called the *difference*. Subtraction problems can be written in two ways:

**subtraction**
*the process of removing one number from another number; the opposite of addition*

```
  54
− 23    or 54 − 23 = 31
────
  31
```

You can check your answer by adding the difference to the number subtracted. If your answer is correct, your total will equal the first number in the equation. To check the above problem, $54 - 23 = 31$, you would add $31 + 23 = 54$.

## Subtracting by Borrowing Numbers

Some subtraction problems require that you "borrow" a number. When beginning a subtraction problem, align the numbers one on top of the other, as you do during an addition problem. Look at the rightmost column. If the number on top is smaller than the number on the bottom, you will have to "borrow" from the column on the left.

Consider the following subtraction problem:

$$\begin{array}{r} 34 \\ -\ 16 \\ \hline \end{array}$$

To subtract a larger number (6) from a smaller number (4), you must borrow 10 from the column to the left to complete the subtraction.

Example:

$$\begin{array}{r} \overset{1}{34} \\ -\ 16 \\ \hline 18 \end{array}$$

By borrowing the one 10 from the three 10s in the left column, 4 becomes 14. The 3 in the left column becomes a 2. When you subtract 6 from 14, you get 8, and 2 minus 1 equals 1, leaving you with an answer of 18.

### Real Life Scenario

*Subtraction in Everyday Life*

1. Paul is an emergency medical technician who has earned 14 vacation days this year. He has already taken 8. How many days does Paul have left?
2. As part of his job, Paul is required to complete 50 hours of continuing education every year. So far this year, he has completed 13 hours. How many hours does he have left to complete his education requirement for the year?
3. Last month, Paul recorded 675 miles traveled in his ambulance. This month, he has traveled 1,220 miles. How many more miles has he traveled this month than last month?

### ✓ Check Your Understanding

1. $2,222 + 99 =$
2. $123,456 + 777 =$
3. $9,689 + 245 =$
4. $68,834 + 8,834 =$
5. $64 + 7 =$
6. $9,888 - 999 =$
7. $90,145 - 326 =$
8. $11,103 - 871 =$
9. $48 - 19 =$
10. $576 - 68 =$

**multiplication**
*mathematical operation that indicates how many times a number is added to itself; a shortcut for addition*

## Multiplication

**Multiplication** is a shortcut for addition. The standard symbol for multiplication is (×). Other ways of expressing multiplication include an asterisk (10 * 10 = 100) or parentheses (10)(10) = 100. The numbers to be multiplied are called the *multiplicand* (the first number) and the *multiplier* (the second number). The answer to a multiplication problem is called the *product*.

$$
\begin{array}{r}
87 \leftarrow \text{multiplicand} \\
\times \quad 15 \leftarrow \text{multiplier} \\
\hline
1305 \leftarrow \text{product}
\end{array}
$$

You will encounter many situations that require the use of multiplication throughout your healthcare career. The following is an example of one such situation.

> Joy is working out the budget for the healthcare facility where she is employed. As part of her budgeting, Joy needs to know how much 12 boxes of latex gloves cost. Joy researches the price for one package and finds it costs $10.35. Joy could determine the cost of 12 boxes of gloves by adding $10.35 together twelve times, but that is time-consuming. Instead, Joy can find the answer using multiplication. The equation Joy must solve is: $10.35 × 12 = ?

To solve such a problem, you might want to memorize some basic multiplication problems. Using a multiplication table is the best way to practice this skill (Figure 10.2). Knowing your multiplication tables allows you to calculate numbers quickly and without error.

To answer the problem above using a multiplication table, you would multiply each digit separately to create partial answers. Then add the partial answers to find the final answer. Note that alignment of the numbers is very important!

$$
\begin{array}{r}
\$10.35 \\
\times \quad 12 \\
\hline
\end{array}
$$

First, multiply the ones digit of the multiplier (2) with each digit in the multiplicand. Because 2 × 5 = 10, you should place a 0 beneath the 5 and 2, and carry the 1 to the tens column, so it appears above the 3. Now, when you multiply 2 × 3, add 1 to the answer (2 × 3 = 6; 6 + 1 = 7). Place a 7 beneath the 3 and 1, and move on to the next digits. The first partial answer is 2,070.

$$
\begin{array}{r}
1 \\
\$10.35 \\
\times \quad 12 \\
\hline
2070
\end{array}
$$

Next, multiply the tens digits. Since you have already multiplied the ones column, place a 0 or X beneath the 0 in the ones column. Multiply 1 with each digit of the multiplicand (1 × 5 = 5, 1 × 3 = 3, 1 × 0 = 0, and 1 × 1 = 1). The second partial answer is 10,350.

$$
\begin{array}{r}
\$10.35 \\
\times \quad 12 \\
\hline
2070 \\
10350
\end{array}
$$

Now, add the two partial answers together to find the product. Because there is a decimal point in the number $10.35, the product also needs a decimal point. To determine the location of the decimal point, count the number of digits to the right of the decimal point in the multiplicand (two). Now, place the decimal point in the product so that there are two places to the right.

$$
\begin{array}{r}
\$10.35 \\
\times \quad 12 \\
\hline
2070 \\
+ \quad 10350 \\
\hline
\$124.20
\end{array}
$$

| | 1 | 2 | 3 | 4 | 5 | 6 | 7 | 8 | 9 | 10 | 11 | 12 |
|---|---|---|---|---|---|---|---|---|---|---|---|---|
| **1** | 1 | 2 | 3 | 4 | 5 | 6 | 7 | 8 | 9 | 10 | 11 | 12 |
| **2** | 2 | 4 | 6 | 8 | 10 | 12 | 14 | 16 | 18 | 20 | 22 | 24 |
| **3** | 3 | 6 | 9 | 12 | 15 | 18 | 21 | 24 | 27 | 30 | 33 | 36 |
| **4** | 4 | 8 | 12 | 16 | 20 | 24 | 28 | 32 | 36 | 40 | 44 | 48 |
| **5** | 5 | 10 | 15 | 20 | 25 | 30 | 35 | 40 | 45 | 50 | 55 | 60 |
| **6** | 6 | 12 | 18 | 24 | 30 | 36 | 42 | 48 | 54 | 60 | 66 | 72 |
| **7** | 7 | 14 | 21 | 28 | 35 | 42 | 49 | 56 | 63 | 70 | 77 | 84 |
| **8** | 8 | 16 | 24 | 32 | 40 | 48 | 56 | 64 | 72 | 80 | 88 | 96 |
| **9** | 9 | 18 | 27 | 36 | 45 | 54 | 63 | 72 | 81 | 90 | 99 | 108 |
| **10** | 10 | 20 | 30 | 40 | 50 | 60 | 70 | 80 | 90 | 100 | 110 | 120 |
| **11** | 11 | 22 | 33 | 44 | 55 | 66 | 77 | 88 | 99 | 110 | 121 | 132 |
| **12** | 12 | 24 | 36 | 48 | 60 | 72 | 84 | 96 | 108 | 120 | 132 | 144 |

**Figure 10.2**   To use a multiplication table, choose one number from the top row and one number from the row on the left-hand side. Identify the cell where these two rows meet— this is the product of your multiplication problem.

## Real Life Scenario

*Multiplying on the Job*

1. Elise is a respiratory therapist. Her supervisor has asked her to work 8 hour shifts for the next 3 weeks (Elise works 5 days a week). How many total hours will Elise work during the next 3 weeks?

2. During each 8 hour shift, Elise sees 13 patients. How many patients will she see in the next 3 weeks? Remember, Elise works 5 days a week.

# Division

**Division** is a process that enables you to find how many times one number is present in another number. Division is the opposite of multiplication. Therefore, memorizing the multiplication table will help you to solve division problems.

**division**
*process of determining how many times one number is present in another number*

The most common symbol for division is (÷). The number that gets divided is called the *dividend*. The number that does the dividing is called the *divisor*. The answer to a division problem is called the *quotient*.

$$5 \leftarrow \text{quotient}$$
$$\text{divisor} \rightarrow 3\,)\overline{15} \leftarrow \text{dividend}$$

Division problems can be written several ways:

$$6 \div 3 \text{ or } \frac{6}{3} \text{ or } 3)\overline{6}$$

Many situations will arise during your career requiring the use of division. The following is an example of how you might use division in a healthcare setting:

> Hazel is the front office medical assistant in charge of buying new chairs for the medical office's reception room. She is given a budget of $745 to purchase five new chairs. What is the most that Hazel can pay for each chair while staying in budget? The equation Hazel must solve is 745 ÷ 5 = ?

To begin, divide 5 into the first digit of the dividend (7). Because 5 goes into 7 only one time, write a 1 above the 7. Next, multiply the 5 and 1, and write the product (5) below the 7. Then, subtract the 5 from the 7, which gives you the remainder of 2.

$$
\begin{array}{r}
1\phantom{00} \\
5\,)\overline{745} \\
\underline{5\phantom{00}} \\
2\phantom{00}
\end{array}
$$

Now, bring the 4 from the 745 down next to the 2. Divide 5 into 24. Because 5 goes into 24 four times, write a 4 next to the 1 in the quotient. Multiply the 4 and the 5 and put the result (20) below the 24. Subtract the 20 from the 24 and write the difference (4) beneath the 20.

```
      14
  5 )745
     5
     ‾‾
     24
     20
     ‾‾
      4
```

Next, bring the third digit (5) down so that it is next to the 4. Divide 5 into 45. Write the answer (9) next to the 4 in the quotient. Because $9 \times 5 = 45$, the difference is 0 and there is no remainder. Hazel has $149 to spend on each chair for the reception room.

```
      149
  5 )745
     5
     ‾‾
     24
     20
     ‾‾
      45
      45
      ‾‾
       0
```

## Remainders

Some numbers do not divide perfectly into others. In such division problems, there is a *remainder*, or number left over after dividing all of the numbers in the dividend by the divisor. A remainder can be expressed by using a lowercase r or as a fraction. For example, a problem with a quotient of 7 and a remainder of 2 would be written as: 7 r.2 or $7\frac{2}{7}$.

Example:

```
      5
  5 )26
     25
     ‾‾
      1
```

Because 2 is less than 5, you should determine instead, how many times 5 goes into 26. Because $5 \times 5 = 25$, and $26 - 25 = 1$, this quotient is 5 with a remainder of 1. This quotient can be expressed as

- 5 r.1;
- $5\frac{1}{5}$; or
- 5.2.

## Real Life Scenario

### Calculating Volunteer Hours and Student Loans

1. Madison is a high school senior who wants to be an LPN (licensed practical nurse). Madison's school counselor recommends volunteering at a hospital to observe the daily responsibilities of an LPN. The volunteer program at the local hospital requires a commitment of 100 volunteer hours to complete the program. If Madison volunteers for 5 hours a week, how many weeks will it take her to complete her volunteer commitment?

2. Steven decides he wants to become an EMT. He will need a student loan to pay for the required classes. The cost of an EMT program is $1,195 with additional fees for textbook rentals of $240. After training, he will have to pay back the loan at $100 a month. How many months will it take Steven to pay back the loan?

 *Check Your Understanding*

1. $100 \times 10 =$
2. $325 \times 35 =$
3. $220 \div 20 =$
4. $1{,}425 \div 5 =$
5. $\$15.20 \times 9 =$
6. $457 \div 3 =$
7. $\$547.89 \times 40 =$
8. $\$546.20 \div 4 =$
9. $\$10{,}439 \times 426 =$
10. $40{,}200 \div 9 =$

# Fractions

Fractions, decimals, and percentages are mathematical concepts that express numbers that are part of a whole (Figure 10.3). These three concepts will be especially important for anyone entering the healthcare field to understand. As you will recall, fractions are one or more parts of a whole number. Fractions are written in the following way:

$$1/2 \text{ or } \frac{1}{2} \qquad 13/15 \text{ or } \frac{13}{15} \qquad 5/7 \text{ or } \frac{5}{7}$$

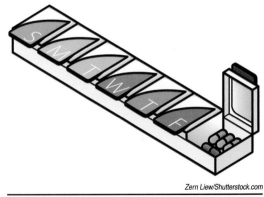

*Zern Liew/Shutterstock.com*

**Figure 10.3** A seven-day pill box represents a fraction. In this image, 1/7 of the pill box is open and 6/7 are closed.

The number written above or before the line is called the *numerator*. The number below or after the line in a fraction is called the *denominator*. The denominator is the number of parts into which the fraction is divided. When reading fractions, you always read the top number first, followed by the bottom number.

$$\frac{\text{Numerator}}{\text{Denominator}}$$

## Fractions with the Same Denominator

**common denominator**
*the number that can be divided evenly by all of the denominators in a group of fractions*

When adding or subtracting fractions with a **common denominator** only the numerator is added or subtracted.

$$\text{Example: } \frac{9}{8} + \frac{6}{8} + \frac{4}{8} = \frac{9+6+4}{8} = \frac{19}{8}$$

If adding the fraction leaves you with a numerator that is divisible by the denominator, the fraction must be reduced. This can be done by dividing the numerator by the denominator.

$$\text{The answer } \frac{19}{8} \text{ must be reduced by dividing } 19 \div 8 = 2\frac{3}{8}$$

Because 8 goes into 19 twice, the answer includes a 2 next to the remaining fraction, which is 3/8. This creates the mixed number of 2⅜.

Subtraction of fractions with common denominators is similar to addition.

$$\text{Example: } \frac{10}{9} - \frac{5}{9} - \frac{4}{9} = \frac{10-5-4}{9} = \frac{1}{9}$$

## Fractions with Different Denominators

To add or subtract two or more fractions that have different denominators, a lowest common denominator must be found.

$$\text{Example: } \frac{1}{2} + \frac{2}{5} + \frac{4}{10} = ?$$

To find the lowest common denominator for 2, 5, and 10, consider the multiples of each number.

Multiples of 2: 2, 4, 6, 8, **10**…
Multiples of 5: 5, **10**, 15, 20…
Multiples of 10: **10**, 20…
10 is the lowest common denominator.

For the first two fractions that do not already have a denominator of 10 (1/2 and 2/5), you need to multiply both the numerator and denominator by the number that will produce a denominator of 10. So the fraction 1/2 will have its numerator and denominator multiplied by 5 to equal 5/10. The fraction 2/5 will have its numerator and denominator multiplied by 2 to become 4/10. The fraction 4/10 already has a common denominator of 10. So the problem becomes:

$$\frac{5}{10} + \frac{4}{10} + \frac{4}{10} = \frac{13}{10} = 1\frac{3}{10}$$

Subtracting fractions is done through the same process used to add fractions. First, find a common denominator, then subtract the numerators, and write the answer using the common denominator.

## Multiplying Fractions

When multiplying fractions, it is not necessary to find a common denominator. Instead, simply multiply across the fraction (numerator × numerator, and denominator × denominator).

$$\text{Example: } \frac{3}{4} \times \frac{2}{3} = \frac{6}{12}$$

$(3 \times 2 = 6 \text{ and } 4 \times 3 = 12) = 6/12$

The fraction 6/12 needs to be reduced (or *simplified*). You are trying to get the smallest possible number for both the numerator and denominator. To reduce this fraction, you would divide 6 into the top number, and 6 into the bottom number (6 goes into 6 once, 6 goes into 12 twice).

The fraction 6/12 becomes 1/2.

## Dividing Fractions

The process of dividing fractions is very unique and requires the use of the reciprocal fraction. To identify a fraction's reciprocal, turn the second fraction in the problem upside down to switch the numerator and denominator. For example, the fraction 5/8 would become 8/5. Then, multiply the first fraction and the inverted second fraction. There is no need for a common denominator.

$$\text{Example: } \frac{3}{4} \div \frac{5}{8} = \frac{3}{4} \times \frac{8}{5} = \frac{24}{20} = \frac{6}{5} = 1\frac{1}{5}$$

Note that the answer was reduced from 24/20 to 6/5 by dividing the numerator and denominator each by 4. The fraction 6/5 was then converted to a mixed number. When dividing mixed numbers, you will need to convert them to fractions first.

**Converting Mixed Numbers to Fractions.** A mixed number is composed of a whole number and a fraction (5½). If you want to convert 5½ into a fraction, you must first multiply the whole number (5) by the denominator of the fraction (2). Now you have solved how many 1/2s there are in 5 (10). Next, add the numerator (1) to give you 11/2. 11/2 is another way of expressing 5½.

## Real Life Scenario

### Using Fractions in Healthcare

1. Dennis has been told that his blood pressure is bordering on high. Dennis' physician has given him a prescription to reduce his blood pressure. The prescription calls for Dennis to take 1/2 a pill daily for 45 days, and then have his blood pressure checked to see if there is improvement. How many pills will Dennis need so he can take half of a pill every day, for 45 days?

2. Leeann is a nurse's aide on the surgical floor of a busy hospital. 1/4 of the patients will have surgery on Monday and will go home on Wednesday. Another 1/4 of the remaining patients will go home on Thursday. If no new patients arrive, what fraction of the patients will be left on the floor on Friday?

 *Check Your Understanding*

Convert the following mixed numbers to fractions.

1. 6½                                   3. 1⅛
2. 7¼

Reduce the following fractions to their simplest form.

4. 6/18                                 6. 14/17
5. 10/80

Complete the following calculations.

7.  1/8 + 4/8 + 3/8 =                13. 1/4 × 2/3 =
8.  1/2 + 1/4 + 3/8 =                14. 1/8 × 5/8 =
9.  1/2 + 3/5 + 2/10 =               15. 5/8 × 3/4 =
10. 7/8 – 5/8 =                      16. 4/8 ÷ 1/8 =
11. 7/16 – 1/8 =                     17. 3/4 ÷ 1/8 =
12. 1/2 – 1/4 =                      18. 9/10 ÷ 1/4 =

# Decimal Fractions

In healthcare, you will be working primarily with decimal fractions (often referred to as *decimals*). Decimals are special types of fractions that most people find easier to use than traditional fractions. Decimal fractions are much easier to write and compute than traditional fractions. Decimals represent parts of the whole. For example, 0.5 is 1/2 of 1 and 0.75 is 3/4 of 1.

Decimal fractions are always expressed in multiples of ten, making them easier to work with. A decimal fraction has a denominator that is a multiple of 10, such as 100, 1,000, or 10,000. When writing a decimal fraction, eliminate the denominator and place a dot, or *decimal point* next to the ones digit. For example, 1/10 becomes 0.1. Both stand for one-tenth.

When there is one number to the right of the decimal point that is read as a tenth. Two numbers to the right of the decimal point are hundredths. Figure 10.4 shows the decimal, fraction, and written-out expression of various parts of a whole using multiples of 10.

| **Expressing Parts of a Whole** | | |
|---|---|---|
| *Decimal* | *Fraction* | *Written-Out* |
| .1 | 1/10 | One-tenth |
| .01 | 1/100 | One-hundredth |
| .001 | 1/1,000 | One-thousandth |
| .0001 | 1/10,000 | One ten-thousandth |

**Figure 10.4** Expressing parts of a whole

Example: 28.74 is a decimal fraction. 28 is the whole number, the (.) is a decimal point, and the numbers to the right of the decimal point represent the decimal itself.

In the healthcare field, it is standard to always place a zero to the left of the decimal point when there is not a digit in that value (for example, 0.95). Putting a zero before the decimal point prevents misinterpretation, such as reading .95 as the number 95. Also, a zero after the last digit to the right of the decimal point is not necessary (1.2, not 1.20).

When writing an equation that features a decimal fraction, you must remember to properly align all of the numbers. Make sure when you add or subtract decimal fractions, you line up the decimal points from each number.

Example:
```
   23.45
    1.40
+ 451.23
  ------
  476.08
```

## Converting a Fraction to a Decimal

You will sometimes need to convert fractions to decimals. Converting a fraction to a decimal is done through a division problem. The first step is to divide the numerator of the fraction by the denominator. If your fraction is 2/3, you should divide 3 into 2.

Example: Change the fraction 7/8 to a decimal number.

```
      0.875
   8 )7.000
      64
      --
       60
       56
       --
        40
        40
        --
         0
```

### Think It Through

Notice that a gas station posts the cost of a gallon of gas on its sign. What kind of numbers do gas stations use to post the cost of a gallon of gas?

Create a long division problem in which the denominator (8) is dividing into the numerator (7). Add a decimal and zeros to the numerator to complete the division problem. You can add as many zeroes as you need.

## Rounding Decimal Fractions

Decimal fractions can be rounded up or down for the specific degree of accuracy required. The rounding off rule states that if the digit to the right of the number you are rounding is 5 or greater, round it up to the next number. If the digit is less than 5, round the number down by deleting any digits that follow the chosen place value. Leave the original digit unchanged.

Let's suppose that a decimal must be accurate to two place values. To round a number such as 17.363 up or down two places, you would first locate the digit two places to the right of the decimal point. In this case, that number is 6. Next, look at the number that comes after the 6, which is 3. Since that number is less than 5, you would round the number off to 17.36. In the case of the number 17.367, the number 7 is greater than 5, so you would have rounded the 6 up to a 7, making the number 17.37.

### *Real Life Scenario*

*Working with Decimal Fractions*

1. Suzanne is a part-time occupational therapist. Her schedule for next week has her working some partial shifts as well as a full shift. Suzanne's schedule looks like this:

   Monday: 5½ hours
   Tuesday: 5¼ hours
   Wednesday: 6½ hours
   Thursday: 3¼ hours
   Friday: 8 hours

   A. Convert the mixed numbers into decimal fractions.
   B. Add the decimal fractions together to find out how many total hours Suzanne will be working next week.

2. Suzanne wakes up on Thursday with a sore throat. She calls her supervisor to tell him she will not be working Thursday, but will be in on Friday. Now how many hours will Suzanne work for the week?

# *Percentages*

The term used to describe part of a whole number is *percentage*. Percent means *per one hundred*. Thirty percent, written as 30%, means 30 parts out of 100 parts. Written as a fraction, it would be expressed as 30/100. A number can be written as a fraction, a decimal, or a percentage (Figure 10.5). To solve mathematical problems, sometimes it may be necessary to convert a percentage to a fraction or decimal fraction.

## Calculating Percentages

To calculate a percentage, you must divide the part by the whole. Then convert the decimal answer to a percentage by moving the decimal point two places to the right and adding a percentage sign (%). This will tell you what percentage represents the part of the whole.

| Fractions, Decimals, and Percentages | | |
|:---:|:---:|:---:|
| **Fraction** | **Decimal** | **Percentages** |
| 3/20 | 0.15 | 15% |
| 1/5 | 0.20 | 20% |
| 5¼ | 5.25 | 525% |

**Figure 10.5** Moving from fractions to decimals and percentages provides a variety of ways to express numbers less than 1.

Example: Grace is in a health occupations class. There are 35 students in the class. A high percentage of the students are interested in a nursing career. The total number of students interested in a nursing career is 28, representing 80% of the students. The calculation to establish this percentage is: 28 ÷ 35 = .80, or 80%.

## Converting a Percentage to a Decimal Fraction

To convert a percentage into a decimal fraction, you must divide by 100 or move the decimal point two places to the left and drop the percent sign.

Examples: 14% = 14.0 = 0.14
29.9% = 0.299

In the same manner, a decimal fraction can be converted to a percentage by multiplying by 100, or by moving the decimal point two places to the right and adding a percent sign.

Percentages are often used in your daily life. For example, you are charged a sales tax on every purchase you make. The sales tax is always a percentage of the total bill. You will also see percentages used during department store sales. The sale price represents a percentage of the original price (Figure 10.6).

Examples: 0.41 = 41%
0.042 = 4.2%

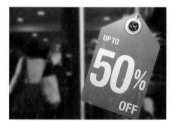

*Bikeworldtravel/Shutterstock.com*

**Figure 10.6** Percentages are often used in department store sales.

### *Real Life Scenario*

*Using Percentages*

1. A box of table salt (sodium chloride) is comprised of 40% sodium. If a box of salt weighs 26 ounces, how many ounces of sodium are in the box of salt?

2. 30 people at Eastridge Hospital had surgery on May 21st—4 were children, 12 were men, and 14 were women. What percentage of the people who received surgery on May 21st were children?

3. Dr. Levin, an orthopedist, has 36 patients who suffer from osteoporosis. This condition causes the bones to become brittle and break more easily than healthy bones. This year, 15 patients had broken hips, 11 had collapsing vertebrae, and 10 had broken wrists. What percentage of Dr. Levin's osteoporosis patients had broken hips this year?

# *Ratios*

**ratio**

*comparison of one quantity with another, similar quantity*

A **ratio** expresses the relationship between two numbers. Ratios can be used to show how many times one number can be found within another number.

The quantities that are compared in a ratio are called the terms, or *components*, of the ratio. The components are written with a colon (:) or the word "to" between them. A ratio can also be expressed as a fraction.

> Example: In Eastridge High School's medical terminology class, there are 15 girls and 10 boys. What is the ratio of girls to boys?
> 15:10 or 15 to 10 or 15/10

As was discussed with fractions, ratios can be reduced. Because both 15 and 10 can be divided by 5, you can use that number to reduce the ratio.

> $15 \div 5 = 3$
> $10 \div 5 = 2$
> The ratio expressed in its lowest terms would be: 3:2 or 3 to 2 or 3/2

A ratio is written in the same order as the words describing it are written. For instance, the newborn nursery in Eastridge Hospital has one nurse for every four newborns, so the ratio of nurses to newborns would be expressed as 1:4. But, if you wish to express how many newborns there are in the nursery for every nurse, you would write the ratio 4:1.

If a ratio is known, you can determine what percentage one of the components is of the whole. To do so, first add the components together to get the total. Then, divide the component for which you want to find the percentage by the total. Your answer will be a decimal fraction and you can determine the percentage by multiplying the decimal by 100.

> Example: In Eastridge Extended Care Hospital, the ratio of male patients to female patients is 1:4. What is the percentage of male patients at the hospital?
> The ratio is 1:4, males to females.
> The total number is 1 male + 4 females = 5.
> The percentage of males in the hospital is 1/5 or 0.2
> Multiply 0.2 by 100 to get the percentage. $0.2 \times 100 = 20\%$

## *Real Life Scenario*

*Ratios in Real Life*

1. Last month at Eastridge Hospital, 32 infants were born. Of these 32 deliveries, doctors performed 8 caesarean sections (surgical removal of a baby). What is the ratio of caesarean sections to normal deliveries expressed in lowest terms?

2. On his flight last week, Jamal sat next to a woman who was coughing and sneezing throughout the entire trip. There were 8 people seated in direct contact with the sick woman. Jamal and two other people became sick a few days later. Of the people exposed to the germs, what was the ratio of those who became sick to those who did not? What percentage of people exposed became sick?

# Proportions

A **proportion** is an equation with a ratio on each side. To use a proportion, the ratios must be equal to each other.

**proportion**
*a statement of the equality of two ratios*

Example: 8:4 = 2:1.

Another way of expressing this is 8/4 = 2/1 or: $\dfrac{8}{4} = \dfrac{2}{1}$

One way proportions are used by healthcare professionals is in determining dosages of medicine.

Example: John is a 150-pound man. The dosage directions for one of John's medications is to give a 150-pound man 10 milliliters (ml) of the liquid medicine. What if John weighed 300 pounds (lb)? What dosage would he be given then? A proportion can be used to find the answer.

$$\frac{150}{10} = \frac{300}{x \text{ (or unknown)}}$$

Cross multiply to begin solving for $x$. Multiply the numerator of the first fraction by the denominator of the second. Repeat this step with the numerator of the second fraction and the denominator of the first. In this case, you end up with:

150$x$ = 3000

To find the value of $x$, divide 3000 by 150.

3000/150 = $x$
$x$ = 20
A 300-pound man would need 20 ml of the medication to receive the proper dose.

## *Real Life Scenario*

*Ratios and Proportions*

1. The Eastridge Hospital Emergency Department reported that 1 out of 6 patients arriving on the second Saturday in December had the flu. If 78 people were admitted, how many of these patients had the flu?
2. If 1:16 patients on a hospital floor need special meals, and there are 64 patients on the floor, how many special meals should the kitchen prepare?

# *Using a Calculator*

Healthcare workers are required to perform math calculations when doing various tasks such as determining medication dosages, working in a healthcare facility's accounting department, or determining the salt content of a low-sodium diet. Even though calculators are on hand in most cases, it is important to understand the fundamentals of mathematics. You may have to solve a problem by knowing how to manipulate the numbers involved if a calculator is not available to you.

You are likely familiar with the calculator's functions, but a brief review of how to add, subtract, multiply, and divide using a calculator follows. Many calculators perform much more complex functions such as graphing, calculus, trigonometric operations.

However, when used correctly, a calculator saves valuable time and ensures accuracy, especially in the case of complex problems. Double-check your answers by performing the calculation at least twice—wrong entries will result in wrong answers.

Entries are made by pressing certain numbers and symbols on the keyboard of the calculator (Figure 10.7). The information entered appears in the display area above the keyboard. It is always helpful to check the display area after entering a number to make sure you've entered the number correctly. Figure 10.8 explains some of the common buttons on a calculator and their uses.

- **Addition.** Enter the first addend of your problem and then press the (+) key. Enter the second addend. Press the (=) key and the sum will appear on the display.
- **Subtraction.** Enter a number and press the (–) key. Next, enter the number to be subtracted from the first number. Then press the (=) key to find the difference.
- **Multiplication.** Enter the multiplicand and press the (×) key. Next, enter the multiplier and press the (=) key. The product will appear on the display.

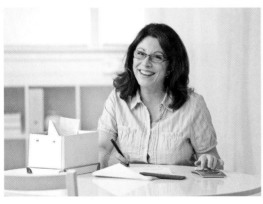

AVAVA/Shutterstock.com

**Figure 10.7** Using a calculator will make it easier to complete math problems while on the job.

| Common Symbols on a Calculator | |
|---|---|
| **Key** | **Function** |
| C | clears all entries |
| CE | clears last entry |
| . | enters a decimal point |
| + | adds |
| – | subtracts |
| × | multiplies |
| ÷ | divides |
| % | calculates percentage |
| = | calculates the final answer |

**Figure 10.8** Common symbols on a calculator

- **Division.** Let's say you want to divide 100 by 20. Enter the dividend (100), press the (÷) key, and enter the divisor (20). After pressing the (=) key, the quotient (5) will appear on the display.
- **Calculating a percentage.** Say you need to identify 20% of 50. Enter 50, press the (×) key, then enter 20, and then press the (%) key. The answer, 10, will appear on the display. If your calculator does not have a (%) key, you can calculate this percentage by multiplying 50 by 0.2.

### *Real Life Scenario*

**Calculator Uses in Healthcare**

1. Karen works in the accounting department of Eastridge Hospital. Her boss has asked her to calculate how many employees make over $50,000 each year. Karen finds that the hospital employs 450 people. 75 employees make over $50,000. What is the percentage of employees who make over $50,000?

2. Gail is studying to become a cardiac care nurse. She learns that the heart pumps about 65 milliliters of blood every time it beats. Gail measures her own pulse and finds that her heart beats 75 times per minute. How many milliliters of blood does Gail's heart pump per minute? per hour?

# *Introduction to Algebra*

**Algebra** is the branch of mathematics that substitutes letters for numbers to solve for unknown quantities. The term *algebra* comes from the Arabic *al-jebr* meaning "reunion of broken parts." Algebra problems are designed to solve a problem with the answer represented by a letter—typically $x$ or $y$. When you learned how to solve for x in the Proportions section of this chapter, you were using algebra. This section will briefly explain how algebra can be used while treating patients.

The mathematics involved in an algebraic equation are like a balancing scale (recall the scale used to illustrate the scale of justice). What is done on one side must be done to the other side to balance the scale. In the case of an algebra problem, what is done to one side of the problem must be done to the other. Moving from arithmetic (simple math including, addition, subtraction, multiplication, and division) to algebra will look something like this:

Arithmetic: $3 + 4 = 4 + 3$
Algebra: $x + y = y + x$

The examples above are **equations**. An equation consists of expressions (collections of numbers and letters) separated by an equal sign. The two sides of the equation must be equal, like a scale that has equal weights on both sides.

When solving an algebra problem, you must first write out the equation and identify the unknown quantity you plan to solve for. Then, use your basic arithmetic skills—addition, subtraction, multiplication, and

**algebra**
*branch of mathematics that substitutes letters for numbers; involves solving for the unknown*

**equations**
*mathematical statements containing expressions composed of both numbers and letters; two sides of an equation are separated by an equal sign and must be equal to one another*

division—to isolate the unknown on one side of the equation. This will help you determine the value of the unknown.

Example: $3x - 5 = 10$

$3x - 5 = 10$

$+5 \qquad +5$

Add 5 to both sides of the equation to isolate the $3x$ on the left.

$3x = 15$

$3 \qquad 3$

Divide each side by 3, so that only the $x$ remains on the left-hand side of the equation.

$x = 5$

To check your answer, plug 5 into the equation where $x$ appears.

$3(5) - 5 = 10$

$15 - 5 = 10$

$10 = 10$

Because both sides of the equation are equal, you know that 5 is the correct answer.

One way algebra is commonly used in healthcare is to calculate medicine dosage. Nurses, in particular, are responsible for performing these calculations and administering the proper amount of medicine to a patient. The following example shows one way of using algebra to calculate the ml (milliliters) amount for a liquid medication administered by injection (Figure 10.9).

To calculate the amount of medicine to administer, use the following algebraic equation:

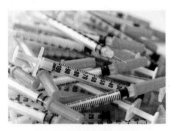

Kidsana Maimeetook/Shutterstock.com

**Figure 10.9** Calibrated syringes are used for medication injections.

$$\frac{D\ (desired\ dose)}{H\ (have\ on\ hand)} \times V\ (vehicle) = x\ (amount\ to\ be\ administered)$$

Example: A vial of medication states that there are 300 mg of the medicine per 0.5 ml. The doctor orders 600 mg of medication to be administered to the patient. How many ml of the medication should the nurse inject?

$$\frac{600\ mg}{300\ mg} \times 0.5 = x$$

$600/300 = 2$

$2 \times 0.5 = x$

$x = 1\ ml$

The nurse should administer one ml of the medicine to achieve the desired dose of 600 mg.

## *Real Life Scenario*

### *Using Algebra to Calculate Vacation Days*

Judy works in the Human Resources Department of Eastridge Hospital. She is told to calculate how many vacation days will be given to new, full-time employees in one year if the employee earns one-and-a-half vacation days every two months. How would you set up an algebraic equation for this calculation? How many vacation days would the employee earn per year?

 *Check Your Understanding*

Solve for $x$.

1. $5x - 5 = 20$
2. $x + 30 = 50$
3. $5x = 100$
4. $400 \times 5 = 2x$
5. $20x - 20 = 400$

# Data Analysis

The healthcare world produces a wealth of information each day. Hospitals need to keep track of inventory to maintain all vital supplies, pharmacies need to be aware of the drugs they have on hand, and health departments need to analyze rates of contagious disease outbreaks such as influenza and venereal disease.

Information like this is commonly stored in databases and spreadsheets and presented in charts and graphs. Charts and graphs allow for analysis of large amounts of information. This analysis is necessary to fully understand the subjects and themes of the information. A common way of analyzing information is the use of basic statistical methods, which are mean, median, and mode.

## Mean, Median, and Mode

The statistical tools of mean, median, and mode are three ways of analyzing data. Each of these statistical tools will help you find a different type of average. To find the **mean**, total all numbers in your information and divide the result by the quantity of numbers you have been given.

**mean**
*mathematical average of data*

> Example: Lori decides to calculate how much she spent taking her beagle to the veterinarian in the past year. Her charges are listed in Figure 10.10.

After adding up the total of each bill, Lori determines she spent $795.00 on vet bills last year. Now she wants to know what the mean amount was for each visit. To calculate the mean, take the total Lori has paid ($795) and then divide by the number of visits (5).

$$\frac{\$795}{5} = \$159$$

| Calculating Mean, Median, and Mode | | |
|---|---|---|
| **Month** | **Services** | **Charges** |
| January | Checkup, shots | $140 |
| March | Office visit, ear examination, ear medicine, nail trim | $165 |
| May | Office visit, allergy testing, hypoallergenic food | $270 |
| July | Office visit, allergy shots | $110 |
| October | Office visit, allergy shots | $110 |

**Figure 10.10**   Calculating, mean, median, and mode

**median**
*the number exactly in the middle of a group of numbers listed in ascending or descending order*

**mode**
*the number(s) that occur most frequently in a set of numbers*

On average, Lori spent $159 per vet visit.

The **median** is the number that falls exactly in the middle of a list of numbers organized in either ascending (*increasing*) or descending (*decreasing*) order.

> Example: As Figure 10.10 shows, Lori spent $110, $110, $140, $165, $270 (in ascending order). The median number is $140 because it is in the exact middle of the values.

In the example above, it was easy to identify the median because there were an odd number of bills. However, if you have an even numbered list (let's say that Lori went to the vet six times), look for the *two* numbers that fall in the middle of the group. Add these two numbers together, and then divide the total by 2 because that's how many numbers were entered into the equation.

> Example: Imagine the numbers in your list are 1, 2, 3, 4, 5, and 6; the median numbers are 3 and 4.

Add 3 + 4 together and you get 7. Now you divide by 2 because there were two median numbers.

> 7 ÷ 2 = 3.5, the median is 3.5

The **mode** is the number(s) that occur most frequently in a set of numbers. Some lists of numbers do not have a mode, while others may have one or more. In the case of Lori's vet bills, the mode is $110.

### Real Life Scenario

*Using Mean, Median, and Mode in Healthcare*

1. Five people who visited the Eastridge Hospital emergency room on Sunday were admitted with the following temperatures:
   98.6°F, 101°F, 105°F, 98.6°F, 98.6°F
   Calculate the mean, median, and mode of these temperatures.
2. Over the course of the past week, the following number of meals was served each day in the Eastridge Hospital cafeteria:
   Monday—145 meals, Tuesday—152 meals, Wednesday—192 meals, Thursday—230 meals, Friday— 230 meals
   Calculate the mean, median, and mode for the number of meals served over the course of those five days.

**spreadsheet**
*a document containing rows and columns of data; useful for organizing numeric values and executing computer calculations*

## Spreadsheets and Databases

A **spreadsheet** is a document that holds information in rows and columns, and is usually created by a computer program. Each row and column contains cells that hold information in the form of words or numbers (Figure 10.11). Spreadsheet programs make it easy to perform mathematical operations on groups of numbers. You can easily add a column; calculate the mean, median, or mode of a column; or perform other mathematical operations on information organized in a column or a row. Inserting formulas into the spreadsheet will enable the user to perform automatic calculations.

A **database** is a detailed collection of related information organized for convenient access, generally on a computer. An example of a database in a physician's office is a specialized database with patient information such as name, address, telephone number, emergency contact number, social security number, health insurance information, and dates of office visits.

**database**
*collection of records such as addresses, phone numbers, and other patient information*

## Charts and Graphs

Charts and graphs are used to display information clearly and quickly. Healthcare environments use charts and graphs extensively. Temperature is often graphed on a patient's chart so the physician can quickly view the fluctuations in a clear, easy-to-read manner.

Many graphs and charts are used throughout the healthcare world, but the examples below depict sample annual cases of influenza in one clinic. The same data is represented in four formats—a simple table, line graph, bar graph, and circle graph (or *pie chart*).

A simple table arranges dates and numbers of influenza cases in a clinic in rows and columns (Figure 10.12). A line graph shows the relationship of two or more numbers. This graph can also show trends across periods of time (Figure 10.13). The bar graph shows comparisons among categories (Figure 10.14). For our purposes, the pie chart in Figure 10.15 presents the number of influenza cases by season.

| Month | Cases of influenza |
|-------|--------------------|
| Jan | 55 |
| Feb | 50 |
| Mar | 45 |
| Apr | 35 |
| May | 26 |
| Jun | 14 |
| Jul | 7 |
| Aug | 6 |
| Sep | 7 |
| Oct | 25 |
| Nov | 31 |
| Dec | 40 |

**Figure 10.12**   A simple table

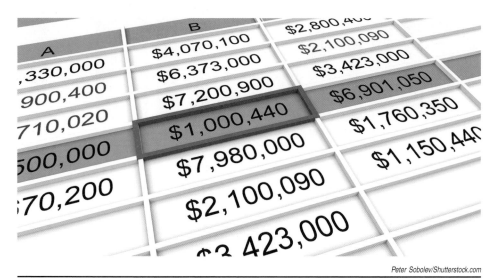

Peter Sobolev/Shutterstock.com

**Figure 10.11**   Spreadsheets are particularly useful for compiling and calculating numerical data.

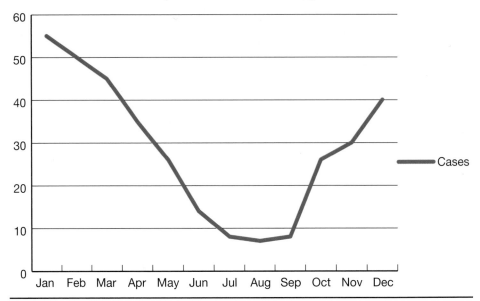

**Figure 10.13**    Line graph

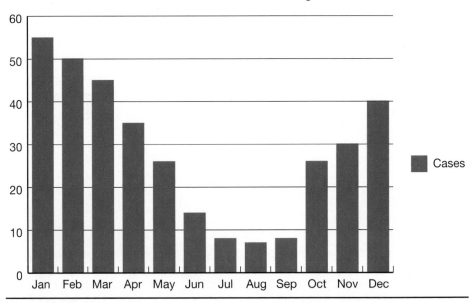

**Figure 10.14**    Bar graph

## Reading Graphs

When you read bar and line graphs, you will see a vertical axis called the *x axis* and a horizontal axis called the *y axis*. In Figure 10.13, the graph's *y* axis represents a clinic's total flu cases. The *x* axis represents the period

**Annual Influenza Cases at Eastridge Clinic**

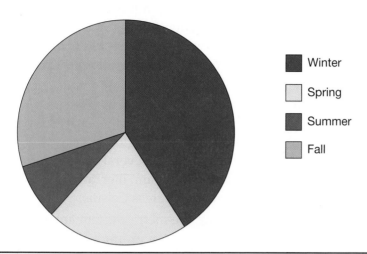

- ■ Winter
- □ Spring
- ■ Summer
- ▨ Fall

**Figure 10.15**  A circle graph is sometimes called a pie chart.

of time in which the cases were recorded (January–December). Data was entered for each month, and the line connecting the data points illustrates the trends in number of flu cases. You can see that in the winter months the flu cases were highest, and in the summer months the number of cases declined.

The bar graph in Figure 10.14 shows the same values represented on the *x* and *y* axes as Figure 10.13. In the case of a bar graph, the number of flu cases per month is easily read. Data trends are also easy to identify by comparing the height of each month's bar.

## *Real Life Scenario*

### *Creating Charts and Graphs*

1. John works in sports medicine. Broken arms account for 1/4 of his patients' injuries, knee injuries make up another 1/4 of the cases, broken fingers account for 1/8 of his cases, 1/8 are elbow injuries, and 1/4 are shoulder injuries. Create a pie chart representing this data.

2. Emile works in the human resources department of Eastridge Hospital. His boss has asked him to make a bar graph showing how many total sick days hospital employees used during each month of the last year. Put the following data into a bar graph:

   | | |
   |---|---|
   | January: 190 | July: 110 |
   | February: 195 | August: 100 |
   | March: 165 | September: 110 |
   | April: 130 | October: 125 |
   | May: 125 | November: 140 |
   | June: 115 | December: 180 |

# *Measurement in Healthcare*

When asked to measure something in the United States, most people use the **English system of measurement**. Today, the United States is one of the very few countries that have not converted to the metric system. The rest of the world has adopted the **metric system of measurement**.

The main differences between the metric and English systems of measurement can be found in the measurement units. The metric system uses units organized by factors of ten. This allows the various types of units to be related. Units of measurement in the English system are not related or consistent. While the English system uses several different units, the metric system has only three basic units: the gram, liter, and meter. In the metric system, temperature is measured in degrees Celsius.

Calculations performed using the metric system are much easier than calculations using the English system. For example, 1,000 meters are found in 1 kilometer; however, there are 5,280 feet in a mile. In the English system, there is no common base, which makes it challenging to use. The relationship between the different units of measure can be confusing because English system units are not based in the powers of 10, as in the metric system. For example, in the English system, the length of a yard was based on the distance from King Henry I's nose to his thumb.

For these reasons, the metric system is universally used in science and medicine. Those who wish to have a career in the health sciences must become comfortable using the metric system by understanding its terminology, including its basic units and its prefixes.

**English system of measurement**

*a system of measurement commonly used in the United States; measurements are based on the inch, pound, gallon, and Fahrenheit degrees*

**metric system of measurement**

*a system of measurement using units related by factors of ten; measurements based on the gram, liter, meter, and temperature measured in Celsius*

**Did You Know?**

### *The History of Measurement*

The English system of measurement was originally based on the human body, nature, and everyday activities. For example, an acre originally was a measure of land based on the amount of land that could be plowed in a day. An inch was the width of a thumb. Such natural measures were fine for a simple, agricultural society. However, as trade and commerce grew, there was a need for more exact measures.

The metric system was developed by the French to create a system that uses units related by factors of ten and only three basic measurements for weight, volume, and length. When moving from one unit to another when using the decimal system, simply move the decimal point to the appropriate power of 10.

## Metric Units

There are three basic units of measurement in the metric system—grams, liters, and meters (Figure 10.16). The gram (g) is the basic metric unit of measurement for weight. Weight is the physical measurement of an object subjected to the force of gravity. Scientists consider mass and weight the same within the gravitational field of Earth. In the English system, weight is measured in ounces and pounds.

The liter is the basic metric measurement of liquid volume. In the English system, volume is measured in cups, pints, quarts, and gallons.

The meter is the metric unit for linear measurement (length). It is slightly longer than the English yard. Inches, feet, and miles are other English units of measurement for length.

| Basic Metric Measurements | | |
|---|---|---|
| **Metric System** | **Measures** | **English System** |
| gram (g) | weight or mass | ounces and pounds |
| liter (l) | volume | cups, pints, quarts, and gallons |
| meter (m) | length | inches, feet, yards, miles |

**Figure 10.16** Basic measurements as represented in the metric and English measurement systems

## Metric Prefixes

To properly use the metric system as a healthcare professional, you will need to recognize a variety of metric prefixes. These prefixes are added to the front of one of the basic units (meters, grams, liters) to indicate the size of a particular metric unit. Figure 10.17 lists the metric prefixes, the related multiple of 10, and an example.

## Converting Measurements

In addition to scientific use, the metric system is being used in industry, governmental agencies, education, and many other important areas in the United States. Being able to convert a measurement from one type to another is a very useful skill to master. As a healthcare professional, you

| Metric Prefixes | | |
|---|---|---|
| **Prefix** | **Multiple** | **Example** |
| nano- | 1/1,000,000,000 | 1 nanometer=1/1,000,000,000 of a meter |
| micro- | 1/1,000,000 | 1 microliter=1/1,000,000 of a liter |
| milli- | 1/1,000 | 1 millimeter = 1/1,000 of a meter |
| centi- | 1/100 | 1 centiliter = 1/100 of a liter |
| deci- | 1/10 | 1 decimeter = 1/10 of a meter |
| deca- | 10 | 1 decagram = 10 grams |
| hecto- | 100 | 1 hectometer = 100 meters |
| kilo- | 1000 | 1 kilogram = 1000 grams |
| mega- | 1,000,000 | 1 megameter = 1,000,000 meters |
| giga- | 1,000,000,000 | 1 gigameter = 1,000,000,000 meters |

**Figure 10.17** Metric prefixes

will likely find yourself converting English measurements to metric measurements more often than converting metric to English. Appendix A in the back of this textbook contains conversion information and calculations.

Consult the metric conversion chart in Appendix A for converting values in the English system to the metric system. Find the English measurement that you wish to convert in the left-hand column. Then, multiply by the number in the middle column to convert to the related metric system value.

Example: 145 pounds = _____ kilograms
140 pounds × 0.45 = 65.25 kilograms

You can also convert from the metric system to the English system. To do so, divide the metric value by the number given in the middle column of the chart. The quotient is the related English system value.

Example: 100 grams = _____ ounces
100 grams ÷ 28.0 = 3.6 ounces

## Extend Your Knowledge

*Examining Food Labels*

Look at the food labels of 10 products you have in your home. How many labels use only the metric system? How many use only the English system? How many represent measurements using both the English and metric systems? Select two labels from each system and convert them to the opposite system. Show your work.

 *Check Your Understanding*

1. Calculate your weight, height, and body measurements (waist, hips, and chest) by converting the English measurements to metric units.

2. Convert the mileage on your car to kilometers.

3. On a recent trip to Canada, you filled your gas tank with 40 liters of gasoline. How many gallons of gasoline did you put in your tank?

4. Convert 100 kilometers per hour into miles per hour.

# *Metric Temperature Measurement*

The **Celsius temperature scale (°C)** is a metric scale used to measure temperature throughout the healthcare world. The Celsius scale is in general use wherever metric units are accepted, and it is used in scientific work everywhere. Many countries have adopted the Celsius scale, but the United States has not. The **Fahrenheit temperature scale (°F)** is the non-metric

**Celsius temperature scale (°C)**

*metric temperature scale; defines the freezing point of water as 0° and the boiling point of water as 100°*

**Fahrenheit temperature scale (°F)**

*the temperature scale commonly used in the United States; the freezing point of water is 32° and the boiling point is 212°*

scale used in the United States to measure body temperature in healthcare settings.

The freezing point of water on the Celsius scale is 0°, and the boiling point is 100°. The Fahrenheit scale is based on a system that is less logical and often more challenging to use. The freezing point of water in Fahrenheit is 32°, and the boiling point is 212°.

Most healthcare facilities have conversion charts that can be used to convert temperatures on one scale to the other and vice-versa. The conversions can also easily be made by using specific formulas.

## Converting Temperatures from Fahrenheit to Celsius

The formula for converting Fahrenheit temperatures to Celsius is: $°C = 5/9 \times (°F - 32)$.

Example:   F = 98.6°

$$C = \frac{5}{9} \times (98.6 - 32)$$

$$C = \frac{5}{9} \times 66.6$$

$$C = \frac{5 \times 66.6}{9}$$

$$C = \frac{333}{9}$$

$$C = 37°$$

## Converting Temperatures from Celsius to Fahrenheit

The formula for converting Celsius temperatures to Fahrenheit is: $°F = 9/5(C) + 32$.

Example:   C = 37°

$$F = \frac{9}{5} \times (37) + 32$$

$$F = \frac{9 \times 37}{5} + 32$$

$$F = \frac{333}{5} + 32$$

$$F = 66.6 + 32$$

$$F = 98.6°$$

## Real Life Scenario

### Converting Temperatures

1. While on vacation in Germany with your family, you become ill and need to visit a doctor. The doctor tells you that your temperature is 39°. Given your location, you assume, correctly, that he has given your temperature using the Celsius scale. Using the appropriate conversion formula, what is your Fahrenheit temperature?

2. You are a nurse at Eastridge Hospital and you have a patient from France. She asks you what her temperature is, and you tell her 103°F. She doesn't understand what this means. Convert her temperature into Celsius using the appropriate formula.

 *Check Your Understanding*

Convert the following Fahrenheit temperatures to Celsius.

1. 98.6°F                                  4. 37°F
2. 100°F                                   5. 40°F
3. 10°F

Convert the following Celsius temperatures to Fahrenheit.

6. 0°C                                     9. 100°C
7. 5°C                                     10. 50°C
8. 37°C

# The 24-Hour Clock

**24-hour clock**

*method of measuring time based on 24-hour-long segments; also called military time*

**12-hour clock**

*expression of time used internationally; based on a 12-hour system in which a.m. and p.m. designations must be assigned to identify the proper time*

In the healthcare world, time is often expressed using the **24-hour clock**, or what is commonly known as *military time*. A clear, concise way of accurately recording time is essential in a healthcare facility. Medical records are legal documents. Time is critical when treatment, medication, and duration of procedures depend on accurate timekeeping.

**The 12-hour clock** (which you typically use in your daily life) has the disadvantage of using just 12 numbers to designate 24 different hours. This means that each of those 12 numbers is used twice a day. Therefore, without the a.m. and p.m. designations, you cannot know for sure what time of day a particular number represents.

In contrast, the 24-hour clock designates every hour with a unique numerical time. When you say that it is 11:00 o'clock, do you mean 11:00 a.m. or 11:00 p.m.? If you are using military time, then those hours are written as 1100 and 2300, respectively. You don't need the a.m. or p.m. designation, and there is no chance for confusion.

Time on the 24-hour clock is always expressed in four digits. The first two digits represent the hours, and the second two digits represent the minutes. A 0 is placed in front of the hours 1 through 9 (01, 02, 03). Do not use colons to separate hours from minutes. Figure 10.18 shows how the 12-hour clock relates to the 24-hour clock.

✔ *Check Your Understanding*

Convert the following 12-hour clock times to military time.

1. 1:35 a.m.                                    4. 10:45 p.m.

2. 3:34 p.m.                                    5. 9:09 a.m.

3. 7:15 p.m.

Convert the following military times to the 12-hour clock.

6. 2345                                         9. 1145

7. 1450                                         10. 0637

8. 0256

| Conversion of the 12-Hour Clock to the 24-Hour Clock | | | |
|---|---|---|---|
| **12-hour clock** | **24-hour clock** | **12-hour clock** | **24-hour clock** |
| 1:00 a.m. | 0100 | 1:00 p.m. | 1300 |
| 2:00 a.m. | 0200 | 2:00 p.m. | 1400 |
| 3:00 a.m. | 0300 | 3:00 p.m. | 1500 |
| 4:00 a.m. | 0400 | 4:00 p.m. | 1600 |
| 5:00 a.m. | 0500 | 5:00 p.m. | 1700 |
| 6:00 a.m. | 0600 | 6:00 p.m. | 1800 |
| 7:00 a.m. | 0700 | 7:00 p.m. | 1900 |
| 8:00 a.m. | 0800 | 8:00 p.m. | 2000 |
| 9:00 a.m. | 0900 | 9:00 p.m. | 2100 |
| 10:00 a.m. | 1000 | 10:00 p.m. | 2200 |
| 11:00 a.m. | 1100 | 11:00 p.m. | 2300 |
| 12:00 p.m. | 1200 | 12:00 a.m. | 2400 |

**Figure 10.18**   Conversion of the 12-hour clock to the 24-hour clock

# Chapter Review and Assessment

## Summary

No matter what healthcare field you decide to enter, you will be required to perform some math calculations when doing your job. In this chapter you reviewed basic math skills such as recognizing types of numbers, and practicing addition, subtraction, multiplication, and division. Fractions, decimals, percentages, basic algebra, ratios, and proportions are also important skills to master, and will be used in your healthcare career.

Analyzing data is another skill for the healthcare worker to practice. You can use the mean, median, and mode, along with charts and graphs to illustrate the relationships among numbers. Data analysis is a critical part of healthcare. Healthcare employees continuously compile statistics about the facility. Compiling this data may include gathering and updating patient information, keeping track of nosocomial infection rates, and tracking on-hand medical supplies.

Although the metric system of measurement is used in healthcare and science disciplines, the majority of the United States continues to use the English system. As you begin your healthcare career you must understand the metric system and its basic units—the gram, liter, and meter. Converting measurements of temperature from the metric, Celsius scale to commonly used Fahrenheit values is another important math skill for all healthcare students to master.

Because of its accuracy, the 24-hour clock (military time) is used in most healthcare settings. Healthcare workers must learn how to read and easily use military time. Maintaining accurate and proper records is dependent on the use of this timekeeping system.

Improving your math skills will not only benefit your career, but it can make things easier in your daily life. People with strong math skills are, for example, better at maintaining a budget than those people who lack math skills.

## Review Questions

### Short Answer

1. What is the difference between the 12-hour clock and the 24-hour clock?
2. Explain how spreadsheets and databases might be used in a healthcare facility.
3. Which measuring system is used throughout most of the world? Why is this measuring system preferred?
4. Explain the concept of a common denominator.
5. What is the base ten system in math?
6. What are the differences between ordinal and nominal numbers?

### True/False

7. *True or False?* The English system is more logical than the metric system.
8. *True or False?* Algebra contains equations.
9. *True or False?* The 24-hour clock is the same as military time.
10. *True or False?* The term percentage means *per 100*.
11. *True or False?* A yard is a metric measurement.
12. *True or False?* If you have a calculator, there is no need to improve your math skills.
13. *True or False?* Addition is the opposite of multiplication.
14. *True or False?* The statistical tool called the *mean* is a mathematical average of data.
15. *True or False?* A zero should be placed before a decimal point if there is no whole number.

### Multiple Choice

16. _____ is the branch of mathematics that substitutes letters for numbers.
    A. Algebra
    B. Arithmetic
    C. Geometry
    D. Statistics

17. Each of the following is a metric prefix *except* _____.
    A. nano-
    B. maxi-
    C. mega-
    D. giga-

18. The three basic statistical terms used to analyze information are _____.
    A. averages, median, sum
    B. median, mean, mode
    C. mean, estimate, prediction
    D. total, mode, sum

19. The mode of a set of numbers is _____.
    A. the average
    B. the sum of the numbers
    C. an estimation
    D. the number that occurs most frequently in a number set

20. The top number of a fraction is called the _____.
    A. denominator
    B. numerator
    C. reciprocal
    D. remainder

21. Which of the following statements about decimal fractions is *true*?
    A. They are a special type of fractions that most people find easy to use.
    B. They are also called decimals.
    C. Decimal fractions represent parts of the whole.
    D. All of the above.

22. Which of the following statements about division is *true*?
    A. Division problems can be written several ways.
    B. The most common symbol for division is (÷).
    C. The number that gets divided is called the dividend.
    D. All of the above.

23. Which of the following is *not* a format of a graph or chart?
    A. Roman graph
    B. bar graph
    C. pie chart
    D. line graph

24. Which of the following statements about multiplication is *false*?
    A. Multiplication is a shortcut for subtraction.
    B. The standard symbol for multiplication is (×).
    C. Other symbols for multiplication are parentheses (1)(8) or an asterisk (*).
    D. The numbers to be multiplied are called the multiplicands.

25. Which of the following statements about the 12-hour clock is *true*?
    A. The 12-hour clock is used in all hospitals.
    B. The military uses the 12-hour clock exclusively.
    C. The 12-hour clock has unique numbers for each hour of the day.
    D. The 12-hour clock is commonly used in our everyday lives.

## Critical Thinking Exercises

26. Some students argue that learning basic math skills such as the multiplication tables is not important because the calculator can do all math calculations for them. Why is it important to learn basic math skills? How will basic math skills be used during your healthcare career?

27. Why is it important for members of a healthcare team to use the 24-hour clock?

28. Do you have a preferred type of graph or table used to express data for analysis? pie chart? bar graph? line graph? simple table? Explain why you find one method better for expressing and analyzing data than the others.

29. Do you think that the United States should begin using the metric system and the 24-hour clock exclusively? Do you think a mathematic change to the metric system will happen in the future? Why or why not?

30. Which type of calculation do you find the most confusing? fractions? percentages? measurement conversions? algebra? basic arithmetic? Why? What can you do to feel more comfortable when performing the calculations that confuse you?

# Additional Practice

## Basic Math Review

*If you are confident in your math abilities and are able to answer these questions correctly, skip ahead to the Data Analysis section. These questions can also be used as review upon completing the chapter.*

### Values

*Identify the value of each digit in the following numbers.*

1. 210
2. 3
3. 203,987
4. 1,244,765
5. 66,789

### Addition

*Find the sum of the following addition problems without using a calculator.*

6. 213 + 456 + 342 =
7. 4,500 + 97 + 456 =
8. 43 + 345 + 1,234,679 =
9. 45 + 678 + 1,908 =
10. A student studying to be a hospital dietician is told by her instructor that a diet should not contain large amounts of salt. The student is asked to track the salt intake in her lunch. She recorded: 1,200 mg in a tuna sandwich, 300 mg in French fries, 320 mg in a milkshake, and 325 mg in a cherry pie. How many mg of salt did the student consume during lunch?
11. 49 + 99 + 52,045 =
12. 669 + 4,000 + 924 =

### Addition Using a Calculator

*Use a calculator to find the sum of the following addition problems.*

13. 998 + 2,346 + 21 + 367 + 1,489 =
14. 22 + 1,345,780 + 7,500 + 236 + 31 =
15. 2,331,498 + 226,560 + 67 + 7,611 + 85,423 =

16. 546 + 3,467 + 237,689 + 34 + 7 + 90,458 =
17. 34 + 345 + 1,234 + 12,608 + 214,896 =

### Subtraction

*Find the difference without using a calculator.*

18. 23 − 12 =
19. 245 − 239 =
20. 1,200 − 36 =
21. 534 − 315 =
22. Dr. James told an obese patient that he needed to enroll in a weight loss program. The patient initially weighed 320 pounds; today the patient weighs 245 pounds. How much weight has he lost?
23. Javier's physician has told Javier that he needs to lose 15 pounds. Javier weighed in at 210 pounds. What does Javier's physician want him to weigh?
24. 10,000 − 9860 =
25. Lizzie's phlebotomy instructor announces that there will be a total of 100 internship hours required to pass the course. Lizzie has already finished 21 hours. How many hours does she have left?

### Subtraction Using a Calculator

*Use a calculator to find the difference in each of the following subtraction problems.*

26. 2,345 − 300 =
27. 4,444 − 666 =
28. 2,890 − 345 =
29. 1,234,589 − 3,467 =
30. 3,590 − 768 =

## Multiplication

*Find the product without using a calculator.*

31. $22 \times 10 =$

32. $56 \times 8 =$

33. $120 \times 60 =$

34. $28 \times 28 =$

35. A registered nurse is giving a patient 225 mg of penicillin 4 times a day. How many mg of penicillin does the patient receive each day?

36. On average, Juanita processes 35 insurance claims per day. How many claims does she process in a two-week period (assuming she works 5 days a week)?

37. $1,466 \times 599 =$

## Multiplication Using a Calculator

*Use a calculator to find the product in each of the following multiplication problems.*

38. $23 \times 234 \times 543 =$

39. $6,846 \times 414 =$

40. $14 \times 6 \times 678 =$

41. $2,234 \times 123 =$

42. $12,375 \times 346 =$

## Division

*Find the quotient without using a calculator.*

43. $120 \div 10 =$

44. $300 \div 5 =$

45. $450 \div 9 =$

46. $240 \div 4 =$

47. $320 \div 7 =$

48. $410 \div 9 =$

49. Ms. Mercer recently suffered a heart attack. She spent six days in the coronary care unit of the hospital. At the end of her hospital stay, her bill was $15,420. How much was Ms. Mercer charged per day?

50. Jesse is training to be a paramedic. He is expected to job shadow a paramedic in the field for a total of 96 hours. How many 12-hour shifts does Jesse have to shadow to reach the required 96 hours?

## Division Using a Calculator

*Use a calculator to find the quotient in each of the following division problems.*

51. $125 \div 15 =$

52. $400 \div 200 =$

53. $1,456 \div 56 =$

54. $54,320 \div 245 =$

55. $23,000 \div 15 =$

## Fractions

*Solve the following fraction equations without using a calculator.*

56. $\dfrac{1}{10} + \dfrac{2}{10} + \dfrac{6}{10} =$

57. $\dfrac{4}{16} + \dfrac{3}{16} + \dfrac{10}{10} =$

58. $\dfrac{5}{9} \div \dfrac{2}{7} =$

59. $\dfrac{4}{5} \times \dfrac{1}{3} =$

60. Triplets were born yesterday at Eastridge Hospital. Each baby was weighed at birth. The three girls weighed: 3½ pounds (lbs), 4¼ lbs, and 3⅛ lbs. How much did they weigh all together?

61. $\dfrac{10}{12} \times \dfrac{1}{6} =$

62. $\dfrac{100}{125} \div \dfrac{25}{5} =$

## Decimals

*Answer the following questions without using a calculator.*

63. $19.55 + 127 + 2,130.02 + 54.5 =$

64. Round off each of the following numbers to the nearest tenth.
    A.  534.67
    B.  45.64
    C.  5.69

65. Round off each of the following numbers to the nearest one-hundredth.
    A. 3.456
    B. 43.333
    C. 57.892

66. A patient has a medical bill for $16,201.99. What is the balance remaining after her insurance company pays $12,961.59?

67. Convert the following fractions to decimal fractions.
    A. 5/16
    B. 43⅖
    C. 4⁴⁄₇

## Percentages

*Answer the following questions without using a calculator. When necessary, round off to the nearest hundredth.*

68. Convert 42% to a decimal fraction.

69. What is 20% of 150?

70. What is 6.5% of 645?

71. Convert 180% into a fraction.

72. Convert 0.657 into a percentage.

73. One study has found that 25% of people who get the flu shot will still get the flu. If 15,230 people got the vaccine, how many people would still get the flu even with the vaccination?

74. In a medical clerical class of 29 students, 12 students want to work in a hospital, 10 students want to work in a doctor's office, 3 students want to work in a clinic setting, and 4 are undecided. What percentage of students wants to work in a hospital?

75. Convert 85% into a fraction.

76. Convert 5¾ into a percentage.

77. Convert 3.1416 into a percentage.

## Ratios

*Answer the following questions without using a calculator.*

78. Convert 1:5 into a fraction.

79. In a chemistry laboratory, a student is asked to create a solution that contains 10 milliliters of a weak acid to 400 milliliters of distilled water. What is the ratio of the weak acid to the distilled water?

80. A student planning to be a dietician is surprised to learn that a gallon of ice cream contains 15 grams of fat, 12 grams of which are saturated fat. What is the ratio of saturated fat to the total fat in the gallon of ice cream?

81. Express the ratio 6:4 two different ways.

82. An instructor grades a health occupations class final. 24 students passed. 4 students failed the class. What is the ratio between the students who passed and those who failed?

## Algebra

*Answer the following questions without using a calculator.*

83. $x + 15 = 45$

84. $3x - 18 = 78$

85. $4x + 2 = 8x$

86. $\frac{1}{4}x + 12 = 220$

87. $\frac{1}{5}x - 10 = 365$

88. Dr. Edward has $x$ number of patients. Dr. Ryan has twice as many patients as Dr. Edward. Dr. Ryan has 42 patients. How many patients does Dr. Edward have? Show your work.

89. A doctor has ordered 70 mg of medication to be given to a patient by mouth. The medicine label indicates that one capsule contains 20 mg of medicine. How many capsules should be given to the patient to reach the required dosage?

90. When working with a patient, a nurse is instructed to give an injection of 75 mg of liquid medication. The medication bottle reads 125 mg/ml. How many ml of the medicine should be injected to achieve the desired dosage of 75 mg?

91. A patient needs 600,000 units of a medication. The medicine bottle states that there are 400,000 units per ml. Identify the proper dosage in milliliters to be given to the patient.

## Data Analysis

*Answer the following data analysis questions using what you have learned in this chapter.*

92. Grace, a patient at Eastridge Hospital, has been running a fever for the past eight hours. Construct a line graph showing Grace's temperature at each hour. Then, look at the resulting graph and explain why this representation of the data might be helpful to a healthcare professional.
    0600–102°F
    0700–102°F
    0800–101.6°F
    0900–101°F
    1000–100.6°F
    1100–100°F
    1200–99.2°F
    1300–99°F

93. Construct a bar graph using the following patient data from Eastridge Hospital.
    2 patients have a temperature of 103°F
    5 patients have a temperature of 99.8°F
    7 patients have a temperature of 101.6°F
    12 patients have a temperature of 98.6°F

## Measurement in Healthcare

*Answer the following questions about metric units, metric prefixes, and measurements using the metric system.*

94. A gram measures _____.
95. A liter measures _____.
96. A meter measures _____.
97. One kilogram is equal to _____ grams.
98. One milliliter is equal to _____ liters.
99. One hectometer is equal to _____ meters.
100. One decagram is equal to _____ grams.
101. One microliter is equal to _____ liters.

## Converting Measurements

*Answer the following questions without using a calculator.*

102. On Stan's hospital chart, the doctor notes that Stan must consume 2 liters of fluid per day. How many milliliters should Stan drink each day?

103. Convert the following measurements to liters.
    A. 769 kiloliters
    B. 77.2 deciliters
    C. 24 hectoliters
    D. 2,456 milliliters

104. The majority of adults have 5,000 to 6,000 ml of blood in their bodies. Convert this quantity to quarts.

105. Convert 68°F to Celsius.

106. Convert 100°C to Fahrenheit.

107. Convert 84°F to Celsius.

108. Convert 120 pounds to grams.

109. Convert 85 pounds to grams.

## The 24-Hour Clock

*Convert the following 12-hour clock times to military time.*

110. 2:30 p.m.
111. 11:30 p.m.
112. 4:15 p.m.
113. 3:30 p.m.
114. 10:00 a.m.
115. 1:45 a.m.

*Convert the following military times to 12-hour clock time.*

116. 0155
117. 1137
118. 0320
119. 1305
120. 1700
121. 2212

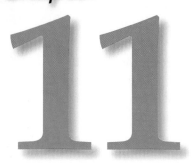

# Chapter

# 11

# *Healthcare Technology*

## Terms to Know

biotechnology
cloning
cloud technology
computer hardware
computer on wheels
  (COW)
computer virus
download
firewall
hackers
healthcare simulation

Internet
malware
podcasts
software
upload
virtual learning
  environment (VLE)
Wi-Fi
word processing
World Wide Web

## Chapter Objectives

- Discuss various hardware components of a computer.
- Explain the most common types of software for computers.
- Understand how the Internet functions and its uses related to medical issues.
- Discuss threats that can derail computer systems.
- Identify ways to ensure confidentiality with patient information on computers.
- Discuss various forms of communication that may be used by healthcare facilities.
- Identify some technologies used in diagnostic services.
- Discuss healthcare developments made possible by biotechnology.
- Explain how future healthcare professionals can use simulators as a learning tool.

No matter what healthcare occupation you choose, technology will play a vital role in your future career. Whether you work as a front office medical assistant, nursing assistant, physical therapist, or physician, technology will be important for your profession (Figure 11.1). Today, medicine and information technology have become increasingly connected, impacting students, healthcare providers, and patients.

Managing information is one of the most important tasks in any healthcare facility. Computers organize and sort information, address patient needs, document care, manage financial data, and provide access to the latest healthcare information via the Internet. Computers also play an indispensable role in almost every aspect of healthcare by storing patient information.

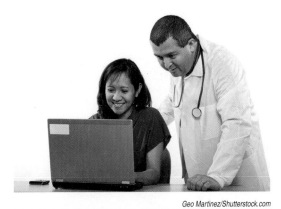

*Geo Martinez/Shutterstock.com*

**Figure 11.1**  Healthcare professionals rely on various computer technologies in order to do their jobs.

Computers have made many contributions to the healthcare industry, including monitoring vital signs of critically ill patients, creating three-dimensional pictures of a patient using sophisticated radiology scans, and helping physicians make accurate diagnoses. Experts predict that the use of computer applications and other technological innovations in modern medicine have only just begun.

Along with this amazing technology in the healthcare world comes several important issues to consider. Serious confidentiality concerns and ethical considerations are being raised as new technology continues to stream into healthcare facilities. Students studying for a career in healthcare must be aware of such privacy and ethical concerns; they must also possess basic computer skills.

## *Basic Computer Technology*

As technology continues to evolve, healthcare workers must adjust rapidly to expanding responsibilities related to the use of technology. It is important for healthcare workers to embrace technology rather than be frightened by it. Healthcare technology will offer endless opportunities to learn new skills and be a part of exciting new paths to improve healthcare for everyone. In any discussion of computers, it is helpful to start with the basics such as computer hardware, software, and peripheral devices.

### Hardware

**Computer hardware** consists of any devices that are connected to the computer (Figure 11.2). Examples of computer hardware include a monitor, keyboard, and mouse:

- **Monitor.** The monitor lets you see what the computer is processing by displaying it on a screen. Today, there are many technologies used

**computer hardware**
*devices such as the monitor or keyboard that are connected to the computer*

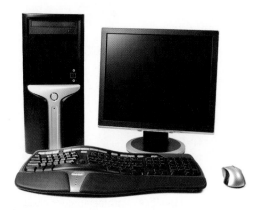

Dmitry Melnikov/Shutterstock.com

**Figure 11.2**   Basic computer hardware includes a monitor, mouse, keyboard, and the tower, which houses the central processing unit (CPU).

to give the monitor display a high resolution, including liquid crystal diodes (LCD) and organic light-emitting diodes (OLED).

- **Central processing unit (CPU).** The central processing unit serves as the "brains" of a computer. All functions of the computer are processed by the CPU. The CPU can be contained in the "tower" of a desktop computer, the base of a laptop computer, or the base of a monitor. The CPU provides the machine's computing power and is the most important element of a computer system.
- **Mouse.** A mouse controls the cursor on the computer screen and allows the user to control the computer's functions by clicking. Some mice have two buttons, each of which has a special purpose, while others have only one. Advancing technologies have offered alternatives to traditional mice, such as external touchpads. These function much like the touchpad on a laptop—the user can "click" by tapping, or double-tapping the touchpad with a fingertip.
- **Keyboard.** A keyboard is a device used to enter text commands into the computer. Keyboards can be plugged into a USB port on the computer, or connect wirelessly. Some computers do not use keyboards, but function with touch screens instead.
- **Printer.** This is a device that prints processed information on paper, creating a hard copy.
- **CDs and DVDs.** CDs and DVDs are physical items that store information to be opened on the computer. These are inserted into computer disk drives located on the CPU.
- **Modem.** This is a device that transmits data to and from a computer by way of a telephone or other communication lines.
- **Router.** This device is attached to a modem, which allows multiple users and computers to share Internet access, files, and data. Some routers are wired and some are wireless.
- **Scanner.** A scanner is connected to a computer and is used to copy documents and photographs. This device converts scanned items into digital files. Scanners are often combined with printers in one machine.
- **Digital Cameras.** Digital cameras have almost entirely replaced film cameras. In these cameras, photos are captured on memory cards rather than film. Digital cameras can be plugged into a computer's USB port, and pictures are transferred onto the computer's hard drive. Webcams are video cameras that are plugged into, or built into, computers and are used for videoconferences or video chatting.

# Inside a Computer

Within the computer, there are several critical devices that allow it to process information. The CPU serves as the computer's brain, and is responsible for running the computer's software. Other devices work with the CPU to process data. Some of these devices include

- **Motherboard.** All hardware in the system is connected to the motherboard, making it the most important component in a computer system.
- **Hard Drive.** The hard drive serves as permanent storage for files and programs.
- **Random Access Memory (RAM).** RAM is memory that plugs into the motherboard.
- **Power Supply.** The power supply sends power to the other hardware systems so they can operate.
- **Disk Drives.** These drives are used to insert CDs, DVDs, or other file storage devices into the computer. A USB flash drive is also used to store data for periods of time (Figure 11.3). A flash drive is sometimes called a *thumb drive*, *keychain drive*, or a *jump drive*. This small unit can be plugged into a computer's USB port. Flash drives can transfer data into or out of the computer.
- **Video Card.** This is part of the computer system that converts code from the CPU so that it can be viewed on the monitor.

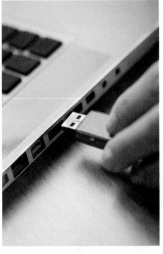

*stefanolunardi/Shutterstock.com*

**Figure 11.3** A USB flash drive is a great tool for saving and transferring small amounts of data.

# Software

**Software** refers to programs and data that are stored digitally within the computer. In contrast, hardware consists of storage, processing, and display devices. Software allows a user to interact with the computer.

Two types of software are *operating system software* and *application program software*. Operating system software directs the computer's hardware. Application program software directs the computer to perform specific tasks. Three commonly used types of software include databases, spreadsheets, and **word processing** programs.

As you learned in chapter 10, databases and spreadsheets are important tools for storing, organizing, and using information. Databases are computer files that contain a collection of related information entered and sorted by category. Patient names and all related medical information can be put into a database, with information such as the patient's medication record that can be pulled out separately. Spreadsheets are documents that may include a combination of text and numbers, and are often used for financial accounting. Microsoft Access is an example of database software, while Microsoft Excel is spreadsheet software.

Word processing programs are some of the most commonly used software. These programs allow the user to enter, edit, save, and print words using a computer. Most word processing programs are able to check and

**software**
*a collection of programs that allow a user to interact with the computer*

**word processing**
*software that allows one to enter, edit, store, and print text through a computer*

correct the grammar and spelling of the entered text. Microsoft Word is a commonly used word processing program.

> **Did You Know?**
>
> ### Software Usage
>
> Did you know that some of the most popular software includes tax preparation software, accounting software, anti-virus software, and word processing software?
>
> What software do you use most often? Your software may vary slightly based on the type of computer you use. Are you an Apple user or a Windows user?

## The Internet

**Internet**
*an electronic communications network that connects computer networks and computer facilities around the world*

**World Wide Web**
*a means of accessing the Internet by using an HTTP web address*

The **Internet** is composed of a multitude of computer networks joined together around the world (Figure 11.4). The **World Wide Web** allows people to access the information available on the Internet (Figure 11.5). Both the Internet and World Wide Web allow healthcare workers to exchange information and access resources at impossibly fast speeds.

When a person accesses the Internet, they are *online*. A user has to have appropriate software and a modem to get online. A connection to the Internet can be provided by a phone line, a cable line, or a digital subscriber line (DSL). You may use a search engine, such as Google, Yahoo, or Bing, in order to find information online.

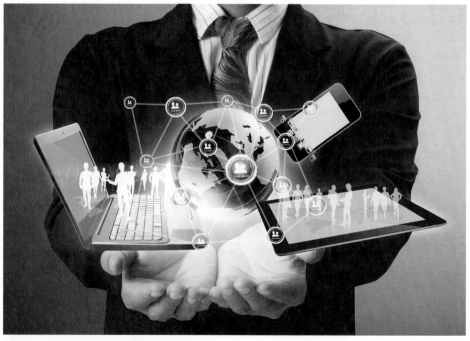

violetkaipa/Shutterstock.com

**Figure 11.4** The Internet is formed by multiple computer networks that are connected to each other.

**Wi-Fi** is a popular technology that enables electronic devices to exchange data wirelessly over a computer network. Many people use Wi-Fi to get online using their smartphone. Wi-Fi is often found in many homes, businesses, and cafés, allowing people to access the Internet wirelessly using a laptop, tablet, or e-reader.

**Wi-Fi**
*technology that enables an electronic device to exchange data wirelessly over a computer network; wireless fidelity*

## Going Online at Work

One thing to remember about going on the Internet when at work is that you are responsible for limiting your use to work-related activities. Your employer will have Internet usage guidelines, and can monitor your time spent online. Do not expect privacy while using the Internet at work. Do not send inappropriate e-mails or visit inappropriate Internet sites. You could lose your job if you do not limit your use of the computer to work-related tasks.

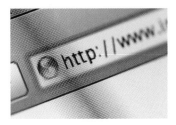

*Volodymyr Krasyuk/Shutterstock.com*

**Figure 11.5** Accessing information on the Internet is easy when browsing on the World Wide Web.

---

**‖Extend Your Knowledge‖**

*Podcasts*

**Podcasts** are audio or video files downloaded and played on a computer, tablet, smartphone, or similar device. Podcasts appear as episodes updated daily or weekly. Podcasts can be entertaining and/or informative. Teachers can use podcasts in instructional settings. There are interesting podcasts that discuss updated medical information. Have you ever seen or listened to a podcast?

---

**podcasts**
*multimedia files that are downloaded and played on a computer, a tablet, or a smartphone*

## Cloud Technology

**Cloud technology** is Internet-based computing, in which programs and data are stored at remote locations rather than on your computer. These remote locations have a high capacity for data, allowing them to store more information than the typical onsite data storage facility. Items stored in the "cloud" can be accessed quickly using a variety of devices such as laptops, tablets, or smartphones.

**cloud technology**
*Internet-based technology that stores programs and data on servers at remote locations instead of your computer*

Cloud technology presents exciting possibilities for the medical community. The transition to electronic medical records has increased the data storage requirements of many healthcare facilities. Facilities must be able to store a large amount of information, but also access it quickly. Healthcare facilities using cloud technology to store data must make certain their cloud storage provider has tough security measures in place. Medical records are sensitive materials, and patient confidentiality must be maintained.

One specific benefit and application of cloud technology in the healthcare world is a physician being able to treat a patient who is on vacation. Any physician should be able to access the patient's medical records from their primary physician via the "cloud." The records could then be updated to include any procedures performed and medication prescribed by the off-site physician.

# Virtual Learning Environments

A **virtual learning environment (VLE)**—which may also be called a *course management system* (CMS) or *learning management system* (LMS)—brings learning materials to students using the World Wide Web. VLEs support student learning outside the classroom at any hour of the day, seven days a week. VLEs allow institutions of learning to educate not only traditional full-time students, but also those who cannot be on campus due to health, geographical, or time restrictions. These systems track student progress, allow students to collaborate with one another, offer assessment programs, and include various communication tools. Blackboard Learning System is a popular VLE.

# Internet Research

As an Internet user, you have access to an overwhelming amount of information. Many reliable healthcare websites exist to provide accurate information, but it is always best to consult your physician before following an online diagnosis or treatment plan. Websites sponsored by US government organizations such as the National Institutes of Health or the Department of Health and Human Services provide valuable healthcare resources. The Centers for Disease Control and Prevention (CDC) is another good government source of information. Health organization websites such as the Mayo Clinic's page may also be worth visiting.

The Internet makes it possible to gather up-to-date data on exciting new research. Are you curious about new advances in treating breast cancer? Do you want your résumé to have a new, modern format? The Internet opens up many prospects for learning, and also makes practical information for everyday living available and easily accessible. Nevertheless, there is also a great deal of misinformation on the Internet.

## Internet Misinformation

While the Internet can be an excellent source of information, it is also filled with quite a bit of misinformation. Some misinformation can be completely inaccurate, misleading, or even dangerous to patients seeking help for a health problem. If you are looking for answers on the Internet, you may want to use the Scientific Method to ask questions about the information you are receiving:

1. What is the purpose of the website? Who sponsors the website?
2. Are there sources listed to read more about the information on the website?
3. How often is the website updated?
4. Where else on the Internet can you find details and verification about the information you are reading?
5. Which people in your life with expertise in the area can you ask about what you are reading on the website?

One of the dangers of such websites is that the person will self-treat a health problem after reading an inaccurate or misleading article online. Some healthcare professionals have become concerned about the information available to their patients online. Health information websites and pharmaceutical companies may have a financial agreement in which the pharmaceutical company sponsors the website. This may lead the hosts of the website to recommend a drug that is not the best treatment option for a particular illness, but is produced by their sponsor.

On the other hand, health information websites can help a person answer questions concerning symptoms of an illness—encouraging that person to consult a physician. The lesson to learn here is that you must be an intelligent consumer and consult a reputable physician who will make a diagnosis and treatment plan.

## *Computer Disruptions*

**Malware** is malicious, or *harmful*, software. Malware is used by attackers to disrupt computer operation, gather sensitive information, or gain access to private computer systems. Commonly used types of malware include worms, Trojan horses, and spyware. Some **computer viruses** are also classified as malware (Figure 11.6). Cookies (small pieces of data left on your computer by the websites you visit) may share your personal information.

### Spyware

Spyware is any software that covertly (without your knowledge) gathers user information through the computer's Internet connection, often for advertising purposes. Spyware can often be a hidden component of software that is free for download on the Internet. Once installed, the spyware can watch user activity on the Internet and send the information to someone else. Spyware can also obtain e-mail addresses, passwords, and credit card numbers.

### Worms and Trojan Horses

A computer worm is a type of malware designed to install itself on a computer. Once installed, the worm sends personal data to another party without the user knowing.

Another serious form of malware, a Trojan horse, initially seems to be useful software. However, this malware does extensive damage once installed or run on a computer. A user can be tricked into opening a Trojan horse because it appears to be legitimate software or files.

Trojan horses vary in their destruction. Some are designed to be annoying rather than destructive and

**malware**
*malicious software used to disrupt computer operation, gather sensitive information, or gain access to private computers*

**computer virus**
*malware designed to copy itself into other programs; may cause the affected computer to operate incorrectly or corrupt the computer memory*

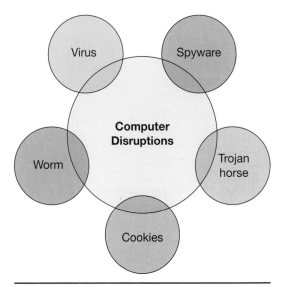

**Figure 11.6**   Computer disruptions come in many forms and various sources.

might, for example, continuously change your desktop icons. Others cause serious damage by deleting files and destroying system information.

## Computer Viruses

Computer viruses are software programs designed to destroy computer information. Viruses replicate (duplicate) themselves, spreading from computer to computer through Internet downloads, e-mails, and other sources. These viruses can destroy files and damage hardware.

Most healthcare agencies store information on large computers and must protect data from viruses through vigilant monitoring. Personal computers and laptops are more difficult to monitor. Comprehensive, reliable anti-virus software is a necessity for all computers. This software must be able to be updated frequently as new viruses are developed every day. Do not **download** attachments from any suspicious e-mails sent by an unknown person or company. Doing so may infect your computer with a virus that is capable of destroying programs and data, and possibly the computer hardware. Viruses can also spread themselves by attaching to your e-mails.

## Avoiding Malware

Unfortunately, these examples of malware are just a few of many computer disruptions that are active today. Computer **hackers** continue to think up new and evolving malware to victimize computer users.

The single most important step that you can take to protect your computer from malware is to install and use well-known anti-virus software. The software will update itself regularly and will constantly monitor your computer for malware. Most anti-malware scanners will provide tools to automate these tasks so that they take place when you are not using your computer. Anti-virus software will protect you when you visit a site that has been hacked and infected.

Avoid fake anti-malware. Do not buy anti-malware software advertised in pop-up ads. Legitimate software isn't sold this way, and these programs can actually load malware onto your machine rather than protect you from it.

Delete e-mails with suspicious attachments and do not open the attachment. E-mail attachments are one of the most popular ways to spread malware. If you don't know what an e-mail is or who it is from, delete the e-mail immediately rather than open it.

Malware often comes from unconventional websites. Download and install software only from websites you know and trust. Symptoms in a computer that suggest a virus or spyware is present include:

- The computer slows down.
- The anti-virus program is turned off.

**download**
*transmission of a file from one computer system to another; usually from a larger computer system to a smaller one*

**hackers**
*people who break into computer systems to access data, steal personal information, and sometimes cause harm to a computer system*

### Think It Through

Have you ever experienced malware on your computer? Are you currently running anti-malware software? Reliable, free software programs are available to protect your machine from malware. Be sure to renew your software when you get a notice that it is expiring. If you are not protected, you are extremely vulnerable to malware.

- The system freezes or crashes.
- The hard drive light is on because the hard drive is constantly working.
- The user receives alerts from a firewall that an unknown program is trying to access the Internet.
- New browser icons appear in the menu.

# Computer Protections

Because new methods of computer disruption are developed daily, your computer needs constant protection from intrusion. While anti-virus software will protect you from some threats, sometimes a higher level of security is required. This is especially true in a healthcare facility that must protect its patients' personal information.

## Firewall

A **firewall** is a software program or a piece of hardware developed to prevent a hacker from accessing personal information on your computer. A firewall filters incoming and outgoing information for potential threats while also preventing security breaches from remote log-ins. Windows operating systems include a built-in firewall that can be kept on at all times. A firewall is also included in some routers and modems.

**firewall**
*software program or piece of hardware developed to prevent a hacker from accessing personal information on your computer or in the healthcare facility computer system*

## Password Protection

Using passwords to control access to the files on your computer helps protect those files and any personal information they may contain. Design strong passwords that cannot be easily guessed by another person. Use at least eight or more characters for the passwords, combining letters and numbers. Including both uppercase and lowercase letters in your password is also helpful. Do not use the same password for multiple accounts, and change your password frequently. When assigned a password in a healthcare facility, you must not share your password with anyone.

### ✓ Check Your Understanding

1. What is the difference between a worm and Trojan horse?
2. List three symptoms of a computer that has been affected by malware.
3. What is the purpose of a firewall?

# Healthcare Computer Systems

Regardless of your position in healthcare, you will almost always use a computer as you complete your tasks. Healthcare facilities usually have large computer systems that require some on-the-job training. You will also be assigned a username to access computer files and will need to create a unique password.

Once you are able to input and find information in the computer system, you will be able to perform such duties as

- ordering supplies and keeping inventories;
- entering treatment notes;
- researching data on the Internet;
- scheduling appointments and tests for patients;
- ordering tests and prescriptions for the pharmacy;
- receiving and entering test results;
- processing patient discharges;
- performing financial calculations; and
- submitting insurance to payers and billing patients.

Many occupations in the healthcare field require several hours a day spent working on a computer. As you learned in chapter 4, it is important to have an ergonomic chair at your desk and to maintain proper body mechanics. Figure 11.7 shows the proper seated position to take when working at the computer. Follow these guidelines to avoid computer-related injuries like carpal tunnel syndrome or repetitive strain injury (RSI).

To prevent RSI, you can obtain a proper desk chair that provides adequate back support. A wrist guard or wrist rest attached to the keyboard can combat injury such as carpal tunnel syndrome. Larger fonts help reduce eyestrain, and performing deep breathing exercises helps to reduce stress, which aggravates RSI.

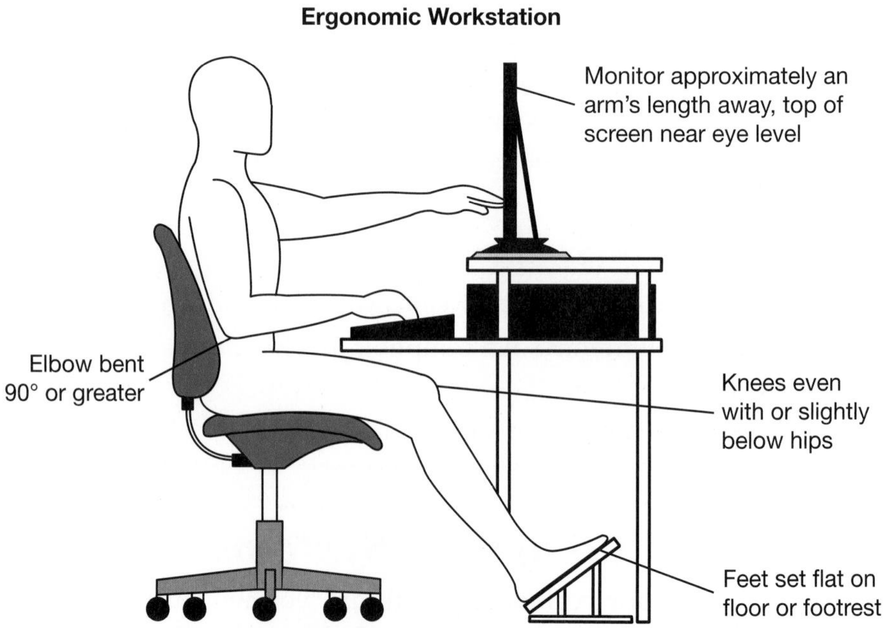

**Ergonomic Workstation**

Monitor approximately an arm's length away, top of screen near eye level

Elbow bent 90° or greater

Knees even with or slightly below hips

Feet set flat on floor or footrest

**Figure 11.7**    Maintaining proper ergonomics will help you to avoid computer-related injuries.

RSI may lead to wrist surgery and, in severe cases, resignation or being laid off from work. The best course of action is to avoid RSI before problems even begin by maintaining proper body mechanics and having an ergonomic workstation.

### Real Life Scenario

#### Repetitive Strain Injury (RSI)

Laura has been a secretary in the radiology department at Eastridge Hospital for four years. Laura spends a significant amount of time working on the computer, and was recently diagnosed with repetitive strain injury (RSI). Her condition is caused by the repetitive motion of keyboarding and sitting in one position for long periods of time in front of a computer. Laura's back and neck ache on the job, and she feels more and more fatigued as her condition worsens. Recently she has been experiencing shooting pains up and down her back. Laura's physician suggested that she take a short walk every hour or whenever possible at work, stretching her neck, back, and fingers.

## Computer on Wheels (COW)

In many healthcare facilities, particularly hospitals, healthcare workers use computers that can be rolled to a patient's bedside or into an examining room (Figure 11.8). These are called **computers on wheels (COW)**. The user is able to access and enter patient information while also having direct patient contact. These computers on wheels are wirelessly connected to the main computer system of the facility.

## Electronic Medical Records

Today, most medical records are stored electronically, rather than in traditional file folders. This allows the information to be available to the facility's staff as well as off-site medical professionals. Test results can immediately be **uploaded** to electronic medical records.

There are many advantages to using electronic medical records (EMRs). Researchers have found that using electronic medical records has reduced medical errors. This is due to the fact that handwritten instructions may be difficult to read, potentially causing errors. Digital transfer means that electronic records can be shared quickly, reducing delays in patient care and making patient information instantly available for the examining physician. Organizing and storing paper records is no longer necessary (Figure 11.9). EMRs are also environmentally friendly because they eliminate the vast amount of paper used with paper record keeping.

**computer on wheels (COW)**
*a mobile computer used to access and enter patient information while moving around the healthcare facility; often rolled into a patient's hospital room*

**upload**
*to transfer data from a smaller device like a personal computer to a larger computer or server*

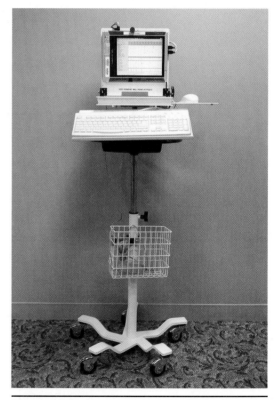

**Figure 11.8** A computer on wheels can be moved between patient rooms, allowing healthcare staff the freedom to enter personal information into electronic medical records from the patient's hospital room.

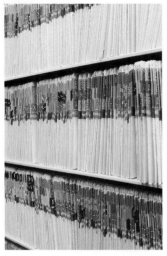

val lawless/Shutterstock.com

**Figure 11.9** Traditional paper medical records required frequent filing, superb organization, and took up a great deal of space in the healthcare facility.

Figure 11.10 illustrates another advantage of the EMR. A pharmacist can enter medication details into the patient's record, which can then be recorded on the permanent medical record, keeping an accurate account of the drugs and dosages ordered.

Converting to electronic medical records can be costly, and some small facilities may have trouble paying for the transition. Another disadvantage associated with EMRs is the potential for a temporary loss of productivity associated with adoption of the EMR system. Electronic medical records may also make patient confidentiality more vulnerable than paper records.

## Maintaining Patient Confidentiality in the Computer Age

Patients expect that their diagnosis, test results, and private information will be kept confidential when they visit a healthcare facility. As you learned in chapter 3, healthcare professionals have a legal and ethical duty to keep patients' medical information private.

### HIPAA

The Health Insurance Portability and Accountability Act of 1996 (HIPAA) was passed by Congress to protect the confidentiality of a patient's medical information. The HIPAA regulations apply to information in patients' medical records in electronic form, as well as in paper form.

Protecting the security of patient information includes watching carefully for threats to computer systems, and protecting precious patient data. There are two main threats that affect healthcare computer systems:

1. threats to the *integrity* of the patient data
2. threats to the *confidentiality* of patient data

### Threats to Patient Information Accuracy

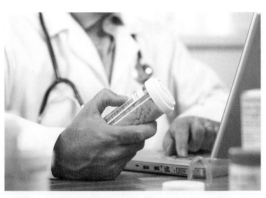

18percentgrey/Shutterstock.com

**Figure 11.10** Using electronic medical records allows a pharmacist to record prescriptions directly into the patient's permanent record.

One of the most common sources of damage to patient data is human inputting errors. Data can be incorrectly entered, and even placed into the wrong patient's medical record. Human beings make mistakes. Sometimes these errors may disclose confidential information to the wrong person.

To avoid making such errors, take extreme care to enter proper results into the healthcare facility computer. Continually check and recheck before you post these results online, send a fax, or before leaving results on a telephone answering machine. (A patient must give permission for a medical provider to leave a voice message containing any personal information.)

Most facilities today protect their information by backing up their computer systems so that computer hardware and software can malfunction, but data is not lost.

Many facilities install privacy screens on computer monitors to limit a computer screen's angle of vision to a front view, preventing visitors from seeing the display. The privacy screen fits directly over the monitor's screen.

## Threats to Confidentiality

Healthcare facilities rely on physical security, software programs, and educated employees to protect private information stored in the hospital computer systems. Computers may be placed where it is hard for outsiders to access them. Passwords and firewalls are used. Remember to never share your password with anyone. Some computers automatically log off when not in use. Despite these efforts, breaches in confidentiality do occur.

Curiosity may motivate an employee without a need to know to access a patient's electronic medical records. Many healthcare computer systems are equipped with monitoring software that records the usernames of those who have accessed patient information. Such access is grounds for discipline and possible termination of employment.

Computer hackers have been known to access information in healthcare facilities and disrupt entire systems. These actions are considered crimes, and efforts are increasingly being made to establish laws against such illegal entry into confidential information. Facility information technology (IT) specialists continually work to put into place systems that make it more difficult for hackers to commit such crimes.

# *Communication Technology*

In this increasingly digital age, it is easy to be constantly connected to others through technology. Smartphones, tablets, e-readers, and other electronic devices make it easy to check e-mail, tweet, surf the web, or play games at school, work, and home. Employees and students who are constantly online experience a decrease in productivity and attention paid to the task at hand. Many classrooms and work environments forbid such activities. Luckily, the healthcare industry has found ways to use this digital revolution to its advantage.

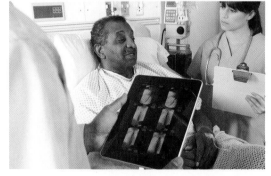

*Monkey Business Images/Shutterstock.com*

**Figure 11.11**   Medical professionals use tablet computers to record and save information while on the go.

## Tablet Computers

Larger than a mobile phone and smaller than a laptop computer, tablets are extremely popular devices (Figure 11.11). Tablets feature a flat touch screen for typing rather than a physical keyboard (although some have attachable keyboards). Tablets are typically used for wireless Internet browsing, e-mail and social media, GPS navigation, reading e-books, downloading applications, and as a media player. Popular for personal use, tablets have also become important tools in education and business. Examples of tablet computers include the iPad and the Surface. Apps such as Pages are available for word processing on some tablets.

## Smartphones

There is an application, or *app*, for practically everything, including healthcare information. Physicians can access patient medical information, disease management programs, prescription history, X-rays, or lab tests with their smartphones.

Apps are also available to provide patients with the healthcare information they need. Not all apps provide reliable information, so the US Food and Drug Administration (FDA) screens and clears certain mobile apps for use. When using any app, make sure you evaluate the source and quality of information just as you would with a website.

Consumers can use their smartphones to research healthcare pricing and obtain information about providers. Individuals can choose a physician in their network based on each provider's ratings. Smartphone users can use an app to follow a diet plan; keep track of prescriptions and set reminders for taking their medications; or manage a disease such as diabetes.

## Electronic Communications with Physicians

Many physicians now use electronics to interact with their patients. Healthcare providers often have a website that allows patients to schedule appointments, ask quick medical questions, renew prescriptions, and view test results. The Internet also offers tools for disease management. For instance, electronic home monitoring equipment can send data to the physician. Studies show that about 20% of office visits per year could be eliminated by online communication between clinicians and patients.

## Telephone Systems

The telephone continues to be used by physicians to provide clinical advice, monitor the effects of certain treatments, help patients monitor themselves, discuss results of tests, relay lab results, and handle prescription renewals. Automated telephone systems provide patients with lists of options for directing calls. Automated call systems can remind patients of appointments and notify them of normal test results.

The latest telephone technology is also being used in many healthcare facilities today (Figure 11.12). Most healthcare workers will be using telephone systems, some relatively simple, but others requiring comprehensive training in order to operate the system properly. Up-to-date phone systems now function wirelessly using transceivers (a combination of a transmitter and a receiver) located throughout the hospital.

In this mini-cellular telephone system, messages are quickly sent to the appropriate caregiver within seconds. Paging systems are built into these telephone networks to locate healthcare workers in and out of the facility without using overhead paging on the facility intercom. If a call is not answered quickly, it is routed to a different extension of the hospital so that the caller is not kept on hold for long periods of time.

Some systems monitor the phone traffic in each area of the hospital. Staffing can be adjusted to provide the most efficient manner of handling calls and messages.

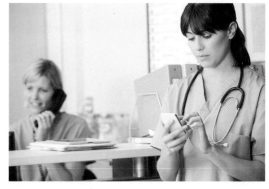
*Monkey Business Images/Shutterstock.com*

**Figure 11.12** Advanced landline telephone systems are used alongside mobile phones in many hospitals to improve call response time and the quality of patient care.

## E-mail

The use of electronic mail (e-mail) in a healthcare facility presents serious challenges. One concern is that the facility remains compliant with HIPAA laws of maintaining confidentiality. A facility's failure to comply with HIPAA regulations can result in heavy fines.

Security measures must be taken when any confidential information is put into an e-mail message. A secure e-mail network must be established, which can be quite expensive for a small facility. Even interoffice e-mails must be secured to follow HIPAA requirements.

With any electronic communications, the patient's confidentiality must be the healthcare employee's first consideration. This is one of the most important ethical and legal considerations to understand before beginning a healthcare career. Evolving technologies present many challenges to maintaining confidentiality. As a result, facilities and employees must continually work to protect patient information.

 *Check Your Understanding*

1. What are the two main threats to healthcare computer systems?
2. How are smartphones used in the healthcare industry?
3. What challenges does e-mail present to the healthcare community?

## *Diagnostic Technology*

In hospital departments such as radiology, the clinical laboratory, and cardiology, highly sophisticated and complex machinery are used. Much of this equipment helps diagnose patient illness. In the past, exploratory surgery may have been used to make a diagnosis. Today, new diagnostic technology often replaces invasive exploratory surgery.

## The Clinical Laboratory

The clinical laboratory is full of many complex machines used to run tests for diagnostic purposes. One of the most advanced machines in a clinical laboratory is an automated cell counter such as a Coulter counter. The Coulter counter performs multiple examinations on small blood specimens in just seconds. Red and white blood cells and platelets are counted, the size of red blood cells is measured, and several other determinations are made. These tests would have taken technologists several hours to complete by hand. Other sophisticated computerized equipment can analyze and produce up to a hundred different blood chemistry results on multiple specimens in minutes (Figure 11.13).

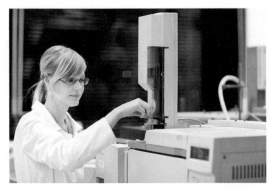

lightpoet/Shutterstock.com

**Figure 11.13**  A laboratory technologist operates a chemistry analyzer.

Operating and troubleshooting these machines takes much training. The operator must recognize when a machine is not functioning at peak performance.

## Diagnostic Imaging

Gone are the days when simple X-ray machines were responsible for all of a hospital's diagnostic imaging. Today, advanced technology plays a huge role in diagnostic imaging. Technicians are trained to operate highly sophisticated, computerized machines such as the PET scan, CT scan, and MRI machines.

Positron emission tomography (PET) scan is done with a computerized machine that scans the body. A small amount of radioactive material called a *tracer* is given to the patient through an IV. The tracer travels through the blood and collects in tissues and organs, making them visible on the PET scan. A PET scan can show how tissues and organs are functioning.

As you learned in chapter 2, the computerized axial tomography (CT) scan is a medical imaging procedure that allows an organ to be seen in a cross direction. This helps physicians find problems (often tumors) without the use of invasive surgery.

Magnetic resonance imaging (MRI) is a test that uses a magnetic field and pulses of radio wave energy to make pictures of structures and organs inside the body (Figure 11.14). MRIs are especially useful when imaging the brain, muscles, heart, and tumors.

Many other departments in the healthcare facility operate complex technology, including intensive and cardiac care units and surgical units. This technology requires extensive training and supervision because new technologies are continually being developed (Figure 11.15). Professionals working with new technology must be flexible and able to learn new procedures quickly.

## Quality Assurance for Diagnostic Machinery

As you learned in chapter 4, quality assurance is a system for evaluating services based on predetermined

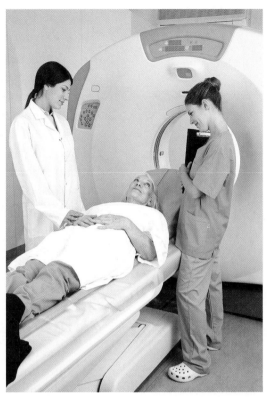

*Robert Kneschke/Shutterstock.com*

**Figure 11.14**  An MRI machine uses a magnetic field and pulses of radio wave energy to make pictures of structures and organs inside the body.

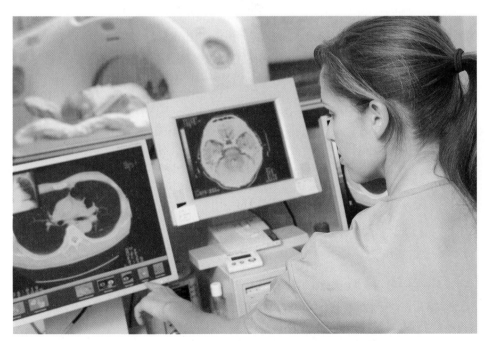

*Monkey Business Images/Shutterstock.com*

**Figure 11.15**  A CT scan technician monitors a patient as the scan is performed.

criteria. In the case of diagnostic machinery, quality assurance is necessary to ensure diagnostic test results are accurate.

When performing tests by hand or with machinery, you must make sure everything is running properly and that reagents being used are free from contamination. The manufacturers of diagnostic machinery provide sample specimens with known test results. These samples can be used to calibrate or measure the machine for accuracy. If the sample does not generate the known result, it is an indication that something is wrong with the machine. Troubleshooting must be done to fix the problem before the machine can be used for further testing.

All quality assurance results are recorded carefully and analyzed during laboratory inspections. Technicians operating advanced machinery must be skilled in both using the machines and testing them for quality assurance purposes. Quality assurance is essential—even sophisticated machines can malfunction.

## *Biotechnology*

Technology that uses biological processes, organisms, or systems to manufacture products intended to improve the quality of human life is called **biotechnology**. Biotechnical advances in the world of medicine have restored, extended, and improved our lives, and will continue to do so in the future.

**biotechnology**
*technology using biological processes, organisms, or systems to develop products intended to improve the quality of human life*

### Biopharmaceuticals

New and exciting advances are being made today in the development of drugs and vaccines (Figure 11.16). Biotechnology and biopharmaceuticals may eventually help us eliminate certain diseases, alleviate pain, and extend our life span. In addition to studying new drugs in clinical trials, scientists are now identifying the previously unknown causes of many diseases. The Human Genome project, which you learned about in chapter 9, strives to find breakthroughs in treatment and possible cures. Biotechnology is making it possible for scientists to design new drugs that are products of genetic engineering (adding new DNA to an organism).

Approved biopharmaceuticals are now treating or helping prevent strokes. Other findings are making a difference in the treatment of multiple sclerosis, heart attacks, leukemia, hepatitis, lymphoma, kidney cancer, cystic fibrosis, and many other diseases. There are now over 900 biopharmaceuticals and vaccines in development to target more life-threatening diseases such as cancer and diabetes.

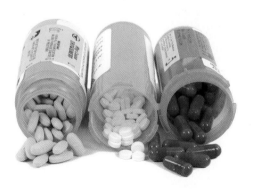

*Brian Chase/Shutterstock.com*

**Figure 11.16** Biopharmaceuticals provide advanced treatment for many diseases and disorders.

# Gene Therapy

Gene therapy is a biotechnological technique for correcting defective genes that cause disease. Gene therapy replaces a defective gene with normal genes. There are thousands of genetic (hereditary) diseases—most of which are caused by a single gene defect. The defective gene (or genes) has been isolated in over two dozen genetic disorders.

Gene therapy is a new technology that has considerable room for growth. Further development of gene therapy will cost millions of research dollars. Hopefully, this investment will enable physicians to effectively treat, or even eliminate, genetic disease.

# Organ Transplantation

Since the 1950s, physicians in the United States have been successfully performing organ transplants. Thanks to improved surgical techniques and new drugs that reduce the chance of rejection, transplants are more successful today than ever before. The organs most commonly transplanted include the

- kidneys;
- liver;
- heart;
- lungs; and
- small intestine.

Unfortunately, because a patient may have to wait a long time to receive an organ transplant, some patients expire (die) before the organ is available. An example of this is a heart patient who is in end-stage heart failure. Ventricular-assist devices that temporarily take the place of a heart are continually being improved to sustain life until an organ is available.

# Bone Marrow Transplants

For patients who have serious blood disorders like leukemia, a bone marrow transplant may be the only effective treatment. Before the bone marrow is transplanted, the patient receives high doses of chemotherapy or radiation to destroy their own unhealthy bone marrow. Then, the patient receives a transplant of either their own healthy marrow, marrow from a relative, or healthy marrow from a person with a similar genetic makeup.

Advances in biotechnology have made this process more successful. Researchers are continually making progress in avoiding graft versus host disease. Graft versus host disease occurs when the transplant recipient's body rejects the donated bone marrow.

# Advances in Prosthetics

Prosthetic limbs replace missing body parts and have been used throughout history (Figure 11.17). A prosthetic toe was discovered in an

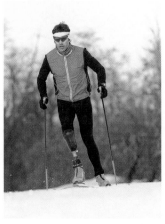

**Figure 11.17** Prosthetic limbs make it possible for people to enjoy physical activities such as skiing.

Egyptian tomb. Today, the science behind prosthetic limbs is advancing thanks to developments in biotechnology.

Some prosthetics are powered by batteries, enhancing the function of the artificial limb. Researchers at Vanderbilt University have been working on a mini rocket-powered prosthetic. Instead of battery packs, these limbs are fueled by a pencil-sized, rocket-powered engine designed to mimic the system that propels the space shuttle into orbit. A rocket-powered arm would be able to move faster and carry heavier loads than a nonmotorized prosthesis.

Bionic limbs are prosthetics whose performance is improved by incorporating electronic devices within the prosthesis. The first bionic lower limb prosthetic enables the knee and ankle joints to operate together. This is a breakthrough for people who have had their legs amputated above the knee. Microprocessors in the prosthesis are programmed to interpret the person's intended movements and make them happen.

Bluetooth technology is also being used to advance prostheses. In the case of double-leg amputees, Bluetooth is used by the prosthetic legs, allowing them to communicate with one another. This enables the amputee to establish a regular gait and pace as he or she walks.

## Robotic Surgery

Robotic surgery is a technique in which a surgeon uses computer-assisted, robotic equipment to perform an operation (Figure 11.18). During robotic surgery, the surgeon uses a computer to remotely control surgical instruments attached to a robot. The patient is generally put to sleep while the surgeon sits at a computer station and directs the movements of a robot.

Robotic surgery is much less invasive than traditional surgery. Small cuts are made to insert the robotic equipment. A thin tube with a camera attached allows the surgeon to view the surgical area on a monitor. As the surgeon conducts the procedure, the robot mimics the surgeon's hand movements.

A variety of procedures can be performed using robotic surgery:

- coronary artery bypass
- gallbladder removal
- hip replacement
- hysterectomy
- mitral valve repair in the heart

## Cloning

**cloning**
*creation of an organism that is an exact genetic copy of another; a clone has identical DNA to its parent*

The latest bioengineering developments have allowed scientists to clone various organisms, or living things. **Cloning** is the creation of an organism that is an exact genetic copy (has the same DNA) of another. Identical twins, born from a fertilized egg that has split in two, are natural clones and have matching DNA. No human beings are known to have

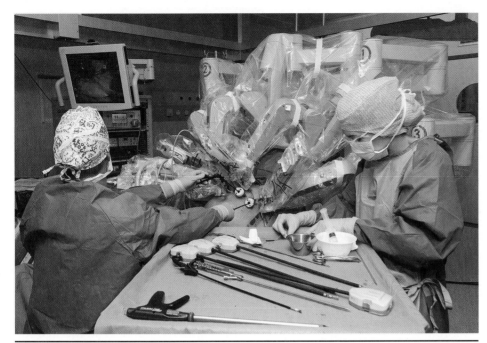

**Figure 11.18** Robotic surgery enables surgeons to perform surgeries like gallbladder removal in a minimally invasive manner.

been artificially cloned, but scientists have successfully cloned many plant varieties, reptiles, and mammals.

## Therapeutic Cloning

Many scientists believe cloning offers possibilities for treating incurable diseases. This type of cloning, called *therapeutic cloning*, does not advocate the birth of human clones.

Therapeutic cloning is performed for the purpose of medical treatment. Potential uses for therapeutic cloning include growing skin, perhaps for burn victims. Therapeutic cloning might also be used to create nerve cells for someone suffering from brain damage.

Cloning is currently a very controversial subject. The ethical issues related to cloning must be considered; the use of cloning technology is up for serious debate.

---

**Did You Know?**

### Dolly Makes History

In 1996, scientists in Scotland successfully cloned the first mammal—a sheep named Dolly. The donor cell was taken from a mammary gland of Dolly's mother. Therefore, Dolly became the clone of her mother. The successful birth of a healthy clone proved that a cell taken from a specific part of the body could recreate the whole individual.

Today, even more animals have been cloned. In fact, a few companies now exist to clone a beloved pet.

## Artificial Organs

Scientists are using biotechnology to explore many healthcare improvements and advancements. Artificial organs such as lymph nodes and kidneys are being developed. Artificial lymph nodes could replace diseased nodes or be used to boost the immune system in people who have diseases such as cancer or HIV. Manufactured kidneys would shorten the wait for those who need a kidney transplant. This life-saving surgery would benefit patients with chronic kidney disease because they wouldn't have to wait for a compatible donor.

## Absorbable Heart Stents

Heart stents are small mesh tubes used to open arteries that have become blocked or narrowed due to coronary artery disease. Stents are inserted into the narrowed artery using a balloon that inflates to expand the stent (Figure 11.19).

Traditional stents are permanently inserted into the body, but a new, absorbable stent is being designed. This stent would release medication to keep the artery from narrowing again and begin dissolving approximately six months after insertion. Within two or three years the stent

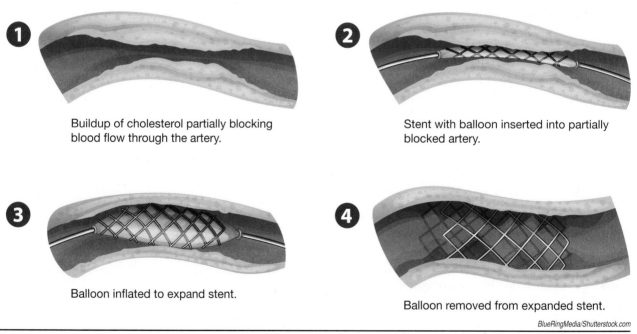

1. Buildup of cholesterol partially blocking blood flow through the artery.

2. Stent with balloon inserted into partially blocked artery.

3. Balloon inflated to expand stent.

4. Balloon removed from expanded stent.

**Figure 11.19**    Inserting a stent

should dissolve completely, leaving a healthy artery. These stents are not yet approved by the US Food and Drug Administration, but are used in other countries.

 *Check Your Understanding*

1. What is biotechnology?
2. What is a bone marrow transplant? Why might a bone marrow transplant be necessary?
3. What is therapeutic cloning?
4. What is the benefit of an absorbable heart stent?

# Simulation in Education

**Healthcare simulation** provides a bridge between classroom learning and real-life clinical experience. A simulator is a machine used to show what something looks like, or to practice a procedure as part of your training (Figure 11.20). Simulator exercises include a range of activities that are all focused on the same purpose—improving the safety, efficiency, and effectiveness of healthcare services. Simulators establish a learning environment in which students can practice necessary skills without risking patient health and safety.

**healthcare simulation**
*learning tools used to show what something looks like or how to perform a procedure*

Thanks to advances in computer technology, simulators are widely used in medical and nursing schools, veterinary colleges, and allied health programs. Some facilities are now setting up simulation laboratories with operating rooms, intensive care rooms, and other areas normally found in healthcare facilities.

Examples of simulations include virtual reality scenarios in which students can interview patients, establish a diagnosis, and practice basic surgical skills. These situations are all possible thanks to the complex, computer-generated environment.

Fully computerized, whole-body mannequins are often part of a simulation. These computerized patients respond to certain medications, and can be used for hands-on procedures such as practicing CPR, drawing blood, assisting in childbirth, and inserting chest tubes and IVs.

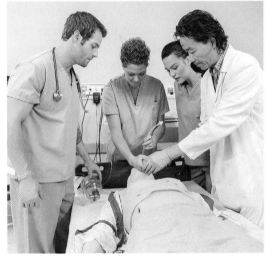
*Tyler Olson/Shutterstock.com*

**Figure 11.20** Healthcare students practice inserting a breathing tube as part of a simulation.

# Chapter Review and Assessment

## Summary

Regardless of which healthcare occupation you choose to pursue, you will be using computers and other complex technology to perform your job duties. Successful healthcare workers are confident in their computer skills and willing to learn the latest technology.

Understanding basic computer technology is helpful when working with computers. Using the Internet effectively to exchange information and access reliable resources will be invaluable skills for an employee. However, it's important to evaluate information online for accuracy and practice safe browsing. Avoid opening e-mails or downloading software from unknown sources as these may contain malware.

It is especially important to protect your computer from viruses and other malware when working in a healthcare facility. Sensitive, confidential patient information must be protected from computer disruptions such as viruses, spyware, and computer hackers. Healthcare facilities often protect their computer systems with complex firewalls, but there are also practices you should adopt to protect your patients' privacy.

In addition to a healthcare facility's computer system, communication technologies are becoming increasingly important for healthcare workers. Along with smartphones, advanced telephone systems have improved the quality of patient care in many facilities. Highly complex diagnostic technology is found throughout many healthcare facilities, making way for new careers as technicians operating complex machines. This equipment also saves time by making diagnoses quickly and accurately.

Biotechnology is opening the doors for many advances in healthcare. Along with this technology comes the development of simulators that allow students to practice key skills without putting the patient at risk. Simulators have become a valuable training tool for many future healthcare professionals.

Developing many of these technologies, specifically in the field of biotechnology, will cost billions of dollars and some will raise serious ethical issues. The healthcare industry is becoming increasingly driven by technology—now is an exciting time to be entering this field!

## Review Questions

### Short Answer

1. Give three examples of computer hardware. Explain the function of each item.
2. Give three examples of computer software. Explain the function of each item.
3. What is the difference between the Internet and the World Wide Web?
4. What is malware?
5. Why is it important for a healthcare facility to maintain powerful firewalls that protect their computer system?
6. Why might a patient need a bone marrow transplant? Describe the science behind this procedure.
7. What are four of the most commonly transplanted organs?
8. How does robotic surgery differ from traditional surgery?

### True/False

9. *True or False?* Maintaining confidentiality of patient records is the duty of all members of the healthcare team.
10. *True or False?* Employers in many workplaces can monitor your activity on the Internet while you are at work.
11. *True or False?* MRI, CT, and PET are all abbreviations for diagnostic imaging procedures.
12. *True or False?* Quality control procedures are limited to the dietary department of the hospital.
13. *True or False?* Scientists have been successful in cloning mammals, plants, and reptiles.

14. *True or False?* Robotic surgery is performed with no human intervention.

15. *True or False?* CPU stands for central progression unit.

16. *True or False?* Medical information found on the Internet is always accurate.

17. *True or False?* Scanners are categorized as software.

## Multiple Choice

18. _____ is *not* a type of computer disruption.
    A. A cookie
    B. A virus
    C. Spyware
    D. Destructo-ware

19. A(n) _____ is a small mesh tube used to expand blocked or narrowed arteries.
    A. stent
    B. dialysis machine
    C. artificial lymph node
    D. MRI

20. The term _____ describes devices that are connected to the computer.
    A. databases
    B. malware
    C. software
    D. hardware

21. Programs and data are stored at remote locations and accessed online when _____ is used.
    A. a USB flash drive
    B. cloud technology
    C. remote saving
    D. a jump drive

22. _____ enable online learning and include student tracking, assessment, and communication tools.
    A. Cookies
    B. Firewalls
    C. Virtual learning environments
    D. Podcasts

23. A computer virus is capable of _____.
    A. destroying hardware
    B. duplicating itself
    C. spreading through e-mails
    D. All of the above.

24. _____ are formed by a machine that scans the body for tracer material, which helps show how tissues and organs are functioning.
    A. CT scans
    B. MRIs
    C. PET scans
    D. All of the above.

25. A computer scanner is _____.
    A. used to listen to police calls
    B. considered software
    C. is never combined with any other device
    D. converts scanned items into digital files

36. Healthcare simulations are used _____.
    A. only in medical schools
    B. for educating patients about upcoming procedures
    C. widely in many schools for training healthcare workers
    D. for demonstrating procedures for the general public

## Critical Thinking Exercises

27. What steps have you taken to protect the data on your computer? Have you ever experienced an intrusion into your computer? If so, what could you have done to prevent this computer disruption?

28. Are your computer skills up to par? Do you feel confident in your abilities to use complex computer systems like the ones found in most healthcare facilities? If not, what can you do to improve your computer skills?

29. What healthcare technology interests you the most? Why?

30. Would you consider donating your organs in the event of a fatal accident? Have you checked the organ donor box on your driver's license? Do you have objections to being an organ donor?

31. Research a controversy that has developed from advances in biotechnology. Examples of controversial topics include cloning, stem cell research, animal testing, and selling organs for transplant.

# Chapter

# 12

# *Employability Skills*

## Terms to Know

compassion
competence
compromise
conflict resolution
cover letter
empathy
enthusiasm
multitasking

networking
patience
prioritizing
professionalism
punctuality
résumé
soft skills
tact

## Chapter Objectives

- Identify what professionalism means in the workplace.
- Describe the characteristics of a professional employee.
- Explain the concept of soft skills and the benefits of having these skills as a healthcare worker.
- Discuss why proper hygiene and appearance are necessary in the workplace.
- List the components of a healthy lifestyle.
- Explain the importance of conflict resolution in the healthcare setting.
- List ways you can prepare for employment.
- Identify a network to help you find employment.
- Create a résumé.
- Explain the importance of a properly completed job application.
- Discuss how to interview for a job.
- Identify ways to keep a job once you are hired.

Reinforce your learning with additional online resources
- **Practice** vocabulary with flashcards and interactive games
- **Assess** with posttests and image labeling
- **Expand** with activities and animations

Companion
G-W Learning

www.g-wlearning.com/healthsciences

**Study on the Go**
Use a mobile device to practice vocabulary terms and review with self-assessment quizzes.

Mobile
G-W Learning

www.m.g-wlearning.com

Whether you are just beginning your health science education, or are ready to apply for the job of your dreams, it is never too early to develop career objectives. In this chapter, you will learn how to find the ideal job and put your skills to the test. First, in an effort to determine your career objectives, ask yourself the following questions:

- How should I be preparing today for my future career?
- What career do I hope to have in five years?
- Can I imagine myself in the same position in ten years or will I want to advance up a career ladder?
- What skills do I need to develop to realize my career goals?

You may need to be employed while going to school to help finance your education. Choosing a job (or even a volunteer position) that can help you develop skills for your future career is a good idea. For instance, if you want to become a physical therapist, you might want to look into a job as a physical therapy assistant. If you are in high school or college and want to explore careers in the medical field, you might want to volunteer in a healthcare facility. If you are ready to begin your chosen career, you need to plan your employment search so that you have the best chance of obtaining a job in a competitive market.

# *Professionalism*

What do you have to learn as a student to understand and practice **professionalism**? Professionalism is an attitude reflected by one's behavior. It is the way you communicate, work, and view yourself and your coworkers. Although it may be early in your healthcare career or education, you still need to have pride in and a great attitude about your job—even if you are still working toward your preferred job.

Having a professional attitude will be a major key to your career success. Every healthcare organization looks for employees who possess skills that will make a difference in the lives of patients. Employees who will contribute positively to the organization are most desirable.

In this chapter, you will learn the skills that companies value and that make you employable. There is much competition for good jobs. Your professional attitude and excellent employability skills will greatly improve your chance of finding and keeping a fulfilling position.

## Personal Characteristics

Successful healthcare workers not only have the skills and knowledge required for their job, but also possess particular personal characteristics that contribute to their success. Certain personal characteristics enable a healthcare worker to better execute responsibilities and improve interactions with everyone in the healthcare facility. Many of these personal characteristics concern interpersonal skills, or a person's ability to establish relationships with others. Such traits are known as **soft skills**. Soft skills include social

**professionalism**
*the conduct or attitude that is required to be the best employee that you can be; contributing positively to an organization*

**soft skills**
*personal characteristics that enable a person to have pleasant, effective interactions with others*

skills such as communicating well, friendliness, and having an optimistic personality. These skills enhance an individual's interactions with others.

It is also important for an employee to recognize social cues. These include being able to read facial expression, posture, and tone of voice, to name a few. Correctly reading social cues, which can sometimes be quite subtle, is important when working with patients who may say they are feeling fine when they are not.

As you begin your healthcare career, you will realize that no two patients are the same, and no two days will present the exact same challenges. **Patience** and **tact** are two skills that will help you navigate the many situations you will encounter throughout your career. These skills are especially important when addressing patients who may be angry, sick, or frightened.

Another helpful trait for healthcare workers to possess is **enthusiasm**. Have you ever worked with someone who was very negative about his or her job and complained constantly? Imagine a person with such an attitude working closely with a sick patient. If you are enthusiastic about your work, your positive attitude will affect the people around you—including fellow workers, supervisors, and patients.

When you become a healthcare worker, you should embrace your role and do the absolute best you can. Errors in healthcare can be serious and should be avoided whenever possible. However, should an error occur, a supervisor should be notified immediately so that the error can be corrected if possible and the patient not harmed.

### Courteous Behavior

You will work closely with a variety of people throughout your healthcare career. Being courteous to coworkers and patients will improve the quality of these relationships. Kind words, **compassion**, and **empathy** go far to build the trust of others. Demonstrate a good attitude and offer patients, visitors, and staff members a sincere smile whenever possible.

One important aspect of a courteous attitude is respect. It is important to respect your coworkers and patients. Avoid using offensive language, gossiping about your patients or coworkers, telling off-color or racist jokes, and other disrespectful behavior. A healthcare facility is no place for prejudice of any kind, and it is important that you respect the diversity of others (Figure 12.1). Show every patient, visitor, and staff member respect, regardless of his or her age, race, religion, or appearance.

**patience**
*a soft skill that will help you interact with coworkers and patients*

**tact**
*the ability to avoid giving offense through your words and actions*

**enthusiasm**
*an excited and positive attitude that you can bring to your work*

**compassion**
*deep awareness and concern for the suffering of others coupled with the desire to relieve this suffering*

**empathy**
*the act of identifying with and understanding another person's feelings or situation*

### Real Life Scenario

*Developing Empathy*

Ricky is a twenty-year-old student nurse. He recently began working in the geriatric department at Eastridge Hospital. Prior to this assignment, Ricky had little experience with the elderly. Ricky admits to his supervisor that he has trouble relating to his patients and finds some of them to be very difficult. How can Ricky overcome this problem?

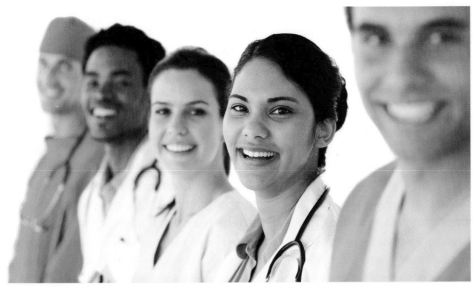

*wavebreakmedia/Shutterstock.com*

**Figure 12.1**   Celebrate and respect diversity in the workplace.

### Being a Team Player

Healthcare careers generally require employees to work cooperatively with others. When you are a team player, you need to put aside personal interests to achieve the common goal. If one of your coworkers asks you for help when you are tired, hungry, or about to go on a break, that is the time to put aside your own needs for a few minutes and be a team player. A big part of working in healthcare is putting the needs of others—specifically patients—before your own. This is why healthcare professions are often called the "helping professions."

### Trustworthy Employees

Trustworthy employees are reliable, responsible, and competent. They are often good at **multitasking** and **prioritizing** their responsibilities to ensure all tasks are completed on time. To be a competent, trustworthy employee, you must possess the ability to do your job well. **Competence** is gained through training and experience. If you prove that you are competent, you will gain the trust of your supervisor, coworkers, and patients.

Dependability is another quality of the trustworthy employee. You cannot be dependable without arriving on time for every scheduled shift. **Punctuality** is extremely important in the healthcare field (Figure 12.2). Arriving late could mean that a patient's procedure has to be delayed or rescheduled, paperwork may be filed past its deadline, or another employee may have to extend his or her shift to cover your absence. Poor attendance or frequently arriving late to work may affect your performance and lead to disciplinary actions or dismissal. Being both dependable and punctual will help you become a successful, trustworthy employee.

**multitasking**
*the ability to do more than one thing at the same time*

**prioritizing**
*to make decisions about the best order in which to perform multiple tasks so that the most important tasks are completed first*

**competence**
*the ability to do your job well*

**punctuality**
*being on time for work, appointments, and any other commitments*

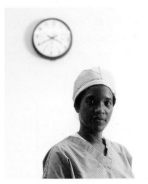

*Blend Images/Shutterstock.com*

**Figure 12.2**   Arrive at work at least five minutes early.

**Think It Through**

What do you think are some legitimate reasons for missing work? Can you think of some reasons that a supervisor would not accept? Have you ever had a job in which you had to work with a short staff because someone called in sick when they were really not?

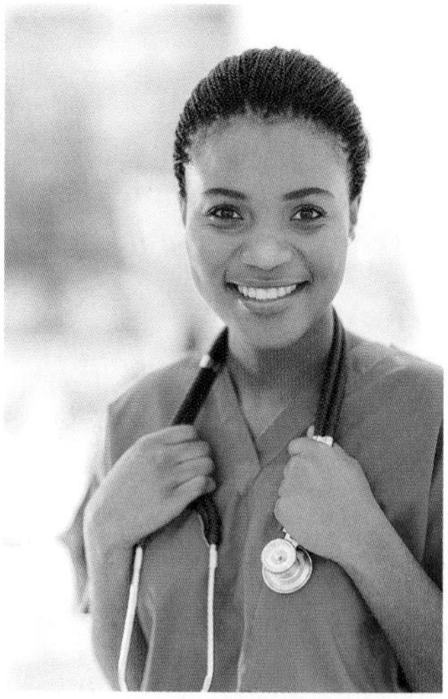

michaeljung/Shutterstock.com

**Figure 12.3** Being enthusiastic about your work may make you more successful.

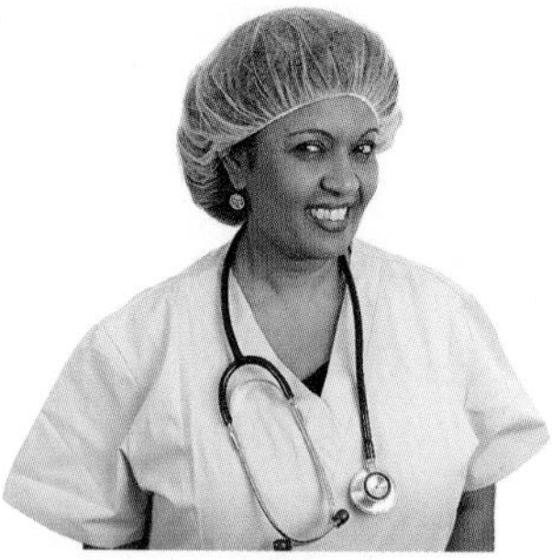

Lisa F. Young/Shutterstock.com

**Figure 12.4** You may be required to wear a hairnet to ensure hygienic conditions in certain areas of the healthcare facility.

### *Attitude Is Everything*

In the healthcare industry, a positive attitude can be the key to professional success. Employers often seek out self-motivated individuals who do not need to be directed to a task, but take the initiative to get things done without being asked. An energetic, ambitious employee with a good attitude is an asset to any organization (Figure 12.3).

Some situations may test your professionalism, such as being asked to learn new tasks or receiving criticism, but you should always maintain a good attitude. Employees who are open to learning new things are more employable than those who are resistant to learning new procedures, computer software, or moving into new positions within the healthcare facility. Also, when received properly, criticism is often constructive—it can be used to improve your job performance. Try to have a good attitude about any criticism your supervisor may provide. Everyone makes mistakes, and it's important to recognize any areas that may need improvement.

## Appearance and Hygiene

A well-groomed healthcare worker in appropriate dress can have a positive psychological effect on those he or she encounters while at work. People who are well-groomed pay attention to the details of their personal appearance. Before beginning your first day on the job, be sure to consult your facility's dress code. Different healthcare facilities may have variations in their dress codes. The following appearance and hygiene tips apply to all healthcare facilities:

- Take daily showers or baths. Be sure to wash your hair and style it appropriately for your job. Many positions require long hair to be pulled back or pinned up and off the collar for both safety and cleanliness (Figure 12.4).
- Brush your teeth at least twice a day, and be sure to floss (Figure 12.5). Good oral hygiene has been proven to prevent cardiovascular disease.
- Get plenty of sleep. Being well-rested will leave you feeling energized and may give you the appearance of someone who is excited to be at work.
- Wear deodorant.
- Depending on the facility's rules and the person's job, men's facial hair may not be allowed. Beards and mustaches need to be washed regularly and neatly combed and shaped. Scraggly facial hair does not create a professional appearance.
- Avoid using perfume, aftershave, or cologne. Patients with breathing problems and those sensitive to strong odors may be adversely affected by perfumes and colognes.
- Makeup should be conservative and applied moderately.
- Limit any jewelry worn on the job to a watch, engagement ring, wedding band, and small stud or hoop earrings. Jewelry may cause injury

to your patient or to yourself (an angry or struggling patient may grab your jewelry). Jewelry can also transmit bacteria. Healthcare workers required to wear gloves on the job may want to leave rings with stones at home because the stone may tear the glove.

- Fingernails should be kept clean and short to avoid scratching the patient. If nail polish is worn, it should be clear.
- Many healthcare jobs require employees to wear an identification name badge, and a uniform or laboratory coat. These items must be worn as they identify the employee as a member of the healthcare team. Uniforms and lab coats must be kept clean and in good repair. For any healthcare job that does not require a uniform, you should dress according the facility's dress code.
- Wear sensible, closed-toe shoes. If you are going to be on your feet all day, low heels and a comfortable shoe are a must.

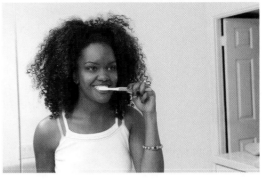

*bikeriderlondon/Shutterstock.com*

**Figure 12.5** Maintaining good oral hygiene has many health benefits.

### ✔ *Check Your Understanding*

Which clothing and accessories do you think are appropriate in a healthcare environment? Which are inappropriate? Have you had a dress code at any other jobs you have held in the past?

## Conflict Resolution

Good interpersonal skills and a respectful attitude do not ensure you will get along with every person you encounter. Some interpersonal conflicts may be unavoidable in a stressful work environment. When people are rushed and under pressure, they don't always practice the best communication skills. Personalities may clash and you may not always get along with your coworkers. To keep the work environment a pleasant and productive place, you should resolve any conflicts that arise on the job.

Conflict often occurs because personalities clash, and responsibilities and roles are misunderstood. Regardless of the reason, conflict can lessen the morale of a healthcare worker. Are you good at **conflict resolution**? It is important that you know how to handle conflict so it does not become a destructive force in your workplace.

A healthcare facility can be a fast-paced, stressful environment. A doctor may be impatient to get laboratory results back and yell at a laboratory secretary who has trouble finding the results in the computer. During stressful periods, it is important to remember that everyone is doing their best to get their job done. In such situations, a professional may not treat a worker in an assistant-level position with proper respect, which can cause conflict.

**conflict resolution**
*methods for alleviating or eliminating sources of conflict*

When conflict does arise in the workplace, there are a few options available for resolving the issue. Traditionally, the supervisor is responsible for managing conflict in the workplace. In healthcare facilities, employees often work as a team. Conflict within the team can destroy team efforts. Often, minor conflict can be resolved without the intervention of the supervisor if the individuals involved work through their issue together. The following list includes some potential solutions to conflict in the workplace:

1. Treat coworkers with respect—especially if you disagree with them on something. If a conflict does arise, talk with the person privately, and be honest and calm as you express your feelings about the situation. If your efforts are unsuccessful, talk to your supervisor about the problem. He or she may want the people involved in the conflict to have a discussion. Make sure all workplace conflicts stay professional instead of personal.

2. Do not take sides when two coworkers have a conflict. Taking sides divides the team and may prevent you from doing your job well. It is also a mistake to confront a supervisor as a group with a complaint.

3. Remember that the goal of your healthcare career is delivering outstanding care to the patient. Any conflicts you might have should not get in the way of that mission.

**compromise**
*settlement of differences where each side makes concessions*

4. Some facilities have procedures for handling conflict to reach a solution that everyone can accept. Often, **compromise** must be achieved for conflict to be resolved. Holding on to rigid views without being open to hearing a solution is not professional behavior.

5. Listening to each other and agreeing to work toward a solution are key elements in solving interpersonal problems. It's important that you are open to compromise and attempt to find a solution. Do not bring other complaints into the conflict, but rather, focus on one problem at a time.

You may experience conflict at some point in your healthcare career. With clear communication that focuses on active listening, and the ability to resolve conflict in a positive manner, your team will be stronger. Successful resolution of conflict will also allow you to provide professional patient care.

### Real Life Scenario

#### Dealing with Conflict

Paula and Melissa are nursing assistants who often work together at East-ridge Hospital. Paula feels like she often does Melissa's duties for her. When there is an unpleasant mess to clean up, Melissa tends to disappear. Melissa takes long breaks, and Paula has trouble finding Melissa when she needs help. Melissa also avoids dealing with difficult patients. What should Paula do? Should Paula talk to Melissa? Should Paula approach her supervisor instead of speaking with Melissa? Have you ever worked with someone like Melissa?

# Preparing for Employment

There are many factors for an employer to consider in a potential hire. Each position is different and requires a specific set of skills to perform the job. Just knowing how to do the job isn't always enough—your personality is important as well. What basic qualities are desirable in a new employee?

- The employer wants a skilled employee, capable of doing the job.
- The employer wants a dependable person who can prove that he or she has been a reliable team member in other jobs. This can be confirmed by checking the potential employee's past employer references.
- The employer wants someone who makes a good first impression, takes pride in his or her appearance, and is well spoken.
- The employer needs to see someone with a good attitude that conveys enthusiasm about the potential position. Asking informed questions about the position or the healthcare facility shows enthusiasm and interest in the job.

## The Résumé

Your **résumé** summarizes your educational background, work experiences, and other qualifications for employment. A résumé can be sent to an employer along with a cover letter or given to an employer with a completed job application. The résumé gives an employer a starting point to assess your potential as an employee.

**résumé**
*a document that summarizes your education, work experiences, and other qualifications for employment; can be printed or submitted electronically*

### Preparing Your Résumé

In some cases, you will be able to submit a hard copy of your résumé, rather than sending it to the employer electronically. When printing your résumé, use a standard, 8 1/2 by 11 inch paper in white or off-white. Avoid using colored or patterned paper—this can detract from the information you are presenting.

All information must be neatly organized with evenly spaced margins. Be sure to review your résumé carefully for spelling, punctuation, and grammar errors! Include all of the important facts about your work history, schooling, and any extracurricular activities. Ask your school counselor or a teacher to read your résumé, and accept their constructive criticism.

Today, many employers ask you to submit your résumé electronically. Known as an *e-résumé*, this digital file is sent to potential employers via e-mail or by uploading it onto the employer's website or a job search website. Detailed instructions for creating electronic formats of your résumé can be found online.

## Extend Your Knowledge

### Résumé References

Online resources are available to help you format and organize your résumé. Your school likely has similar resources available to you. Consult your school's counselor if you have questions when preparing your résumé.

## What to Include on Your Résumé

A résumé alone will not get you a job, but a poorly written résumé may rule you out for an interview. It is very important to make your résumé concise. Most employers will not read through several pages of non-essential information. A well-prepared résumé should not exceed one page of text.

Figure 12.6 is a sample résumé you may use to guide you as you create your own résumé. The format of your résumé may vary, but this sample represents a very traditional approach in which the information is presented in a specific order.

**Job Objective.** The first section of a résumé is the job objective (or *career objective*). This allows the employer to immediately see which position you seek. There are probably many jobs available throughout the facility, and you may be rejected if your objective is poorly written or does not match the job opening.

Depending on the facility, job names or descriptions might be slightly different. You might have to change your job objective to match each position to which you are applying. Double check your job objective before sending your résumé to each prospective employer.

**Education.** Your education is one of the most important features of your résumé, so this section should follow the job objective. The last school that you attended should appear first on the list. For each school, list the name, location, and dates attended. Also, state the diploma or degree you earned (or will earn, including your anticipated date of graduation), and what program you studied. If you did well, you might want to include your grade point average (GPA).

**Work Experience.** List your most recent job first. If you have a sparse work history, include part-time jobs, summer jobs, or volunteer experience, even if such positions were not in a related field. Volunteer positions show an interest in your community. Including positions that may be unrelated lets the employer know that you are responsible and may have transferable skills.

Include your employer's name and location for each job listed. Also, include a brief description of your responsibilities, emphasizing any tasks that might relate to the job for which you are applying. Use the past tense when describing a job that you no longer have. Use the present tense if the experience is current.

**Honors and Activities.** In this section, list the school and community organizations and activities in which you have participated. Offices held and honors received are also very important. If volunteer activities are not related to the position you are seeking, include them here.

**Special Skills and Related Courses.** This section is an optional addition to your résumé. However, if you have a personal qualification that demonstrates

**Lauren E. Castle**
22145 E. Rollins Avenue
Charlottesville, VA 22909
Home: 434-555-4356
Cell: 434-555-2681
E-mail: lcastle@e-mail.com

**Objective**
To obtain a position as a phlebotomist in a healthcare facility.

**Education**
Phlebotomy Technician Certification (CPT)
Atlantic Technical Institute for the Health Sciences, December 2015

Eastridge High School, June 2012

**Experience**
August, 2013–Present
Laboratory Aide, Jefferson Clinic, Charlottesville, VA
- Prepare specimens for testing at clinic laboratory
- Wash glassware used for laboratory testing
- Answer phones on weekends

October–December, 2013
60-Hour Externship, County Hospital, Charlottesville, VA
- Performed 100 phlebotomies under supervision
- Prepared specimens for testing in the main clinical laboratory
- Worked in satellite laboratories connected to hospital
- Gained exposure to on-the-job duties of a phlebotomist
- Learned to gain trust and confidence of patients

**Special Skills**
Familiar with two hospital-based computer programs: FREEmed and Vitera. I also possess excellent people skills, am highly organized, and able to prioritize multiple tasks.

**Figure 12.6**   A sample résumé

a job-related skill or ability, you can list it here. These skills may include a language you speak fluently, computer skills that haven't been mentioned before, or courses related to the position for which you are applying.

# The Cover Letter

You will also need a **cover letter** to accompany your résumé (Figure 12.7). Cover letters should be personalized for each position for which you apply, and are sometimes called *letters of application*.

The appearance of the letter is very important. Use the same paper that you used for the résumé, with a standard font size and style. Your letter should include a return address, date, inside address, salutation, body, and

**cover letter**
*a letter that accompanies a résumé to provide additional information about the applicant's skills and experience*

**Lauren E. Castle**
22145 E. Rollins Avenue
Charlottesville, VA 22909
Home: 434-555-4356
Cell: 434-555-2681

—— Return address

Date —— December 1, 2015

Ms. Penny Jones
Clinical Laboratory Director
Mt. Ross Medical Center
23145 Club Drive
Richmond, VA 23218

—— Inside address

Salutation —— Dear Ms. Jones:

The phlebotomist position you advertised in the *Richmond Reporter* on November 29 is exactly the kind of position I am seeking. Your ad emphasizes good people and organizational skills. As you can see by my résumé, I am qualified for this position.

For the past three years, I have worked in a clinical laboratory environment, giving me a well-rounded knowledge of how the laboratory functions. I have performed laboratory tasks such as specimen preparation, front desk tasks, phlebotomies, and have had experience multitasking. I frequently interact with patients and their families, and I feel very comfortable working with others.

As the enclosed résumé states, I am proud to have received my phlebotomy technician certification from a very fine college and completed my training as second in my class. I gained much knowledge and experience at my externship, and I received excellent evaluations while in the program. As a skilled phlebotomist, I can offer your laboratory a strong work ethic and the ability to successfully interact with patients.

—— Body

I would like very much to meet with you and hope you will contact me by phone or e-mail to schedule an interview for the phlebotomist position.

—— Complimentary close

Sincerely yours,

*Lauren Castle*

Signature ——

Lauren Castle

Enclosure

**Figure 12.7**    Make sure your cover letter includes all the important components shown here.

complimentary close. Again, make sure your letter is neat and clean and is free of spelling or grammatical errors. As with the résumé, a poorly constructed, misspelled cover letter may result in a potential employee never being called for an interview.

When you are writing a cover letter, keep it short and focused. As with a résumé, you do not want to overload the potential employer with too many facts. Find out to whom you should direct the letter—a human resources representative, hiring manager, or perhaps supervisor for the posted position. This information may be online, or you can call the company and ask for the name and title of the appropriate person.

When writing your letter, restrict its length to about three paragraphs. In the opening paragraph, identify the job or type of work you seek, and explain how you learned about the position.

In the next paragraph, tell why you are right for the job. Briefly explain how your education and previous positions have prepared you for this work. Refer the potential employer to your included résumé for more detail.

Finish your cover letter by asking for an interview and thanking the employer for considering you for the position. Make sure the employer knows where you can be reached.

# The Job Search

Future job projections are favorable for those who wish to begin a career in healthcare, an industry that is one of the fastest growing in the United States. To obtain a job, you need to know how to begin the search and understand the job market. Job hunting takes work. How do you find potential employers? There are many sources to explore to find available jobs.

## Friends and Relatives

Friends and relatives can be effective sources for job leads. Make sure they are aware of your specific skills and background. They may know of jobs that fit your skills. Providing them with a résumé can be helpful.

## Networking

**Networking** involves developing contacts with people who are interested in your future employment and can help you search for jobs. These people should be familiar with your abilities and interests. After developing such a network, you may be in the position to help others looking for work. Networking works best when there is benefit to all involved.

There are many ways to build your network. Joining a professional or student organization may put you in touch with those who share your interests. You may meet local employers who participate as speakers in career and technical student organizations. Another option is volunteering in a workplace, such as a healthcare facility, where you can meet potential employers.

**networking**
*a process for developing contacts and relationships with people who are interested in your future employment*

There are also exciting networking possibilities online. LinkedIn, a social networking website for people seeking professional positions, will put you in contact with other people in your chosen field. These websites are expanding all the time, offering another option for employers to view your qualifications.

---

### Extend Your Knowledge

*Networking and You*

Have you tried networking? If so, who do you consider to be some members of your network? If you have not yet established a network, how can you begin?

---

## Resources at Your School

Many schools have a job placement office or a counselor who can help you find jobs in your community. Your school counselor may be able to review your résumé. Many schools also have a variety of online resources.

Your instructors can often guide you toward job opportunities. Instructors often place students in internships that may lead to job offers. Sometimes employers work directly with schools to fill open positions.

Your instructor knows your skills, and can attest to your excellent attitude in class, attendance record, and personal achievements. It is very important to make a good impression on your instructors; these individuals can be a valuable networking source as well.

## Online Job Search

Many people have successfully found jobs on the Internet. There are thousands of employment options available online. If you do not have a computer at home, most public libraries and schools provide Internet access.

Good places to start your Internet job search are government websites sponsored by the United States Department of Labor, Employment, and Training Administration. These sites display a great deal of information about the job market, listing job openings by type, title, and location. Another effective government source for researching careers is The Occupational Outlook Handbook.

## Direct Employer Contact

Many people use direct employer contact to find jobs. Make a list of possible employers by doing an Internet search, looking through the Yellow Pages, or by contacting the Chamber of Commerce. You can also ask those in your network for contacts. Record the names, addresses, and phone numbers of employers who have job openings.

Next, contact the person who is responsible for hiring in each company. Such a person is often found in the human resources department of the facility. A human resources representative will know the available jobs and how to apply. Online postings for facility job openings are common today. Some facilities may have an automated job line that will list jobs available at the present time. You can access the job line information through a telephone extension for the facility.

## Professional and Trade Journals

Many healthcare organizations and related trades publish their own magazines and journals. Some of these journals may be found as online publications, and many include advertisements for job openings. Some journals advertise both national and international job possibilities. Some national trade journals also list job opportunities by state. Journals and magazines published by state and local chapters of an organization provide local job leads. These journals are also valuable resources because they contain up-to-date information about the latest developments in a given field.

## Government and Private Employment Services

State employment offices are found in most large cities and towns. Many of these offices have an online presence as well. These offices are able to help job seekers find job openings within and outside government. You can find the nearest state employment office by searching online, or looking in your local telephone directory under the name of your state. For, example: "Florida (state of), Employment Service." This service is free, but you must fill out an application at a state employment office. There are also some county job centers.

When visiting employment offices, you will be interviewed by an employment counselor to determine your skills and interests. Then you may be matched with positions that fit your profile. Once you have chosen a field, you will be directed to the potential employer(s) that may want to hire you. Only a small percentage of job seekers will find a job this way, so it is best to explore many sources to find the job you want.

Private employment agencies are businesses that help match employers and job seekers. These agencies charge the job seeker or the employer for this service. For most entry-level jobs, the job seeker can expect to pay the employment agency. For most high-paying, professional jobs the fee is often paid by the employer. Ask your school counselor to recommend a private agency. Some agencies specialize in certain jobs. As with the similar government agencies, only a small percentage of people find jobs this way.

## *The Job Application*

Some employers may only require you to submit your résumé when applying for a job, while others will ask that you also fill out an application. You may fill out several applications during your job search. It may be helpful to carry a personal fact sheet, especially when you are completing an application away from your records. The personal fact sheet includes all of the personal and professional information you will need to complete a job application (Figure 12.8). Carry the fact sheet with you at all times when applying for jobs. The fact sheet is for your own personal use during this process.

Do not submit an incorrect or sloppy application form. Read the entire application before beginning to fill it out. Carefully fill out the form using black or blue ink. Do not fill out the sections marked for employer use only. If the application asks you to print, do so. Answer questions on both sides of the form, if it is two-sided.

If a question does not apply to you, write "*does* not *apply*" in the space provided. You may wish to omit your Social Security number. If so, write "will provide if hired" on the application.

If a question asks about wages or salaries, it may be best to write "open" or "negotiable." You do not want to limit your options. When filling out the employment history, remember to include part-time jobs. There may be questions asking you for the reason you left a job. Carefully draft your response to this question. Do not write negative comments about yourself or your former employer.

When handing in your application, you may want to include a résumé as well. The résumé may not be required, but it will provide additional details the human resources staff may find useful.

There are certain questions that cannot be asked on job applications or in a job interview (Figure 12.9). Knowing these questions can help you protect your rights. If you find a discriminatory question on an application, you can write "not clear" or "decline to answer."

## *The Job Interview*

Any job interview requires preparation and research. This could be one of the most important moments of your life—preparation is key! There are several things you can do before your interview to ensure you are properly prepared:

- Research the company or healthcare facility where you are interviewing—doing so shows that you are interested in what they do.
- Make a list of intelligent questions to ask your interviewer. These questions might be specific to the position or to the healthcare facility as a whole.

---

## Personal Fact Sheet

**Education**

| | Name | Location | Date Attended | Date Graduated | GPA |
|---|---|---|---|---|---|
| Junior high school | _____ | _____ | _____ | _____ | _____ |
| High school | _____ | _____ | _____ | _____ | _____ |
| College | _____ | _____ | _____ | _____ | _____ |
| Technical school | _____ | _____ | _____ | _____ | _____ |
| Other | _____ | _____ | _____ | _____ | _____ |

**Work Experience**

Employer _____

Address _____
    (street address)          (city)          (state)          (zip)

Telephone _____ Employed from _____ to _____
                                (mo./yr.)          (mo./yr.)

Job title _____ Supervisor _____

Starting salary _____ Final salary _____

Job duties _____
_____
_____

Employer _____

Address _____
    (street address)          (city)          (state)          (zip)

Telephone _____ Employed from _____ to _____
                                (mo./yr.)          (mo./yr.)

Job title _____ Supervisor _____

Starting salary _____ Final salary _____

Job duties _____
_____
_____

**Skills** _____

**Honors and Activities** _____
_____

**Hobbies and Interests** _____
_____

**References**

Name/Title _____

Address _____

Telephone (daytime) _____ E-mail _____

Name/Title _____

Address _____

Telephone (daytime) _____ E-mail _____

Name/Title _____

Address _____

Telephone (daytime) _____ E-mail _____

**Figure 12.8** Your personal fact sheet is a helpful reference to take with you when applying for jobs or interviewing.

- Be sure to bring relevant materials with you—a pen, your résumé, the completed application, and your list of questions.
- Decide what you are going to wear and lay it out the night before.
- Practice before the interview—think of how you might answer questions commonly asked during interviews (Figure 12.10).
- Make sure you know where to go for the interview and arrive at least 5 to 10 minutes early. Never arrive late for an interview.

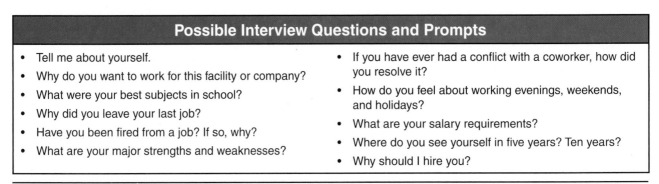

| Illegal Questions for Job Applicants | | | |
|---|---|---|---|
| *Subject* | *Questions* | *Subject* | *Questions* |
| **Race or national origin** | What is the color of your skin, hair, or eyes? What is your race? What nationality are you? What is your ancestry? What language do you and your family speak at home? Is English your first language? What is your place of birth? Are you a naturalized citizen? | **Personal/family** | What is your age? What is the date of your birth? Do you have a current photograph to attach to your application? Do you have any children, or are you planning to have children? What child care arrangements do you have? |
| **Religion** | What is your religion? What church do you attend? What religious holidays do you observe? Who is your religious leader? | **Sex and marital status** | Are you single, married, divorced, or widowed? Do you prefer to be addressed as Miss, Ms., or Mrs.? |
| **Disabilities** | Do you have any disabilities? | **Organizations** | To what organizations or clubs do you belong? |

**Figure 12.9**    Certain questions should not be asked during a job interview.

| Possible Interview Questions and Prompts |
|---|

- Tell me about yourself.
- Why do you want to work for this facility or company?
- What were your best subjects in school?
- Why did you leave your last job?
- Have you been fired from a job? If so, why?
- What are your major strengths and weaknesses?

- If you have ever had a conflict with a coworker, how did you resolve it?
- How do you feel about working evenings, weekends, and holidays?
- What are your salary requirements?
- Where do you see yourself in five years? Ten years?
- Why should I hire you?

**Figure 12.10**    Rehearsing answers to these prompts and questions will help prepare you for a job interview.

- When you arrive for the interview, other employees may see you and judge your appearance and behavior. Act professionally at all times.
- Do not bring anyone with you to an interview, including children, parents, friends, spouses, or significant others.

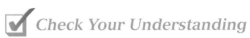 *Check Your Understanding*

Prepare answers to each of the questions presented in Figure 12.10. Discuss your answers with a family member, friend, or teacher. What do you think are the most effective responses to each question?

# Dressing for the Job Interview

Think very carefully about what you want to wear to the interview. Your clothes and appearance will influence the employer's impression of you, just as your general appearance leaves an impression on patients and coworkers.

## *What to Wear*

Dress one step above what will be worn on the job. If you are interviewing for a summer job with the recreation department, you might dress in a casual manner with clothes that are clean, neat, and ironed. Make sure your shoes are in good condition—polished if necessary.

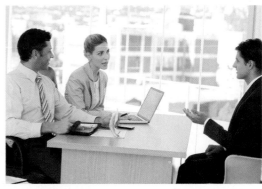

*wavebreakmedia/Shutterstock.com*

If you are interviewing for a position with a great deal of responsibility, it's important to dress more professionally (Figure 12.11). Men should wear a long-sleeved shirt with a tie. You may also want to wear a suit, sport coat, or blazer, if appropriate. Women in this position should wear a two-piece skirt or pant suit in a conservative color (navy, black, or brown). A blouse should be tailored with sleeves. Shoes should have a low heel with the toes covered. When in doubt, lean more toward professional than casual dress.

**Figure 12.11** Dressing professionally and appropriately for a job interview may improve your chances of being hired.

## *What Not to Wear*

When you are interviewing for a healthcare position, remember that the healthcare profession requires conservative dress. Because the healthcare employee is exposed to patients with a wide range of ages and points of view, piercings, tattoos, short skirts, cleavage, high heels, tight pants, and heavy makeup are not appropriate. Do not wear tee shirts with pictures or sayings on them, regardless of the job for which you are applying. No tattoos should be visible, and jewelry should be removed with the exception of small earrings.

Men should wear very little jewelry except perhaps a conservative watch and their wedding band. Do not wear athletic shoes, sandals, or boots. Cologne should not be worn.

Women should avoid wearing too much makeup—less is more. Jewelry should be small and conservative, and perfume should not be worn. Short, tight clothing is not appropriate for a job interview. Organize your purse before the interview—you will look unprofessional and disorganized if you have to dig around in your purse to find an item.

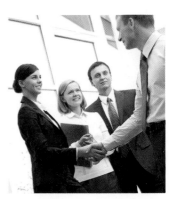

*Pressmaster/Shutterstock.com*

# The Handshake

The first impression your potential employer will get from you is your overall appearance. The second impression may come when he or she shakes your hand. A firm handshake communicates confidence when coupled with direct eye contact (Figure 12.12). Do not get too close to the other

**Figure 12.12** Direct eye contact and a firm handshake make a good impression on an employer.

person during a handshake. Present your hand, not your fingertips. Don't extend your hand first. Not everyone wants to shake hands.

 *Check Your Understanding*

> For the next week, practice shaking hands with family and friends. Make sure you grasp hands firmly, but do not squeeze too hard. Why might you hesitate to squeeze an elderly patient's hand too firmly?

## Conducting Yourself during the Interview

Many employers use phone interviews to decide which applicants they would like to bring into the office for an in-person interview. In this case, a phone interview is your first contact with an employer. These interviews are used to screen applicants before bringing them on-site, so you want to make a good impression. Take the call in a location where there is no outside noise (crying children, ringing phones, or background talking). Remember to speak slowly, clearly, and with confidence. Your attitude will come through on the phone as it does in person.

For an in-person interview, there is quite a bit more to consider. Do not sit until you are invited to do so by the interviewer. If you are already seated when an interviewer enters the room, stand to greet him or her. Introduce yourself if the interviewer has not stated your name. Smile and try to appear relaxed, even though you will probably be nervous.

When you are offered a seat, sit in a comfortable position, do not slouch, and lean forward slightly. Put your hands in your lap. If you cross your legs, cross them at your ankles rather than your knees. Avoid doing anything distracting, such as chewing gum, shifting nervously in your seat, playing with your hair, or avoiding direct eye contact. Keep the conversation positive throughout the interview. Do not mention reasons why it would be hard for you to take this job, such as child care problems or transportation challenges.

It may seem like the interviewer is asking you hard questions to get you to say the wrong thing. If you receive a question that you aren't prepared for and that surprises you, take a moment to think about your answer. Interviewers are interested in your ability to think on your feet. They are not interested in someone who gets flustered easily and is unable to come up with a reasonable answer.

When the interviewer has finished questioning you, you may be asked if you have any questions. Questions you might ask can include specific questions about the company, or more general questions:

- What opportunities could this job present for me to learn and grow professionally?
- What is a typical workday like?

- What does the interviewer like about working for this particular company?
- When does the interviewer think the decision will be made about the job?

Do not ask about salaries on a first interview. If you will refuse a job that pays less than a certain amount, you can state the required amount in your cover letter. However, if you are even somewhat flexible regarding salary, it is best not to discuss compensation until you are offered a position. The employer will most likely promise to contact you in the future about the job. If you do not get the job, you may not get a call at all.

### *Real Life Scenario*

#### *Responding to Questionable Questions*

Brianna has an interview with an employer for a part-time job in a long-term care facility over the summer. She is excited because if she gets this job, it will be a stepping stone for a career in this facility when she finishes her education.

Brianna's interviewer, Mr. Stone, asks her about her last name, which is Sanchez. He says he is curious about the origin of her name—specifically if it is Spanish, Mexican, or Filipino. Brianna recognizes that it is illegal for Mr. Stone to ask such a question. How should she handle this situation?

## After the Interview

Within two days of your interview, you should send a follow-up letter. This brief note, written in a business-like manner, should thank the interviewer for his or her time. Draft another letter to thank anyone who referred you to the position. They may be pleased to get your feedback about how your interview went and to hear if you were offered a job.

If you go on many interviews, but are not offered any jobs, consider the following questions:

- Are you really qualified for this job? Maybe the jobs require more experience and training. You may have to start in an entry-level position that does not require experience.
- What is the job market like for the position you are seeking? Maybe you need to apply for jobs in neighboring towns or move to an area where there are more opportunities.
- Was your application filled out completely and properly? Did the application look neat? Did you cross out answers and attempt to write over the first answers? Did you read the application directions carefully?
- Did you present a résumé that was clear and appropriate for the jobs you wanted? Was the résumé neat and restricted to one page?
- Were you tired or excessively nervous during the interview? Did you project enthusiasm? Not asking questions about the job or seeming distracted during the interview could tell the interviewer that you are not really interested in the job.

- Did you lack confidence during the interview? Did you apologize for any trouble that you might have doing the job?
- Were you courteous with the interviewer? Did you get defensive when asked about your past employment?
- Were you late to an interview? Did you properly thank the interviewer?

## *The Job Offer*

It is thrilling to be offered your first job in the healthcare world after training is over. Depending on where you live, jobs could be scarce, so you might feel very fortunate to receive a job offer. It is important to remember that your first job will likely be a stepping stone to a better-paying position with more responsibility.

When applying for an entry-level position in a healthcare facility, you should be able to obtain salary information by contacting the facility's human resources department. You need to be realistic about the compensation and recognize that an entry-level job may lead to a better opportunity in the future. However, if you have a family to support and cannot get by on the specified salary, do not apply for the job knowing you will turn down an offer.

Make sure you know what will be expected of you when you are offered a job. If specific information is not given to you by the employer such as work hours, salary, and other expectations not mentioned in the job description, ask realistic questions about the job. Remember to be enthusiastic and optimistic about the job.

### Rejecting the Job Offer?

If after an interview you realize that the job is not a good fit for you, you will probably not accept an offer. Politely thank the interviewer and briefly explain why you feel you are not right for the job. Be direct, but polite. Although this specific position did not work out, you may want to apply for another job at the facility in the future.

The process of searching for, applying for, and interviewing for a job calls for careful preparation. The process will be time-consuming and often stressful. It is important to be properly focused and organized before you take this final step that began with your education. Your time is valuable, and so is the time of potential employers. An informed and efficient job search is critical for beginning a successful career.

## *The Art of Keeping a Job*

You have studied your options for pursing a healthcare career and have completed the necessary coursework and training to begin your career. You carefully prepared a successful job search strategy, and you obtained your dream job. Now, how do you keep your new job? Here are a few suggestions that can help you be a valuable employee:

- **Show up on time.** Arriving early is even better than being on time. Always give yourself plenty of time to get to work in case of complications. Employers do not want to hear about your alarm clock not going off, your car battery dying, or the impossible traffic. Lack of punctuality may lead to disciplinary actions or dismissal.
- **Always look professional.** Wrinkled, dirty clothes and unwashed hair will not make a good impression on your employer. Pay attention to your grooming, hygiene, and appearance.
- **Present a positive attitude.** Complaining about your fellow employees, resisting any new tasks, and bringing your personal problems to the job are all signs of a bad attitude. Embrace any new task that you are asked to perform. Try as hard as you can to get along with other employees and keep personal drama out of the workplace.
- **Use appropriate language with patients and fellow employees.** Sarcasm shouldn't be used in the healthcare facility. People who do not use or understand sarcasm may be confused and even offended by it. Swearing is not tolerated in a healthcare facility, and using offensive language may be reason for termination.
- **Maintain appropriate relationships with coworkers.** You might think that flirting is harmless, but someone might feel your flirting is sexual harassment. You do not want to make fellow employees or even patients feel uncomfortable. Overt sexual behavior can be punished by termination and even criminal charges.
- **Keep busy.** If your assigned task is finished, ask your supervisor for another. Help a coworker if you see that he or she is struggling to finish a task. Look around to see what needs to be done, and do it without direction or complaint.
- **Do not argue with a supervisor.** Some new employees feel like they know a better way to do a task than how it is being done in the workplace. You need to prove yourself as an excellent employee before you can make suggestions. Do not correct your supervisor, especially in front of others. You are not in the position to point out mistakes.
- **Try to smile as much as possible.** Smiling more will show everyone that you are happy with your new job. You will also seem much more approachable and pleasant to be around (Figure 12.13).

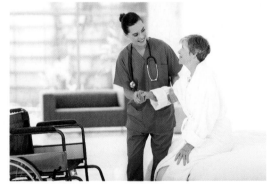

michaeljung/Shutterstock.com

**Figure 12.13** A positive attitude and smile will improve your relationships with coworkers and patients.

# Chapter Review and Assessment

## Summary

If you have a professional attitude and appearance, you will be one step closer to becoming an excellent employee with a promising career future. Evaluating your personal characteristics may help you determine which area of healthcare will be best for you. Soft skills can improve your interactions with patients, visitors, and staff members, and make you a better employee. Correctly recognizing social cues adds to your effectiveness when dealing with others. Learning how to find compromise and resolution in conflict will make you an asset to your professional team.

Preparing for the job search can be time-consuming. There are many sources for job leads including networking and Internet searches. Your school may have invaluable resources to help you get leads for job openings.

Creating a well-written cover letter and résumé are necessary first steps to take when applying for jobs. As you fill out job applications, it's crucial to include accurate, complete information. Doing so improves your chances of getting an interview. Interviewing, whether in person or by phone, requires specific skills to present yourself in a positive light. Be confident in yourself and your ability to do the job.

Professional attitudes combined with employability skills will help you find a fulfilling job that fits your personal needs. These attitudes and skills will take a great deal of effort, but you will be rewarded for the time spent. Once you have your long-sought job, do everything in your power to keep the job by having a great attitude on the job.

## Review Questions

### Short Answer

1. List four personal characteristics of someone who acts in a professional manner.

2. List five aspects of personal appearance necessary to maintain a professional appearance in the workplace.

3. Name three steps that should be taken to conduct a successful job hunt.

4. Explain the importance of properly completing a job application.

5. If a question on a job application form does not apply to you, what should you do?

6. Name three questions that federal law prohibits employers from legally asking you during a job interview.

7. Identify three ways to keep a job once you are employed.

### True/False

8. *True or False?* Perfume should be worn while interacting with patients.

9. *True or False?* Conflict resolution is something *only* your supervisor needs to know.

10. *True or False?* Chewing gum during a job interview is unacceptable.

11. *True or False?* A firm handshake is important when interviewing.

12. *True or False?* Only a small number of jobs are found through government and private employment services.

13. *True or False?* You should feel free to ask about a potential salary as soon as you are interviewed.

14. *True or False?* Soft skills include friendliness, optimism, and the ability to communicate well with others.

15. *True or False?* Making direct eye contact with a potential employer is a sign of dominance and should be avoided.

16. *True or False?* It is important to address your cover letter to a specific person instead of "To Whom It May Concern."

17. *True or False?* Employees in healthcare facilities never work as a team.

## Multiple Choice

18. Which of the following behaviors are considered unacceptable at work?
    A. Calling in sick when you have a respiratory infection.
    B. Arriving at work at least five minutes early.
    C. Wearing closed-toe, comfortable shoes.
    D. Occasionally leaving your facility identification badge at home.

19. Which of the following resources are helpful when looking for a job?
    A. direct employer contact
    B. school resources
    C. friends and family connections
    D. All of the above.

20. Which of the following are considered unprofessional in the workplace?
    A. using coarse language
    B. gossiping
    C. wearing sloppy clothes
    D. All of the above.

21. When being criticized by an employer, you should do all the following *except* _____.
    A. Resist being defensive.
    B. Listen carefully to what your employer is saying.
    C. Help determine a way to improve your performance.
    D. Question the validity of the criticism.

22. _____ is the ability to avoid giving offense through your words and actions.
    A. Compassion
    B. Empathy
    C. Tact
    D. Competence

23. All of the following items should be included in a cover letter *except* _____.
    A. the correct name of the person who will read the cover letter
    B. a clearly written statement of the job you are seeking
    C. a short statement about your likes and dislikes
    D. a phone number where you can be reached

24. What should you remember when filling out a job application?
    A. Read the entire application over before you begin.
    B. Use black or blue ink.
    C. Answer each question honestly.
    D. All of the above.

25. Which of the following would be inappropriate to include in the special skills section of your résumé?
    A. computer programs with which you are familiar
    B. languages you speak fluently
    C. gardening expertise
    D. ability to multitask

26. A well-written résumé should include each of the following *except* _____.
    A. a clear objective
    B. work experience
    C. education
    D. travel experiences

## Critical Thinking Exercises

1. What aspects of practicing professionalism in attitude and appearance can be challenging for you, if any?

2. Have you ever interviewed for a job that you didn't get? What might have been the reasons for not getting the job?

3. What would you do if a potential employer acted unprofessionally during a job interview?

4. Do you have a job-seeking network? If not, how can you assemble one?

5. What career advising or placement services does your school offer? If you are still a student, see if these services can help place you in a job that will enhance your skills for future employment.

6. Do you have a potential employer that you would like to target when you finish your preparation for your career? What are some ways you can begin to prepare for this future employment?

# Metric Conversion Tables

| Conversion Table: US Customary to SI Metric* | | |
|---|---|---|
| **When You Know** ⬇ | **Multiply By:** ⬇ | **To Find** ⬇ |
| **Length** | | |
| inches | 25.4 | millimeters |
| inches | 2.54 | centimeters |
| feet | 0.3048 | meters |
| feet | 30.48 | centimeters |
| yards | 0.9 | meters |
| miles | 1.6 | kilometers |
| **Weight** | | |
| ounces | 28.0 | grams |
| ounces | .028 | kilograms |
| pounds | 0.45 | kilograms |
| short tons | 0.9 | tonnes |
| **Volume** | | |
| teaspoons | 5.0 | milliliters |
| tablespoons | 15.0 | milliliters |
| fluid ounces | 30.0 | milliliters |
| cups | 0.24 | liters |
| pints | 0.47 | liters |
| quarts | 0.95 | liters |
| gallons | 3.8 | liters |
| cubic inches | 0.02 | liters |
| cubic feet | 0.03 | cubic meters |
| cubic yards | 0.76 | cubic meters |
| **Area** | | |
| square inches | 6.5 | square centimeters |
| square feet | 0.09 | square meters |
| square yards | 0.8 | square meters |
| square miles | 2.6 | square kilometers |
| acres | 0.4 | hectares |
| **Temperature** | | |
| Fahrenheit | $5/9 \times (F - 32)$ | Celsius |
| Celsius | $(9/5 \times C) + 32$ | Fahrenheit |

*Note: For all but temperature, when you know the metric measurement, divide by the same numbers given above to determine the US customary measurement.

| BMI Calculation | US Customary | SI Metric |
|---|---|---|
| | $BMI = \dfrac{wt\ (lb)}{ht\ (in^2)} \times 703$ | $BMI = \dfrac{wt\ (kg)}{ht\ (m^2)}$ |

# Image Credits

| | | | | |
|---|---|---|---|---|
| **Figure 1.16** | Body Scientific International, LLC | | **Figure 9.14** | Body Scientific International, LLC |
| **Figure 2.4** | Goodheart-Willcox Publisher | | **Figure 9.15** | Body Scientific International, LLC |
| **Figure 2.7** | Goodheart-Willcox Publisher | | **Figure 9.17** | Body Scientific International, LLC |
| **Figure 4.3** | Goodheart-Willcox Publisher | | **Figure 9.19** | Body Scientific International, LLC |
| **Figure 4.9** | Goodheart-Willcox Publisher | | **Figure 9.20** | Body Scientific International, LLC |
| **Figure 4.12** | Goodheart-Willcox Publisher | | **Figure 9.21** | Body Scientific International, LLC |
| **Figure 4.13** | Goodheart-Willcox Publisher | | **Figure 9.22** | Body Scientific International, LLC |
| **Figure 4.14** | Goodheart-Willcox Publisher | | **Figure 9.23** | Body Scientific International, LLC |
| **Figure 5.11** | USDA | | **Figure 9.24** | Body Scientific International, LLC |
| **Figure 6.5** | Goodheart-Willcox Publisher | | **Figure 9.25** | Body Scientific International, LLC |
| **Figure 8.3** | Goodheart-Willcox Publisher | | **Figure 9.26** | Body Scientific International, LLC |
| **Figure 8.6** | Body Scientific International, LLC | | **Figure 9.27** | Body Scientific International, LLC |
| **Figure 8.7** | Body Scientific International, LLC | | **Figure 9.30** | Goodheart-Willcox Publisher |
| **Figure 8.8** | Body Scientific International, LLC | | **Figure 9.35** | Goodheart-Willcox Publisher |
| **Figure 8.9** | Body Scientific International, LLC | | **Figure 10.1** | Goodheart-Willcox Publisher |
| **Figure 8.10** | Body Scientific International, LLC | | **Figure 10.2** | Goodheart-Willcox Publisher |
| **Figure 8.11** | Body Scientific International, LLC | | **Figure 10.13** | Goodheart-Willcox Publisher |
| **Figure 8.16** | Body Scientific International, LLC | | **Figure 10.14** | Goodheart-Willcox Publisher |
| **Figure 9.5** | Body Scientific International, LLC | | **Figure 10.15** | Goodheart-Willcox Publisher |
| **Figure 9.6** | Body Scientific International, LLC | | **Figure 11.6** | Goodheart-Willcox Publisher |
| **Figure 9.7** | Body Scientific International, LLC | | **Figure 11.7** | Goodheart-Willcox Publisher |
| **Figure 9.8** | Body Scientific International, LLC | | **Figure 11.8** | ©Ed Kashi/VII/Corbis |
| **Figure 9.9** | Body Scientific International, LLC | | **Figure 11.18** | ©Salvatore Di Nolfi/epa/Corbis |
| **Figure 9.10** | Body Scientific International, LLC | | **Figure 12.6** | Goodheart-Willcox Publisher |
| **Figure 9.11** | Body Scientific International, LLC | | **Figure 12.7** | Goodheart-Willcox Publisher |
| **Figure 9.12** | Body Scientific International, LLC | | **Figure 12.8** | Goodheart-Willcox Publisher |
| **Figure 9.13** | Body Scientific International, LLC | | | |

# Glossary

**12-hour clock**   expression of time used internationally; based on a 12-hour system in which a.m. and p.m. designations must be assigned to identify the proper time

**24-hour clock**   method of measuring time based on 24-hour-long segments; also called military time

## A

**acronyms**   words formed from the first letters or parts of other words

**active listening**   the act of listening intently to not only hear the words being spoken, but to understand the complete message being sent

**active reading**   reading with extreme concentration and focus to ensure you are fully present and aware of what you are reading; note taking and reading out loud are sometimes part of active reading

**addition**   the process of combining two or more numbers to obtain their total value

**adjective**   a word that modifies or describes a noun or pronoun

**advanced directive (AD)**   a legal document in which a patient gives written instructions about healthcare issues in the event that the patient becomes unable to make such decisions in the future

**adverb**   any word that tells how, when, where, or how much

**Affordable Care Act**   passed into law in 2010 for a major regulatory overhaul of US healthcare

**algebra**   branch of mathematics that substitutes letters for numbers; involves solving for the unknown

**anatomical position**   a standing position in which the feet are parallel and the arms and hands are at the sides, palms facing out

**anatomy**   the study of the structure of the body

**anesthesia**   loss of feeling with or without the loss of consciousness

**antibiotics**   drugs that slow the growth of, or destroy bacteria; used to treat infections

**antibody**   a protein produced by the immune system; circulates in the plasma in response to the presence of foreign antigens

**antigen**   any foreign substance, either outside or inside the body, that causes the immune system to produce antibodies

**arbitration**   a cost-effective alternative to litigation

**arteriosclerosis**   hardening of arteries as a result of plaque buildup on an arterial wall

**associate's degree**   a two-year college degree, often offered through a community college and awarded after completing 60 credit hours or more when on a semester system

**atherosclerosis**   buildup of plaque on the inner lining of an arterial wall over time

**auditory learner**   one who learns best by listening; lectures, discussion, and talking things through are helpful tools for this learner

**autoclave**   a machine that employs hot, pressurized steam to kill all microorganisms and their spores on a surface

## B

**bachelor's degree**   a four-year college degree awarded after 120 credit hours or more when on a semester system

**bacteria**   small, one-celled organisms that cannot be seen by the naked eye; can be pathogenic (cause disease)

**base ten system**   numbering system used for counting that is based on multiples of ten

**biohazard sharps container**   a puncture-resistant container used for disposing of waste-contaminated sharps, including needles, scalpels, glass slides, and broken glassware

**biopsy**   a small piece of tissue removed from the body for examination

**biotechnology**   technology using biological processes, organisms, or systems to develop products intended to improve the quality of human life

**bloodborne pathogens**   infectious microorganisms in human blood that can cause disease

**body cavities**   spaces in the body that contain organs; the human body is divided into the dorsal and ventral cavities

**body mass index (BMI)**   weight in kilograms divided by height in meters squared; a method of determining caloric nutritional status

**body mechanics**   term for the proper use of body movements to prevent injury during tasks that require lifting or moving

**body planes**   imaginary planes, or flat surfaces, that divide the body into sections; include sagittal, coronal, and transverse planes

**body system**   a group of organs working together to perform various functions and maintain homeostasis

**bone marrow**   soft, spongy, blood-forming tissue found inside bones

# C

**caduceus**   an emblem of medicine in the United States

**cancer**   an abnormal growth of cells in the body that multiply rapidly and invade normal tissue

**capitalization**   the use of an uppercase letter for the first letter of a word, and lowercase for the remaining letters; used for proper nouns

**carcinoma**   cancerous tumor derived from epithelial cells

**career ladder**   term for the progression from an entry-level position to higher levels of pay, skill, and responsibility

**carpal tunnel syndrome**   a painful, progressive hand and arm condition caused by compression of a key nerve in the wrist; can be caused when wrists are not supported during keyboard use

**cell membrane**   the outer layer of a cell that holds the cell together

**Celsius temperature scale**   metric temperature scale; defines the freezing point of water as 0° and the boiling point of water as 100°

**Centers for Disease Control and Prevention (CDC)**   federal agency in the United States responsible for protecting public health and safety by promoting awareness, control, and prevention of disease, injury, and disability

**central nervous system (CNS)**   part of the nervous system that includes the brain and the spinal cord

**certification**   recognition given for completing a course of study

**chain of infection**   the visualization of the sequence of events allowing infection to invade the human body

**chromosome**   threadlike structure found in the nucleus of most living cells; carries genetic information

**civil law**   directives that pertain to disputes between individuals, organizations, or a combination of the two in which monetary compensation is awarded; also known as *tort law*

**cloning**   creation of an organism that is an exact genetic copy of another; a clone has identical DNA to its parent

**cloud technology**   Internet-based technology that stores programs and data on servers at remote locations instead of your computer

**combining form**   term that describes a word root and a combining vowel used to form medical terms

**combining vowel** letter used to combine two word roots, or a word root and a suffix; usually an *o*

**common denominator** the number that can be divided evenly by all of the denominators in a group of fractions

**compassion** deep awareness and concern for the suffering of others coupled with the desire to relieve this suffering

**competence** the ability to do your job well

**complex sentence** sentence with an independent clause joined by one or more dependent clauses

**compound sentence** sentence containing two independent clauses joined by a conjunction

**comprehension** an understanding of what you have read or heard

**compromise** settlement of differences where each side makes concessions

**computer hardware** devices such as the monitor or keyboard that are connected to the computer

**computer on wheels (COW)** a mobile computer used to access and enter patient information while moving around the healthcare facility; often rolled into a patient's hospital room

**computer virus** malware designed to copy itself into other programs; may cause the affected computer to operate incorrectly or corrupt the computer memory

**confidentiality** the practice of allowing only certain individuals the right to access information; ensures that others do not have the personal information of others

**conflict resolution** methods for alleviating or eliminating sources of conflict

**conjunction** a word that joins other words, phrases, clauses, or sentences

**consonants** all letters of the English alphabet except *a, e, i, o,* and *u*

**contraction** a shortened form of a word or term; one or more letters are omitted and replaced with an apostrophe to create one word

**cover letter** a letter that accompanies a résumé to provide additional information about the applicant's skills and experience

**criminal law** directives that pertain to a crime in which the guilty party is punished by incarceration and possible fines

**critical thinking** a process of actively and skillfully analyzing and evaluating information to draw a conclusion

**cytoplasm** transparent, gel-like substance inside of every cell; cellular activities occur here

# D

**database** collection of records such as addresses, phone numbers, and other patient information

**decimal numbers** numbers expressed with a decimal point; values left of the decimal are whole numbers and values to the right are fractions

**decoding** the process used to break down words into recognizable units as part of a word

**dementia** a disorder featuring a progressive loss of memory and other intellectual functions

**deoxyribonucleic acid (DNA)** genetic material shaped like a double helix; part of all living cells

**diabetes** an incurable metabolic disease that results in an increased level of glucose, or sugar, in the blood

**diagnostic-related groups (DRGs)** a system that categorizes patients according to their diagnosis

**diagnostic services** a healthcare pathway offering careers in implementing procedures to determine causes of diseases or disorders

**differentiation** process through which cells of the body vary according to their specific function

**disinfection**   term for the use of antimicrobial agents on nonliving objects or surfaces to destroy or deactivate microorganisms

**division**   process of determining how many times one number is present in another number

**doctorate**   a degree awarded after two to six years of education beyond the bachelor's degree; available in many disciplines

**do not resuscitate (DNR) document**   a legal document made by a patient, which states that CPR or other advanced cardiac life support should not be performed if a patient stops breathing or a patient's heart stops

**download**   transmission of a file from one computer system to another; usually from a larger computer system to a smaller one

**durable power of attorney**   a legal document that grants another person the authority to make legal decisions for you; the Durable Power of Attorney for Health Care includes patient instructions for healthcare decisions and gives another person the power to enforce such decisions

**duty of care**   a legal obligation for healthcare personnel to take reasonable care to avoid causing harm to a patient

**dyslexia**   a learning disorder characterized by problems processing words; often causes difficulties when learning to read

## E

**electronic medical records (EMR)**   digital versions of a paper chart that contains a patient's medical history

**emancipated minor**   a person under 18 years of age who has legally established that he or she does not live with parents

**empathy**   the act of identifying with and understanding another person's feelings or situation

**endocrine glands**   glands that secrete chemical substances called hormones, which regulate body functions; part of the endocrine system

**English system of measurement**   a system of measurement commonly used in the United States; measurements are based on the inch, pound, gallon, and Fahrenheit degrees

**enthusiasm**   an excited and positive attitude that you can bring to your work

**epidemics**   diseases that affect many people and spread rapidly by infecting a certain area or population

**equations**   mathematical statements containing expressions composed of both numbers and letters; two sides of an equation are separated by an equal sign and must be equal to one another

**ergonomics**   term for simple practices meant to minimize physical effort and discomfort and maximize efficiency

## F

**Fahrenheit temperature scale**   the temperature scale commonly used in the United States; the freezing point of water is 32° and the boiling point is 212°

**fire triangle**   term for the three elements needed to start a fire: fuel, heat, and oxygen

**firewall**   software program or piece of hardware developed to prevent a hacker from accessing personal information on your computer or in the healthcare facility computer system

**fractions**   numbers composed of a numerator on top and a denominator on the bottom; indicates part of a whole

**fungi**   organisms that include disease-causing microorganisms such as yeasts and molds

## G

**Good Samaritan laws**   laws that protect people from legal action after voluntarily giving emergency medical aid while using reasonable care

**grammar**   the study of how words and their components combine to form sentences

**guardian**   a court-appointed person who may make decisions for a patient who is mentally or physically incapable of making such decisions

# H

**hackers**   people who break into computer systems to access data, steal personal information, and sometimes cause harm to a computer system

**hand hygiene**   hand washing with a detergent or antimicrobial soap and water, or by applying an alcohol-based hand rub; considered the single most important way to prevent the spread of infection

**healthcare simulation**   learning tools used to show what something looks like or how to perform a procedure

**health informatics services**   career field considered to be a bridge between medicine and technology, and which provides critical support to all other medical services; includes positions such as medical clerical worker, human resource workers, and medical records workers

**Health Insurance Portability and Accountability Act (HIPAA)**   an act approved by the US Congress in 1996 and fully enforced in 2006; created a law including a privacy provision for patient health records

**health maintenance organizations (HMO)**   managed care organizations that provide prepaid, comprehensive healthcare at a flat rate and for a fixed period of time through a network of participating healthcare professionals and hospitals; policyholders select a primary care physician (PCP) and referrals from the PCP must be obtained to see a specialist

**Hippocratic Oath**   a promise of professional behavior made by physicians beginning their careers; promises ethical and honest practice of the medical profession

**homeostasis**   state of internal balance achieved by adjusting the physiological systems of the body

**hormones**   chemicals secreted by endocrine glands to regulate body functions

**hospice**   a type of care designed to relieve pain and reduce suffering in terminally ill patients

**hospital emergency codes**   signals used in hospitals to alert staff to various emergencies; examples include code red (fire) and code blue (cardiac arrest)

**human reproduction**   process that occurs when the male sex cell and female sex cell unite to create a new human being

**hypothesis**   an idea or a suggestion often developed to explain something, the cause of which is unknown

# I

**immunity**   ability to resist pathogens

**incident reports**   reports used in a healthcare facility to document both safety and non-safety related incidents that are not part of a routine operation in the facility

**infection control**   term that describes any efforts made to avoid the spread of infection in a healthcare facility

**inflammation**   term for redness, swelling, pain, tenderness, and heat affecting an area of the body; often a result of tissues reacting to injury

**informed consent**   a form given to a patient by a physician explaining the benefits and risks of a procedure; the patient accepts the risk by signing the informed consent form

**interjection**   a word, phrase, or clause that expresses emotion

**Internet**   an electronic communications network that connects computer networks and computer facilities around the world

**isolation rooms**   rooms in a healthcare facility used to contain contagious diseases as well as protect immune-compromised patients from disease

# J

**job shadowing** a job exploration tool that involves following an employee completing the tasks of a job you find interesting

**joints** physical point of connection between two bones; *articulation*

# K

**kinesthetic learner** one who learns through experiencing and doing things; labs, field trips, and study breaks can be helpful for this learner

# L

**learning styles** different ways that people learn; three basic types include visual, auditory, and kinesthetic; most people have a mixture of all three

**licensure** recognition given by a state agency when a person meets the qualifications for a particular occupation; given after the person passes a licensure examination; required in order to practice

**ligaments** tough bands of fibrous tissue that connect bone to bone

**lymph** colorless fluid from the body's tissues that carries white blood cells; collects and transports bacteria to the lymph nodes for destruction; carries fats from the digestive system

**lymphocyte** white blood cell that destroys pathogenic microorganisms

# M

**malignant** term that describes a tumor that is threatening to life; *cancerous*

**malpractice** any misconduct or lack of skill that results in patient injury; also known as professional liability

**malware** malicious software used to disrupt computer operation, gather sensitive information, or gain access to private computers

**master's degree** academic degree awarded by a college or university to those who complete from one to two years (depending on the degree) of prescribed study beyond the bachelor's degree

**material safety data sheet (MSDS)** a sheet that accompanies every chemical used in a hospital and which contains important information regarding that chemical

**mean** mathematical average of data

**median** the number exactly in the middle of a group of numbers listed in ascending or descending order

**Medicaid** a program jointly-funded by state and federal taxes that provides medical aid for low-income individuals of all ages; managed by the states

**medical ethics** standards concerned with whether a healthcare worker's actions are right or wrong

**medical law** standards concerned with whether a healthcare worker's actions are legal or illegal

**medical specialties** specific areas of focus practiced by medical professionals, which are often named according to a body system

**Medicare** a federal health insurance program for persons 65 or older and disabled individuals

**metabolism** term for the chemical processes occurring within a living organism that maintains life

**metastasis** the spread of cancerous cells from their place of origin to other parts of the body via the bloodstream

**Methicillin-resistant *Staphylococcus aureus* (MRSA)** an antibiotic-resistant bacterium responsible for a difficult-to-treat infection; sometimes prevalent in hospitals, prisons, schools, and nursing homes

**metric system of measurement** a system of measurement using units related by factors of ten; measurements based on the gram, liter, meter, and temperature measure in Celsius

**microscope** an instrument that uses a lens to magnify objects too small to be seen with the naked eye

**mixed numbers** whole numbers followed by a remaining fraction

**mnemonic devices** learning techniques such as rhymes, catchphrases, and acronyms used to help remember and retain information

**mode** the number(s) that occur most frequently in a set of numbers

**morphology** term for the form and structure of an organism

**motivation** a process by which one initiates, guides, and maintains goal-oriented behavior

**multiplication** mathematical operation that indicates how many times a number is added to itself; a shortcut for addition

**multitasking** the ability to do more than one thing at the same time

**myocardial infarction (MI)** heart attack

# N

**National Healthcare Skill Standards Project** system developed by the United States Department of Education to address a critical shortage of highly skilled healthcare professionals

**needlesticks** any accidental puncture of the skin by a needle; can be dangerous in a healthcare setting because the puncture can cause a potentially serious infection

**Needlestick Safety and Prevention Act** law enacted in 2000; mandates that OSHA require employers to identify, evaluate, and introduce safe medical devices to avoid needlesticks

**negligence** performing an act that a reasonable person would not have done, or not doing something that a reasonable person would have done in the same or similar circumstance that results in harm to a patient

**neoplasm** a tumor; can be either malignant or benign

**networking** a process for developing contacts and relationships with people who are interested in your future employment

**nominal numbers** numbers that name or identify something

**nonverbal communication** any form of communication that does not involve speech, including gestures, the way one sits, eye contact (or lack of), and facial expressions; *body language*

**nosocomial infections** hospital-acquired infections

**noun** a word representing a person, place, or thing

**nucleus** the "brain" of a cell; directs all activities and contains genetic information

# O

**Occupational Safety and Health Administration (OSHA)** a government agency put in place to oversee employee safety in the workplace

**ombudsman** a member of the healthcare team who ensures that patients are not abused and that their legal rights are protected

**ordinal numbers** numbers that place objects in a series in order

**organs** two or more groups of tissues working together to perform specific functions

**OSHA Bloodborne Pathogens Standard** a standard applied to all patients receiving care in any healthcare facility; lists potentially infectious materials and mandates that healthcare workers should always proceed as if the materials are infectious

**OSHA Hazard Communication Standard** a standard that ensures that employees are educated about chemical hazards in the workplace

# P

**paragraph** part of a written composition, which consists of a collection of sentences related to one topic

**parasite** organisms that live in or on another organism

**parts of speech** collective term for eight classifications of words that denote each word's function; in English these include noun, pronoun, verb, adjective, adverb, conjunction, preposition, and interjection

**pathogens** disease-producing microorganisms

**patience** a soft skill that will help you interact with coworkers and patients

**Patients' Bill of Rights** summary of a patient's rights regarding fair treatment and appropriate information

**Patient Self-Determination Act** a law passed by the US Congress in 1990 that requires most healthcare institutions to inform a patient about their rights at the time of admission

**percentage** a number divided into 100 parts; expressed with the percent sign (%)

**peripheral nervous system (PNS)** collective term for nerves that lie outside the central nervous system; transmits information from the CNS to all parts of the body

**personal protective equipment (PPE)** equipment worn by workers to protect them from serious workplace injuries or illnesses

**pH scale** system for measuring a substance's acidity or alkalinity; ranges from 0 to 14

**phagocytosis** process in which white blood cells surround, ingest, and destroy a foreign invader

**physiology** the study of the function of the body

**podcasts** multimedia files that are downloaded and played on a computer, a tablet, or a smartphone

**potentially infectious materials (PIM)** materials designated by OSHA that require healthcare workers to proceed as if they are infectious

**preferred provider organizations (PPO)** health insurance organizations that contract with a network of preferred providers from which the policyholder can choose; often involves an annual deductible payment for service, but patients do not have a designated primary care physician and may self-refer to specialists

**prefix** the part of a word that comes before the word root; changes the meaning of the word root

**preposition** a word that connects or relates its object to the rest of the sentence

**prime number** a number that is only divisible by itself and 1

**prioritizing** to make decisions about the best order in which to perform multiple tasks so that the most important tasks are completed first

**professionalism** the conduct or attitude that is required to be the best employee that you can be; contributing positively to an organization

**pronoun** a substitute word for a noun

**proportion** a statement of the equality of two ratios

**protozoa** microorganisms that depend on a host cell to survive and replicate; can cause serious illness

**proxemics** the study of humans' use of space; includes physical territory and personal territory

**psychoanalysis** a method of analyzing and treating mental and emotional disorders through sessions in which the patient is encouraged to talk about personal experience and dreams

**puberty** a stage of life beginning between the ages of 8 and 14; indicates sexual reproduction is possible

**punctuality** being on time for work, appointments, and any other commitments

**punctuation** the practice or system of using certain conventional marks or characters such as commas, question marks, and periods in writing

## Q

**quality assurance** term for the policies that ensure healthcare facilities monitor and evaluate services based on predetermined criteria; corrective action must be taken if the facility's services do not meet the established criteria

## R

**ratio** comparison of one quantity with another, similar quantity

**reasonable care** legal protection for the healthcare worker if proven that the worker acted reasonably as compared to other members of the profession in a same or similar situation

**respiration** the act of supplying oxygen to the cells and removing carbon dioxide; also called breathing

**résumé** a document that summarizes your education, work experiences, and other qualifications for employment; can be printed or submitted electronically

**retention** the ability to preserve information in the mind

**rickettsiae** parasites that normally choose fleas, lice, ticks, or mites as their host organisms; can cause severe infections

## S

**sanitization** term for the use of antimicrobial agents on objects, surfaces, or living tissue to reduce the number of disease-causing microorganisms

**science** system of acquiring knowledge through observation and experimentation to describe the natural world

**scientific method** a method designed to logically formulate, test, and evaluate a problem or hypothesis

**sexual harassment** unwanted sexual advances and other forms of offensive sexual behavior; both men and women can be sexually harassed

**sexually transmitted infection (STI)** an infection transferred from one person to another through sexual contact

**sharps** needles or any other object that could puncture or cut the skin

**simple sentence** sentence that contains a subject and a verb, and which expresses a complete thought; independent clause

**soft skills** personal characteristics that enable a person to have pleasant, effective interactions with others

**software** a collection of programs that allow a user to interact with the computer

**spreadsheet** a document containing rows and columns of data; useful for organizing numeric values and executing computer calculations

**SQ3R reading system** study strategy used to increase comprehension while reading; stands for Survey, Question, Read, Recite, and Review

**standard of care** reasonable and prudent care that a practitioner of similar qualifications would have performed in the same or similar situation

**statute of limitations** the amount of time during which any legal action may be taken; after such time a lawsuit may not be filed

**stem cells** cells in the body that evolve into specific cells in a particular organ system

**sterilization** the act of killing all microorganisms and their spores on a surface; methods of sterilization in a healthcare facility may include hot pressurized steam, dry heat, gas, ionized radiation, and specialized chemicals

**stress** the feeling of being overwhelmed by worry and pressures in your life

**subtraction** the process of removing one number from another number; the opposite of addition

**suffix** the part of a word that is added after the word root to change its meaning

**support services** a sector of the hospital that plays a critical role in providing a clean, safe environment for all who enter a healthcare facility

# T

**tact** the ability to avoid giving offense through your words and actions

**tendons** fibrous tissues that connect muscles to bone

**therapeutic services** career path that offers hands-on experience with patients and focuses on changing the health status of a patient over time

**thesaurus** a resource that identifies words with the same meaning

**time management** the process of planning and controlling the amount of time spent on specific activities to increase efficiency and productivity

**tissues** groups of cells that work together to accomplish the same task

# U

**upload** to transfer data from a smaller device like a personal computer to a larger computer or server

# V

**vaccination** the use of medicines that contain weakened or dead bacteria or viruses to build immunity and prevent disease

**values** the concepts, ideas, and beliefs important and meaningful to a person

**verb** any word describing an action or a state of being

**verbal communication** expressing your thoughts out loud; speaking

**virtual learning environment (VLE)** an online learning system that brings classroom materials to students via the Internet

**viruses** microorganisms much smaller than bacteria that depend on a living cell to survive; cause many serious diseases and illnesses

**visual learner** one who learns through seeing things; charts, color-coded notes, and videos can be helpful tools for this learner

**vocabulary** a set of words known and used by a person

**vowels** five letters in the English language: *a, e, i, o,* and *u* (sometimes *y* is substituted for *i*)

# W

**whole numbers** numbers used for counting; do not contain decimal points or fractions; *integers*

**Wi-Fi** technology that enables an electronic device to exchange data wirelessly over a computer network; *wireless fidelity*

**word elements** the five parts used to form medical terms; includes the word root, prefix, suffix, combining vowel, and combining form

**word processing** software that allows one to enter, edit, store, and print text through a computer

**word root** the body or the main element of a word

**World Wide Web** a means of accessing the Internet by using an HTTP web address

# *Index*